Andrew Cant. Mario Abinun.
III '95.

ADVANCES IN
Pediatric Infectious Diseases®

VOLUME 10

ADVANCES IN Pediatric Infectious Diseases®

VOLUMES 1 THROUGH 7 (OUT OF PRINT)

VOLUME 8

VOLUME 9

Lower Respiratory Viral Infections in Immunocompetent Children, *by Kelly S. Henrickson*

Genital Herpes Simplex Virus and Human Papillomavirus Infection, *by Jonathan M. Ellen, Anna-Barbara Moscicki, and Mary-Ann B. Schafer*

The Role of Newer Oral Cephalosporins, Fluroquinolones, and Macrolides in the Treatment of Pediatric Infections, *by William J. Rodriguez and Bernhard L. Wiedermann*

Pelvic Inflammatory Disease in Adolescents, *by Ellen R. Wald*

Lyme Disease and Babesiosis, *by Peter James Krause and Henry Morton Feder, Jr.*

Cytokines in the Pathogenesis and Treatment of Infectious Diseases, *by Allan S. Lau*

Occult Bacteremia in Children, *by David M. Jaffe*

ADVANCES IN

Pediatric Infectious Diseases®

VOLUME 10

Editor-in-Chief

Stephen C. Aronoff, M.D.

Professor, Department of Pediatrics and Microbiology/Immunology, West Virginia University School of Medicine; Chief, Pediatric Infectious Diseases, West Virginia University Children's Hospital, Morgantown, West Virginia

Mosby

St. Louis Baltimore Boston Chicago London Madrid Philadelphia Sydney Toronto

Mosby
Dedicated to Publishing Excellence

Vice President and Publisher, Continuity Publishing: Kenneth H. Killion
Director, Editorial Development: Gretchen C. Murphy
Development Editor: Kelly Poirier
Project Manager: Denise M. Dungey
Project Supervisor: Maria Nevinger
Sr. Project Editor: Jill C. Waite
Proofreading Supervisor: Barbara M. Kelly
Vice President, Professional Sales and Marketing: George M. Parker
Marketing and Circulation Manager: Barry J. Bowlus
Marketing Coordinator: Lynn Stevenson

Printed in the United States of America
Composition by The Clarinda Company
Printing/binding by The Maple-Vail Book Manufacturing Group

Mosby–Year Book, Inc.
11830 Westline Industrial Drive
St. Louis, Missouri 63146

Editorial Office:
Mosby–Year Book, Inc.
200 North La Salle Street
Chicago, Illinois 60601

International Standard Serial Number: 0884-9404
International Standard Book Number: 0-8151-0313-1

Contributors

Camille N. Bitar, M.D.
Division of Infectious Diseases, Department of Pediatrics, Louisiana State University School of Medicine, and Tulane University School of Medicine, New Orleans, Louisiana

Norman D. Ferrari III, M.D.
Associate Professor of Pediatrics and Internal Medicine; Chief, General Pediatrics and Adolescent Medicine; Associate Dean, Ambulatory Services, West Virginia University School of Medicine, Morgantown, West Virginia

Carol A. Ford, M.D.
Fellow, Division of Adolescent Medicine, Department of Pediatrics, University of California, San Francisco School of Medicine, San Francisco, California

Anne A. Gershon, M.D.
Department of Pediatrics, Columbia University College of Physicians & Surgeons, New York, New York

Neal A. Halsey, M.D.
Professor and Division Director, Division of Disease Control, Department of International Health, The Johns Hopkins University, Baltimore, Maryland

Margaret R. Hammerschlag, M.D.
Division of Infectious Diseases, Department of Pediatrics, SUNY Health Science Center, Brooklyn, New York

Sheldon L. Kaplan, M.D.
Professor and Vice Chairman for Clinical Affairs, Department of Pediatrics, Baylor College of Medicine; Chief, Infectious Diseases Service, Texas Children's Hospital, Houston, Texas

Anna-Barbara Moscicki, M.D.
Associate Professor of Pediatrics, Department of Pediatrics, University of California, San Francisco School of Medicine, San Francisco, California

Lorry G. Rubin, M.D.
Division of Infectious Diseases, Department of Pediatrics, Schneider Children's Hospital of Long Island Jewish Medical Center, New Hyde Park, New York; Long Island Campus for the Albert Einstein College of Medicine, Long Island, New York

Kathleen Ryan-Poirier, M.D.
Assistant Professor of Pediatrics, Division of Pediatric Infectious Diseases, University of Florida, Gainesville, Florida

Mark B. Salzman, M.D.
Department of Pediatrics, Kaiser Foundation Hospital-West Los Angeles, Los Angeles, California

Rosana Schafer, Ph.D.
Research Instructor, Department of Microbiology and Immunology, West Virginia University School of Medicine, Morgantown, West Virginia

James M. Sheil, Ph.D.
Assistant Professor, Department of Microbiology and Immunology, West Virginia University School of Medicine, Morgantown, West Virginia

Russell W. Steele, M.D.
Division of Infectious Diseases, Department of Pediatrics, Louisiana State University School of Medicine, and Tulane University School of Medicine, New Orleans, Louisiana

Arnold Wald, M.D.
Professor of Medicine, University of Pittsburgh, Division of Gastroenterology and Hepatology, University of Pittsburgh Medical Center, Pittsburgh, Pennsylvania

Martin E. Weisse, M.D.
Assistant Professor of Pediatrics, Sections of General Pediatrics and Adolescent Medicine, and Infectious Diseases, West Virginia University School of Medicine, Morgantown, West Virginia

Nevin Wilson, M.D.
West Virginia University, Department of Pediatrics, Section of Allergy and Immunology, Robert S. Byrd Health Science Center, Morgantown, West Virginia

Charles R. Woods, Jr., M.D.
Assistant Professor of Pediatrics, Bowman Gray School of Medicine, Wake Forest University, Winston-Salem, North Carolina

Contents

Mosby Document Express

Copies of the full text of journal articles referenced in this book are available by calling Mosby Document Express, toll-free, at 1-800-55-MOSBY.

With Mosby Document Express, you have convenient 24-hour-a-day access to literally every journal reference within this book. In fact, through Mosby Document Express, virtually any medical or scientific article can be located and delivered by FAX, overnight delivery service, international airmail, electronic transmission of bit-mapped images (via Internet), or regular mail. The average cost of a complete delivered copy of an article, including copyright clearance charges and first-class mail delivery, is $12.

For inquiries and pricing information, please call the toll-free number shown above.

Atypical Pneumonias in Children

Margaret R. Hammerschlag, M.D.
Division of Infectious Diseases, Department of Pediatrics, SUNY Health Science Center, Brooklyn, New York

In 1901 Osler noted in the fourth edition of *The Principles and Practice of Medicine* that "the most widespread and fatal of all acute diseases, pneumonia, is now Captain of the Men of Death."[1] Over 90 years later, pneumonia remains preeminent as a clinical entity in all age groups.

As with other infectious diseases, the epidemiology has changed with the advent of effective chemotherapy. Whereas *Streptococcus pneumoniae* and other bacteria were probably the most prevalent organisms responsible for acute pneumonia in the preantibiotic era, nonbacterial pneumonias are now the most prevalent infections, especially in children and adolescents. A number of terms have been used to differentiate these pneumonias from the "classic" or "typical" acute pneumonia, with pneumococcal pneumonia being the prototype. These include atypical pneumonia, interstitial pneumonia, and community-acquired pneumonia. Since a wide array of organisms may cause atypical pneumonia, including *Mycoplasma pneumoniae, Chlamydia* species, rickettsia, and viruses, specific diagnosis remains a prerequisite for appropriate therapy. Recent studies suggest that these "atypical" pathogens, including the newly described *Chlamydia pneumoniae* (TWAR), may play a greater role in respiratory infections in children than previously thought.

The topic of atypical pneumonia and specifically *M. pneumoniae* pneumonia has been presented in great detail recently.[2–4] This chapter will provide some review but will concentrate on new data relating to these infections, especially *C. pneumoniae,* where comprehensive culture and serologic studies in children have only recently been presented. The release of two new macrolide antibiotics has also prompted renewed interest in these infections.

EPIDEMIOLOGY OF PNEUMONIA IN CHILDREN

Historically, with the development of systematic bacteriology in the late 19th century, it was thought that pneumonias were all caused by bacteria. However, during the 1918 influenza pandemic many postmortem examinations were done, and although a variety of different bacterial species were isolated (*Haemophilus influenzae* and others), there were cases in which no bacteria were found. Some had a distinctive histopathologic appearance, and it was concluded that they were due to a nonbacterial agent. Influenza A virus was isolated in 1933 by Smith, Andrewes, and Laidlaw[5]; subsequently, *Chlamydia psittaci* and *Coxiella burnetii* (Q fever) were identified. *Mycoplasma pneumoniae* was recognized as an etiologic agent of atypical pneumonia in the 1940s but not identified as *Mycoplasma* until 1962. *Legionnella* was identified in the late 1970s and *C. pneumoniae* in 1986.

A series of studies of pneumonia in children conducted in the late 1960s and early 1970s defined the epidemiologic and clinical patterns of illness. These studies came from disparate geographic areas and populations, but the findings have been similar. The sites included a large health maintenance organization (HMO) in Seattle, Washington, a pediatric group practice in Chapel Hill, North Carolina, Chapel Hill Memorial Hospital, and Cook County Hospital. In outpatients, *M. pneumoniae* and respiratory viruses predominated and accounted for approximately 50% of cases.[6–11] Bacterial infections were infrequent (<5%) in children who were not admitted to the hospital.[7, 11] Possible explanations for the remaining 50% cases of unknown cause may include bacteria, problems with specimen collection and transport, and agents that were not identified at that time, especially *C. pneumoniae*. The relative frequency of the agents to be discussed are presented in Table 1.

TABLE 1.
Frequency of Etiologic Agents of Atypical Pneumonia in Children

Agent	0–1 yr	1–5 yr	6–16 yr
Mycoplasma pneumoniae	–*	++	+++
Chlamydia pneumoniae	–	+++	+++
Chlamydia psittaci	–	+	+
Coxiella burnetii	+	+	+
Legionella	+	+	+

*– = no reported cases; + = rare to infrequent; ++ = frequent; +++ = very frequent.

Annual incidence rates of pneumonia in childhood have a rough inverse correlation with age that ranges from 40 per 1,000 in children under 5 years of age to 7 per 1,000 in children 12 to 15.

MYCOPLASMA PNEUMONIAE

Mycoplasma pneumoniae is probably the most frequent cause of atypical or nonbacterial pneumonia in children and adults. Two of the greatest misconceptions in pediatrics and medicine relate to *M. pneumoniae*. The first is that it is uncommon in young children, and the second, that specific therapy does not affect the clinical course of the disease. We shall present data that we hope will clarify these points since if a diagnosis is not considered, it will not be made and the disease certainly not appropriately treated.

THE ORGANISM

Members of the genus *Mycoplasma* are pleomorphic organisms that lack a cell wall; instead, they are bounded by a triple-layered unit membrane.[2] Like bacteria, mycoplasmas will grow on cell-free media and multiply by primary fission. However, unlike bacteria, since they lack a cell wall, they are not susceptible to antibiotics that interfere with cell wall synthesis, e.g., β-lactams. In electron microscopic studies the organism appears filamentous and has a terminal organelle containing an electron-dense core that appears to be an attachment factor.[12] The organism attaches to respiratory epithelial cells by slipping in between the cilia. Studies of exfoliated human tracheal epithelial cells and hamster tracheal organ culture demonstrate that *M. pneumoniae* causes cell injury after attachment. Cellular injury leads to ciliostasis, which may account for the prolonged paroxysmal cough that often occurs.[13]

EPIDEMIOLOGY

Mycoplasma pneumoniae infections are ubiquitous; they occur in urban and rural communities and temperate and tropical countries.[14–16] In urban areas, *M. pneumoniae* infection tends to be endemic and punctuated by epidemics at 4- to 7-year intervals.[10, 14] Outbreaks may also occur in institutional settings such as military bases, schools, and summer camps.[17–20] During these epidemics the proportion of pneumonia attributable to *M. pneumoniae* may reach 50%. The incidence of overt disease caused by *M. pneumoniae* is dependent on the prevalence of the infection in the population and appears to be related to age. Longitudinal studies, especially those of Foy et al. of the Group Health HMO in Seattle, found that the rate of endemic *M. pneumoniae* pneumonia was highest in children 5 to 9 years of age (4 per 1,000 per year), the next highest rate being in children 10 to 14 years of age (3 per 1,000 per year).[14] In children less than 5 years of age, the rate of *M. pneumoniae* infection was about 2 per 1,000 per year, which is about twice the rate observed for adolescents and adults. It may appear that *M. pneumoniae* is less frequent because at this age pneumonias caused by various viral pathogens are very frequent; thus pneumonia due to *M. pneumoniae* proportionally occurs less often. Pneumonia attributable to *M. pneumoniae* appears to be uncommon in infants less than 6 months of age. Infections in younger children are less likely to produce pneumonia.

Although studies from Seattle and Chapel Hill found that illness caused by *M. pneumoniae* is seen infrequently in children under 5 years of age, recent studies from Japan and the United States suggest that this may not be so.[21, 22] In a 1988 study from Japan, the peak age of lower respiratory illness due to *M. pneumoniae* was 3 to 4 years.[21] Recently, as part of an antibiotic treatment study, cultures and serology for *M. pneumoniae* were obtained from 260 children, 3 through 12 years of age, with radiographically proven pneumonia.[22] These children were seen at 29 sites in 20 states. *Mycoplasma pneumoniae* infection, by culture and/or serology, was identified in 14% of the children 3 through 6 years of age as compared with 22% of the children over 6 (Table 2). Although the infection was more frequent in the older children, it was still present in a respectable portion of the younger ones. Seven children in this study were coinfected with *M. pneumoniae* and *C. pneumoniae*. Clinically they could not be differentiated from those children who had *Mycoplasma* or *Chlamydia* infection alone. Coinfections with *M. pneumoniae* and other agents has been described.[23, 24] Only 1 child in this study had a positive blood culture for *S. pneumoniae*.

This apparent difference in age patterns of disease may also be related to differences in child-rearing practices. Japanese children entered preschool at an earlier age than American children at the time that the previous studies were conducted. However, the number of young children now being cared for in day care facilities or attending preschool in the United States has increased significantly. A study in 1975 from a day care center in North Carolina demonstrated that young children had primary asymptomatic carriage and experienced repeated infections.[25] A recent study from Denmark suggests that the previously regular 4-year cycles of epidemics of *M. pneumoniae* pneumonia seen for over 30 years ceased

TABLE 2.
Prevalence of *Mycoplasma pneumoniae* and *Chlamydia pneumoniae* Among Children With Community-Acquired Pneumonia*

	Total	Age	
		≤6 yr	>6 yr
No. (%)	260	161	99
Mycoplasma pneumoniae			
Culture/PCR†	28 (11)‡	16 (10)	12 (12)
Serology	44 (17)	22 (14)	22 (22)
Chlamydia pneumoniae culture	42 (16)	24 (15)	18 (18)

*Adapted from Hammerschlag MR, Roblin PM, Cassell G, et al: Role of infection with *Chlamydia pneumoniae* among children with community-acquired pneumonia in the USA (abstract 1377). Presented at the 32nd Interscience Conference on Antimicrobial Agents and Chemotherapy, New Orleans, 1993, p 371.
†PCR = polymerase chain reaction.
‡Numbers in parentheses are percentages of children.

as children began to be enrolled in day care centers at an earlier age.[26]

Because isolation rates of *M. pneumoniae* during both epidemic and endemic periods do not vary greatly by season as do those of common respiratory viruses, a greater proportion of patients with *M. pneumoniae* pneumonia is seen during the summer months.

The incubation period for *M. pneumoniae* infection is approximately 3 weeks for community and family outbreaks.[27] An epidemiologic clue is a respiratory illness that spreads slowly but intensively in a family, often with different manifestations in different family members, i.e., one child may contract pneumonia, and the parent may have pharyngitis. In families, 65% to 84% of children and half of the adults may become infected.[28] In point source outbreaks, the incubation period may be shorter, 1 to 2 weeks.[4]

CLINICAL MANIFESTATIONS

Mycoplasma pneumoniae pneumonia is considered to be the "classic" primary atypical pneumonia. However, *M. pneumoniae* infections cannot be readily differentiated clinically from pneumonia of other causes, especially *Chlamydia pneumoniae*. Generally the onset is gradual, over several days to weeks, in contrast to most viral illnesses such as influenza where the onset is more abrupt. Constitutional symptoms predominate, especially headache and malaise.[3] Patients may also have pharyngitis. The cough is usually dry initially and may be paroxysmal, eventually becoming productive of mucoid or mucopurulent sputum. The signs of *M. pneumoniae* infection tend to be minimal even though the patient feels very ill. Fever is frequent and 80% or more patients will have abnormal chest findings of rales or wheezes on auscultation. Ear pain may be due to otitis or bullous myringitis. The symptoms and signs vary according to the stage of illness. Since the onset is gradual, a patient may not come to the physician until a few days or a week has passed. The constitutional symptoms of headache and malaise along with fever may be at their maximum at this stage of the illness. Chest radiography may show an infiltrate at this time even though the results of the chest examination itself may be normal. By the second week the patient should be producing sputum, and the physical examination findings will be more consistent with pneumonia. Untreated disease will continue for 2 or more weeks.

These signs and symptoms are not specific. There is considerable overlap with other infections, especially *C. pneumoniae*. Pneumonia can be associated with respiratory failure. *Mycoplasma pneumoniae* may disseminate and cause multisystem disease. Rashes ranging from maculopapular eruptions to erythema multiforme may occur. The development of erythema multiforme following pneumonia is very suggestive of *M. pneumoniae* infection.[29] Pleural effusions may occur in as many as 20% of cases of confirmed *M. pneumoniae* pneumonia and appear to be more common in children. *Mycoplasma pneumoniae* has been isolated from pleural fluid in three pediatric cases from Japan and a 12-year-old boy from Toronto.[30] *Mycoplasma pneumoniae* is also one of the most frequent identifiable causes of acute chest syndrome in children with sickle cell disease[31] and may be increasing in importance since most of these children receive pneumococcal and *H. influenzae* vaccines and penicillin prophylaxis. Patients with sickle cell disease may also have severe disease associated with greatly elevated white blood cell (WBC) counts, prolonged fever, respiratory distress, and pleural effusion.[3,4] Severe *M. pneumoniae* infection has also been described in patients with humoral and cellular immunodeficiencies.[4] Two reports from France described three children with acquired immunodeficiency syndrome (AIDS) and pneumonia in whom *M. pneumoniae* was isolated from bronchoalveolar lavage (BAL) washings.[4] All responded well to appropriate antibiotic treatment; the disease did not appear to be unusually severe. It is of interest that in two of these children no complement fixation antibody was detectable. The role of *M. pneumoniae* in pneumonia in both children and adults with AIDS needs to be further defined; there are no population-based studies that have used culture techniques.

LABORATORY FINDINGS

The chest x-ray findings in *M. pneumoniae* are also variable and by themselves nonspecific. Four patterns have been described that when taken in context with other clinical features may be diagnostic. They are bronchopneumonia, plate-like atelectasis, nodular infiltration, and hilar adenopathy. The latter two findings are relatively uncommon and may be confused with other diseases, especially tuberculosis. The WBC count is usually under 10×10^9 cells/L. The erythrocyte sedimentation rate may be elevated during the acute illness. Other nonspecific tests that may be positive include the direct Coombs' test, antinuclear antibodies, and nontreponemal tests for syphilis.

DIAGNOSIS

Mycoplasma pneumoniae can be isolated from the throat or nasopharyngeal cultures of individuals with pneumonia. Asymptomatic respiratory carriage has been reported but appears to be uncommon. Recent experience in the multicenter pneumonia treatment study suggests that the throat is a superior site.[22] *Mycoplasma pneumoniae* grows on cell-free media, either broth or agar. Usually the specimen is collected, placed in transport media, and agitated and the swab discarded. An aliquot is then inoculated into liquid *Mycoplasma* media, incubated, and examined for a decline in pH or increased turbidity, which usually occurs in 8 to 15 days. These specimens are then subcultured onto agar media. The typical fried egg appearance of *M. pneumoniae* colonies can be seen after an additional 5 to 14 days' incubation. Culture confirmation is done by hemadsorption, hemolysis, or fluorescent antibody staining with specific *M. pneumoniae* antisera.[2] *Mycoplasma pneumoniae* culture is an involved process that may take 2 to 3 weeks to complete, which makes it not very useful for prospective management of patients. In addition, *Mycoplasma* culture is not widely available. The lack of a rapid, specific test for *M. pneumoniae* infection is one of the major reasons why it is probably the most underdiagnosed respiratory infection in children. Fortunately, there are new highly specific nonculture tests currently under development, especially DNA amplification tests, i.e., polymerase chain reaction (PCR). The use of PCR for culture confirmation shortens the time for culture by 1 week or more.[22]

Nonculture Tests

Because of the length of time needed for isolation of *M. pneumoniae,* there has been intermittent interest in the development of nonculture methods. In the 1970s there was some work with counterimmunoelectrophoresis, but it proved to be cumbersome, relatively insensitive, and not as commercially available as test kits.

A direct hybridization test, GenProbe Rapid Diagnostic Method (GenProbe, San Diego, Calif), had been commercially available for several years until it was withdrawn from the market in 1992. Original evaluations of the test found it to be very sensitive for detecting *M. pneumoniae* in sputum samples but less sensitive for detecting the organism in throat swabs. When sputa and throat specimens were obtained from the same patient, *M. pneumoniae* was detected in twice as many sputum samples as throat swabs.[32] This obviously presents a significant problem for diagnosis in children since very few children with pneumonia will produce sputum. A recent study from the same Finnish investigators evaluated the GenProbe test by using nasopharyngeal aspirates in a group of 216 children (mean age, 3.3 years) with acute lower respiratory infection.[33] Of these 216 children, 19 (9%) were positive by either probe or serology, 7 being positive by both methods. If serology is used as the reference method, the sensitivity and positive predictive value of the probe was 54%; however, the specificity and negative predictive value were 97%. Performance of the test also appeared to be age related. The probe detected 9 of the 10 infections in children less than 4 years of age but detected only 4 of 9 infections in older children. A problem with this study was the lack of a comparison of the probe and culture as in previous studies. Obviously, the performance of the test is related to the number of organisms present, which appears to be greatest in sputum, less in nasopharyngeal aspirates, and much less in throat swabs. It is possible that the sensitivity would have been lower if culture were included as a comparative method. A major drawback of the probe was that it was radioisotopic, which was the ostensible reason for its withdrawal.

Polymerase chain reaction offers the potential of increased sensitivity and rapidity when compared with culture. Several PCR assays have been evaluated, but with limited clinical material. The primers used include variable regions from the 16s RNA gene. In a study from Japan,[34] PCR had a sensitivity of 73% and a specificity of 94% vs. culture in detecting *M. pneumoniae* in a group of symptomatic children. Polymerase chain reaction did not detect *M. pneumoniae* in specimens from healthy controls, although one was culture-positive. Theoretically, PCR should be 100% sensitive and specific. The major reason for culture-positive/PCR-negative specimens is the presence of DNA polymerase inhibitors in clinical specimens, especially blood. If a kit were commercially available, this would represent a major advance in the diagnosis of *M. pneumoniae* infection.

Serology

Serology is probably the most frequently used method to diagnose *M. pneumoniae* infections. The cold agglutinin test remains a fairly sensitive and specific test for the diagnosis of *M. pneumoniae* pneumonia. The cold agglutinin reaction measures an IgM autoantibody that agglutinates human erythrocytes at 4°C. Approximately 30% to 75% of patients with *M. pneumoniae* pneumonia will be positive for cold agglutinins (≥1:32).[2] A specific serologic response to *M. pneumoniae* will develop in 72% to 92% of patients with pneumonia and positive cold agglutinins. Although other infections may be associated with cold agglutinins, data suggest that most cold agglutinin–positive pneumonias are due to *M. pneumoniae*. The height of the cold agglutinin response is directly proportional to the severity of pulmonary involvement, and the higher the titer, the more likely the infection is due to *M. pneumoniae*.

Since cold agglutinins usually appear by the end of the first week or the beginning of the second week of illness and disappear by 2 to 3 months, they can be used to provide a rapid diagnosis of *M. pneumoniae* pneumonia. The "bedside" cold agglutinin test, when done correctly, can be very useful. A positive "bedside" test result correlates with a laboratory cold agglutinin titer of 1:64 or greater.[35, 36] Using this "bedside" test, Griffin found that 85% of patients with pneumonia who had a positive test had diagnostic complement fixation titers.[36] The methodology of this test has been described in detail elsewhere.[2, 35, 36] Briefly, 0.3 to 0.4 mL of blood or a volume equal to the volume of the anticoagulant is added to a standard prothrombin (blue-topped) or hematology (lavender-topped) tube, placed on wet ice for several minutes, and examined for the development of agglutination; upon warming the reaction should be reversed. One should run a control as well. There is some debate as to whether tubes containing sodium citrate (blue topped) or ethylenediaminetetraacetic acid (EDTA; lavender topped) are superior, although there are no data available regarding the sensitivity and specificity of the rapid test when EDTA-containing tubes are used. The volume of blood appears to be important.

There are a number of specific serologic tests for *M. pneumoniae*. The most frequently used and widely available are complement fixation and enzyme-linked immunosorbent assay (ELISA). Most of the major epidemiologic studies of *M. pneumoniae* infection conducted in the 1960s and 1970s used the complement fixation test.[6–11] In patients with *M. pneumoniae* pneumonia, the complement fixation antibody usually peaks 1 to 3 weeks after the onset of infection.[3] A fourfold rise in complement fixation antibody titer is felt to be diagnostic. Since *M. pneumoniae* infection has a relatively long incubation period, complement fixation antibody may be present in significant titer at the time of the acute illness. Thus demonstration of a fourfold rise is important. Young children may have lower antibody titers, or detectable antibody may not develop. Kleemola et al.[34] found that serology, using the complement fixation test, detected only 40% of the *M. pneumoniae* infections in a group of children less than 4 years of age.

The complement fixation test is based on the glycolipid antigen.[2] This antigen cross-reacts with a variety of other microorganisms, plants, and body tissues. Whether these cross-reactions result in false-positive results with the *M. pneumoniae* complement fixation test is not known. Complement fixation antibody persist for several years following acute infection; thus obtaining paired sera is necessary to confirm acute infection.

Recently, many laboratories began using ELISAs for *M. pneumoniae* serology. This assay appears to be more sensitive and specific than the complement fixation test.[2] The ELISA uses the P1 protein surface antigen from purified *M. pneumoniae* organisms. The ELISA also allows for detection of IgG and IgM antibodies.

TREATMENT

The conventional wisdom has been that it really does not matter whether antibiotics are given to patients with *M. pneumoniae* infection, including pneumonia, because the morbidity is low and, unless treatment is started very early in the course of the infection, no clinical response will be seen. However, there are data, mainly from studies conducted in the 1960s, that show that treatment significantly reduces the morbidity of pneumonia caused by *M. pneumoniae*, even if started late in the course of the illness. Antibiotic therapy for *M. pneumoniae* infection is largely empirical because of the absence of a rapid, sensitive diagnostic test.

Tetracyclines and erythromycin are active against *M. pneumoniae* in vitro (Table 3). Erythromycin is approximately 300-fold more active than tetracycline. Rasch and Mogabgab in 1966 demonstrated that treatment with either erythromycin or tetracycline reduced the duration of fever, days in the hospital, and time to clear the chest radiograph as compared with no treatment or treatment with penicillin.[37] Similar results have been reported by other investigators. Foy et al. also reported that treatment did not affect the antibody response.[14] Most of the studies from this period relied on serologic diagnosis, i.e., a fourfold rise in complement fixation titer; thus microbiologic efficacy would not be assessed. A study conducted at Keesler Air Force Base by Shames et al. evaluated the effect of the therapy on recovery of *M. pneumoniae* from pharyngeal washings.[33] The clinical and radiologic responses to treatment were similar regardless of whether or not *M. pneumoniae* was isolated from throat washings at the end of therapy. Subsequently, Smith et al. demonstrated the persistence of *M. pneumoniae* after antibiotic treatment in experimental infections in adult volunteers.[39] Despite persistence of the organism, all of the subjects improved clinically. There are no published studies of treatment of *M. pneumoniae* infection in children that have used culture in addition to serology.[40]

TABLE 3.
In Vitro Activity of Various Antibiotics Against *Mycoplasma pneumoniae* and *Chlamydia pneumoniae*

Drug	*M. pneumoniae* MIC* (μg/mL)	*C. pneumoniae* MIC (μg/mL)
Erythromycin	<0.002–0.004	0.06–0.25
Tetracycline	0.25	0.06–0.125
Doxycycline	0.25	0.06–0.25
Azithromycin	<0.001–0.004	0.06–0.25
Clarithromycin	≤0.004–0.125	0.004–0.03
Ciprofloxacin	0.5–8	1.0
Ofloxacin	0.5–8	0.5–2
Sulfamethoxazole	—	>500

*MIC = minimal inhibitory concentration.

The recent introduction of two macrolide antibiotics, clarithromycin and azithromycin, has stimulated interest in the treatment of *M. pneumoniae* infections. Clarithromycin, a synthetic macrolide, has Food and Drug Administration (FDA) approval for use in adults, and a pediatric suspension will be available shortly. Clarithromycin is better absorbed and has a higher peak level in serum, excellent tissue penetration, and a half-life twice that of erythromycin.[41] Clarithromycin is similar in activity to erythromycin against *M. pneumoniae* in vitro[42] (see Table 3). Azithromycin differs from erythromycin by the incorporation of a methyl-substituted nitrogen atom into position 9a of the 14-member macrolide ring.[41] For this reason, azithromycin is classified as an azalide. The insertion of this nitrogen atom significantly alters the chemical, microbiologic, and pharmacologic properties. Overall, azithromycin has activity similar to erythromycin against *M. pneumoniae* in vitro,[43] but it differs dramatically in pharmacokinetics. Azithromycin is distributed widely in tissue and has a serum half-life of 68 hours and a half-life in tissue of 5 days.[41] This allows for once-daily dosing and a shorter duration of therapy.

Several studies comparing clarithromycin and azithromycin with erythromycin for the treatment of atypical pneumonia in adults have been published.[42–46] Most of these studies based the diagnosis of *M. pneumoniae* infection on serology alone by ELISA, and the number of evaluable patients with *M. pneumoniae* infection was small. Clarithromycin, azithromycin, and erythromycin were equally effective, with 80% to 100% clinical cure and resolution of chest radiographs. Microbiologic efficacy was not assessed.

Data on treatment of *M. pneumoniae* infection in children are more limited. Foy et al.,[14] in a study of 95 children less than 15 years of age, found that treatment with erythromycin or tetracycline, when given in the first 5 days of illness, reduced the duration of cough from a mean of 18.4 days in nontreated or penicillin-treated controls to 11.9 days. If treatment was started 6 days or more after the onset of symptoms, the mean duration of cough was similar to that in controls. A similar experience was reported by Broome et al.,[20] who described an explosive outbreak of *M. pneumoniae* infection in a boys' summer camp. When erythromycin was administered within 4 days of the onset of symptoms, the duration of cough was significantly shorter when compared with children who were treated after 4 days. Disease in the majority of the patients in both these studies was diagnosed serologically; thus microbiologic efficacy could not be assessed. The multicenter pneumonia treatment study described earlier compared clarithromycin

TABLE 4.
Bacteriologic Response to Treatment in Culture-Positive Children With Community-Acquired Pneumonia

	Pathogen Eradication	
Drug	***M. pneumoniae***	***C. pneumoniae***
Erythromycin	4/4 (100%)	12/14 (86%)
Clarithromycin	9/9 (100%)	15/19 (79%)
Total	13/13 (100%)	27/33 (82%)

with erythromycin for the treatment of pneumonia in 260 children aged 3 through 12 years. The study was randomized and double blinded. A total of 28 children had positive cultures or PCR for *M. pneumoniae*, 14 were evaluable, 9 received clarithromycin, and 4, erythromycin. The organism was eradicated in all patients at the end of treatment, and all were clinical cures (Table 4).[47] These results differ dramatically from results in early studies in adults where the organism persisted after treatment. Studies in children with azithromycin suspension are currently under way.

CHLAMYDIA PNEUMONIAE

Chlamydia pneumoniae, also known as TWAR, was first described as a respiratory tract pathogen by Grayston and colleagues in 1986.[48] Subsequently, much work has been done to characterize this organism and the diseases with which it has been associated. *Chlamydia pneumoniae* is rapidly becoming appreciated as a frequent cause of atypical pneumonia in children and adults. The first isolates of *C. pneumoniae* were serendipitously obtained during trachoma studies in the 1960s.[49] TW-183 was isolated from the eye of a child with suspected trachoma in Taiwan, and IOL-207 was isolated at the Institute of Ophthalmology in London from the eye of another child from Teheran with trachoma. Subsequently, serologic studies of an outbreak of mild pneumonia among schoolchildren in rural Finland in the late 1970s suggested that an organism related to TW-183 was the cause.[50] Following the recovery of a similar isolate from the respiratory tract of a college student with pneumonia in Seattle, Grayston and colleagues applied the designation TWAR after their first two isolates, TW-183 and AR-39.[49]

THE ORGANISM

The genus *Chlamydia* is a group of obligate intracellular parasites with a unique developmental cycle consisting of morphologically distinct infectious and reproductive forms. All members of the genus have a gram-negative envelope without peptidoglycan, share a genus-specific lipopolysaccharide (LPS) antigen, and use host adenosine triphosphate (ATP) for the synthesis of chlamydial protein. The genus contains three species, *C. psittaci*, *C. trachomatis*, and *C. pneumoniae* (TWAR strain) (Table 5). All three species are capable of causing pneumonia in man. On the basis of inclusion morphology and staining characteristics in cell culture, TWAR was initially considered to be a strain of *C. psittaci*. Subsequent analyses, however, have demonstrated that this organism is distinct from both *C. psittaci* and *C. trachomatis*, and it has been recognized as a separate species of *Chlamydia*. Initial ultrastructural studies demonstrated what appeared to be a unique elementary body morphology distinct from *C. trachomatis* and *C. psittaci*.[51] The elementary bodies had a pear-shaped appearance caused by a loose periplasmic membrane, whereas the elementary bodies of *C. trachomatis* and *C. psittaci* are round. However, ultrastructural studies of IOL-207 and other strains of *C. pneumoniae* isolated in the United States, Finland, and Japan revealed round elementary bodies similar in appearance to those of the other two chlamydial species.[52, 53] Restriction endonuclease pattern analysis and nucleic acid hybridization studies suggest a high degree of genetic relatedness (>95%) among the *C. pneumoniae* isolates examined thus far.[54]

TABLE 5.
Staining Characteristics of Chlamydial Species

Stain/Antibody	*C. pneumoniae*	*C. psittaci*	*C. trachomatis*
Iodine	−	−	+
Anti-LPS*	+	+	+
Anti–*C. trachomatis* MOMP	−	−	+
Anti–*C. pneumoniae* MOMP	+	−	−

*LPS = lipopolysaccharide; MOMP = major outer membrane protein.

EPIDEMIOLOGY

Chlamydia pneumoniae appears to be a primary human pathogen. Attempts to identify zoonotic reservoirs have been unsuccessful. The mode of transmission remains uncertain but is probably via infected respiratory secretions. Acquisition of infection by droplet aerosol has been described during a laboratory accident.[55] In vitro studies have demonstrated that *C. pneumoniae* will survive small-particle aerosolization and will remain viable on formica counter-tops for 30 hours and in tissue paper for 12 hours.[56] These observations suggest that several mechanisms of transmission, including fomites, are possible.

Outbreaks of *C. pneumoniae* pneumonia have occurred in enclosed populations such as military recruits.[57, 58] Spread of infection has been documented among family members in the same household.[59] Serologic surveys have documented a rising prevalence of antibody to *C. pneumoniae* with increasing age: in 10% of children 5 to 10 years of age and reaching 30% to 45% by adolescence.[49] Several studies from the early 1980s found a serologic association between serologic evidence of *C. trachomatis* infection and community-acquired pneumonia and pharyngitis in adults.[60, 61] With the advent of specific serologic tests for *C. pneumoniae* it has become clear that these seroconversions were attributable to *C. pneumoniae*, not *C. trachomatis*. Recent serosurveys from Europe, the United States, and Japan have found that over 50% of adults have IgG antibody to *C. pneumoniae* as determined by the microimmunofluorescence (MIF) assay, thus suggesting that infection is common and frequently subclinical.[62–65]

Data from both Sweden and Norway have suggested that a number of cases of "psittacosis" diagnosed serologically with the complement fixation test but with no history of bird exposure were probable due to *C. pneumoniae*.[66, 67] One example was an outbreak of suspected psittacosis in a boys' boarding school in England that involved 24 children and adults.[68] The illness was very mild and characterized by pharyngitis and flu-like symptoms, including headache, fever, and cough. No avian source was identified. The cases occurred over a 3-month period, thus suggesting person-to-person spread, which is very uncommon in psittacosis when secondary cases are very severe. Subsequently sera were tested for *C. pneumoniae* antibody and found to be positive.[69]

The proportion of community-acquired pneumonias associated with *C. pneumoniae* infection has ranged from 6% to 19%, varying with geographic location and the age group examined.[22, 70–74] Infection in children under the age of 5 years has been rare in Seattle and Scandinavia, whereas in a study of Filipino children under the age of 5 years who had lower respiratory tract infection, nearly 10% had either acute or chronic antibody to *C. pneumoniae*.[70] Most of these studies were based on serology alone. In Brooklyn, based on isolation of the organism in culture, we have found that the proportion of lower respiratory tract infections associated with *C. pneumoniae* increased from 9% in children under the age of 5 years to 19% in the 5- to 16-year-old age category.[71] In the multicenter antibiotic treatment study previously described, we also obtained cultures for *C. pneumoniae*. Forty-two (16%) of the 260 children enrolled were culture-positive.[22] The prevalence of *C. pneumoniae* infection in children 3 through 6 years of age and those 6 through 12 years of age was similar (see Table 2). Seven children were coinfected with *C. pneumoniae* and *M. pneumoniae*. The only child in the study who had a positive blood culture for *S. pneumoniae* was also culture-positive for *C. pneumoniae*. Chirgwin et al.[71] also reported several coinfections with *C. pneumoniae*, *S. pneumoniae*, and *H. influenzae* type b. The latter was a 5-year-old boy with bronchopneumonia who had a positive blood culture and who responded promptly to treatment with ampicillin. In these cases, *C. pneumoniae* may not be the primary cause of the pneumonia but might disrupt the normal clearance mechanisms and enable other pathogens to invade. *Chlamydia pneumoniae* has been found to inhibit ciliary motion of bronchial epithelial cells.[75]

In approximately 50% of the children reported by Chirgwin et al. and in the pneumonia treatment study, no antibody was detectable by MIF.[22, 71] These children tended to be younger ($\leq$12 years of age) than the children who did have a serologic response. This would suggest that serosurveys of pediatric populations may actually underestimate the prevalence of infection in young children.

In studies to date, acute infection with *C. pneumoniae* does not appear to vary by season. There are reports of cycles in Seattle and Scandinavia lasting several years during which the incidence of new infection with *C. pneumoniae* waxes and wanes.[76] In contrast, the infection appears to be endemic in Brooklyn, which may be a function of the greater population density.

Chlamydia pneumoniae appears to be capable of causing prolonged, often asymptomatic respiratory infection. Reports from Brooklyn, Norway, and Sweden suggest that asymptomatic carriage may in fact be relatively common.[77–80] A recent study from Sweden documented asymptomatic nasopharyngeal infection in 11 of 234 (4.7%) subjectively healthy adults between 18 and 75 years of age.[79] *Chlamydia pneumoniae* has also been isolated from 2 of 41 (4.9%) healthy children seen for camp or school physical examinations.[80] Persistent nasopharyngeal infection with *C. pneumoniae* following acute respiratory infection has been documented in adults and children for periods of up to 11 months.[77] It is not known what role asymptomatic carriage plays in the epidemiology of *C. pneumoniae* infection.

CLINICAL MANIFESTATIONS

The spectrum of disease associated with *C. pneumoniae* is expanding. Most infections are probably mild or asymptomatic. Longitudinal serologic data obtained from military recruits in Finland suggest that only about 10% of infections result in clinically apparent pneumonia.[49] Initial reports emphasized mild atypical pneumonia clinically resembling that associated with *M. pneumoniae:* fever, malaise, cough, and frequently headache and pharyngitis. In several subsequent studies, however, pneumonia associated with *C. pneumoniae* has been associated with severe illness and even death, although the role of pre-existing chronic conditions as contributing factors in many of these patients is difficult to assess. In some cases, however, *C. pneumoniae* appears to be clearly implicated as a serious pathogen even in the absence of underlying disease. We have isolated *C. pneumoniae* from the respiratory tract and pleural fluid of a previously healthy 19-year-old boy with severe pneumonia complicated by respiratory failure and pleural effusions.[81] Rumbach et al. recently reported a similar case, a 45-year-old man in whom severe pneumonia with respiratory failure developed after pneumonectomy for squamous cell carcinoma. *Chlamydia pneumoniae* was the only pathogen isolated from BAL fluid.[82]

The role of host factors remains to be determined. Although *C. pneumoniae* has been detected in BAL fluid from 10% of a group of patients with AIDS and pneumonia, its clinical role in these patients is uncertain because most were coinfected with other well-recognized pathogens such as *Pneumocystis carinii* and *Mycobacterium tuberculosis.*[83] Gaydos and colleagues[84] recently identified *C. pneumoniae* infection by PCR in 11% of a group of immunocompromised adults with human immunodeficiency virus (HIV) infection, malignancies, and other immune disorders including systemic lupus erythematosus (SLE), sarcoidosis, and common variable immunodeficiency. *Chlamydia pneumoniae* appeared to be responsible for 6 of 31 (19%) episodes of acute chest syndrome in children with sickle cell disease in our population.[31] Five of these children also appeared to be significantly clinically compromised by the infection with severe hypoxemia ($Po_2 < 80$ mm Hg). We have also isolated the organism from three patients with cystic fibrosis who were initially evaluated for acute pulmonary exacerbations.

One of the most exciting recent developments suggests an association between *C. pneumoniae* infection and reactive airway disease. We have seen several patients with culture-documented *C. pneumoniae* infection who have had significant bronchospasm. In one patient asthmatic bronchitis was diagnosed, and the patient received systemic and topical steroids. She did not improve until her chlamydial infection was treated.[77] Hahn et al.[85] reported an association between serologic evidence of acute *C. pneumoniae* infection and wheezing in adults seen for lower respiratory tract illness. However, they were able to isolate the organism from only 1 of 365 patients. As part of a preliminary study in children, we isolated *C. pneumoniae* from 13 of 118 (11%) children 5 to 15 years of age who were initially evaluated for either new or acute exacerbations of asthma.[80] Treatment of the infection appeared to result in both clinical improvement and improvement in pulmonary function test scores. It is also of interest to note that only 5 of the children with confirmed infection had detectable IgG antibody to *C. pneumoniae*. One child who was noncompliant with his antibiotic therapy was culture-positive on five occasions over a 3-month period. In addition, no anti–*C. pneumoniae* antibody was ever able to be detected. The potential of *C. pneumoniae* to cause prolonged, persistent infection may produce chronic inflammation and trigger bronchospasm in susceptible individuals.

DIAGNOSIS

Culture

Diagnosis of *C. pneumoniae* infection has been based on isolation of the organism and on serology. Initial studies suggested that *C. pneumoniae* was very difficult to isolate in tissue culture as compared with *C. trachomatis*. Most investigators originally used HeLa 229 cells pretreated with dextran diethylaminoethyl (DEAE).[86] Specimens required multiple passages in tissue culture, the inclusions were very small and difficult to see, and in general the yield was very poor. *Chlamydia pneumoniae* grows more readily in other cell lines, specifically HL and HEp-2 cells.[87, 88] Omission of pretreatment with dextran DEAE results in much larger inclusions, and specimens need only be passed once. These new methods have greatly simplified and increased the sensitivity of culture and should be within the capacity of any laboratory that performs *C. trachomatis* culture.

The best site for sampling appears to be the nasopharynx rather than the throat. As part of the multicenter pneumonia treatment study, duplicate specimens were obtained from the nasopharynx and throat from a number of children. *Chlamydia pneumoniae* was present in all of the nasopharyngeal cultures but in only 50% of the throat specimens. Nasopharyngeal cultures can be obtained with Dacron-tipped, wire-shafted swabs. Specimens for culture should be placed in appropriate transport media, usually a sucrose-phosphate buffer with antibiotics and fetal calf serum, and stored immediately at 4°C. Viability may decrease if specimens are held at room temperature. If specimens cannot be processed within 24 hours, they should be frozen at −70°C until culture can be performed. After 72 hours' incubation, culture confirmation can be performed with either genus-specific (anti-LPS) or *C. pneumoniae* species-specific fluorescent antibody staining (see Table 5). Inclusions do not contain glycogen and will therefore not stain with iodine. If a genus-specific antibody is used, *C. pneumoniae* should be confirmed by differential staining with a *C. trachomatis* antibody; if the latter is negative, then the isolate is either *C. pneumoniae* or *C. psittaci*. If there was no avian exposure, psittacosis would be highly unlikely.

Nonculture Methods

Direct detection of elementary bodies in clinical specimens by fluorescent antibody stains is sometimes possible.[48] Similarly, chlamydial antigen has been detected in some clinical specimens with an enzyme immunoassay (EIA). All the currently available EIAs will detect *C. pneumoniae* as well as *C. trachomatis* since they use polyclonal or genus-specific monoclonal antibodies. Chirgwin et al.[71] obtained nasopharyngeal specimens from 91 patients with pneumonia for testing with Chlamydiazyme (Abbott Laboratories, North Chicago). Although there were no false positives, the EIA detected only 2 of 15 (15%) patients who were culture-positive for *C. pneumoniae*.

It appears that the number of organisms present in pneumonia is considerably lower than the number found in genital chlamydial infections. DNA amplification methods, e.g., PCR, may be necessary. Initial reports of the use of PCR appear to be promising.[89, 90] In a preliminary study we examined nasopharyngeal specimens from 43 symptomatic and 58 asymptomatic individuals by culture and PCR.[91] Polymerase chain reaction had a sensitivity vs. culture of 84% and a specificity of 99%. Some of the false negatives may have been due to substances present in clinical specimens that inhibit polymerase. It may still be some time before PCR for *C. pneumoniae* will be available in clinical laboratories.

Serology

Most investigators to date have relied on serologic diagnosis using the MIF test and the complement fixation test. The complement fixation test is genus specific and has largely been used for the diagnosis of lymphogranuloma venereum and psittacosis. Most individuals with oculogenital *C. trachomatis* infections will not have detectable complement fixation antibody. Originally, Grayston et al. found that fewer than one third of hospitalized patients with *C. pneumoniae* infection had complement fixation antibody.[49] However, in a recent report of a small outbreak of *C. pneumoniae* infection among University of Washington students, all seven patients with pneumonia had complement fixation titers of 1:64 or greater.[92]

Grayston et al.[49] have proposed a set of criteria for serologic diagnosis of *C. pneumoniae* infection that is being used by many laboratories and clinicians. For acute infection the patient should have a fourfold rise in IgG titer, a single IgM titer of 1:16 or greater, or a single IgG titer of 1:512 or higher. Past or pre-existing infection is defined as an IgG titer of 1:16 or higher but less than 1:512. Grayston et al. further propose that the pattern of antibody response in primary infection may differ from that seen in reinfection. In initial infection, the IgM response appears about 3 weeks after the onset of illness, and the IgG response appears at 6 to 8 weeks. In reinfection, the IgM response may be absent and the IgG response occurs earlier, within 1 to 2 weeks.[49] Because of the relatively long period until development of a serologic response in primary infection, the antibody response may be missed if convalescent sera are obtained too soon, i.e., earlier than 3 weeks after the onset of illness. However, it is important to realize that these criteria have some limitations. These criteria, especially those for use of a single sample, have not been correlated with the results of cultures and are based mainly on data from adults. We have seen the antibody response in primary infection take over 3 months. We have also seen acute culture-positive infection without seroconversion, and this appears to be more common in young children. Results from the multicenter pneumonia treatment study and our asthma study found that approximately 20% of children with culture-documented *C. pneumoniae* infection had serologic evidence of acute infection.[22] Almost 50% had no detectable antibody in the MIF test. These children tended to be 10 years of age or younger. However, results of immunoblotting reveal that these children do have antibody to a variety of *C. pneumoniae* proteins but that fewer than 30% react with the major outer membrane protein (MOMP), which suggests that the problem resides with the MIF test itself.[93]

Background rates of seropositivity can also be very high in some populations. As part of a study of the prevalence of asymptomatic *C. pneumoniae* infection among objectively healthy adults, we obtained cultures and sera from 72 health care workers at our institution. Although none were culture-positive or positive by *C. pneumoniae*–specific PCR, 83% had IgG titers of 1:32 or higher, and 17% had serologic evidence of "acute infection," i.e., an IgM titer of 1:16 or greater and/or an IgG titer of 1:512 or higher.[94] Similar results were reported by Kern et al. among firefighters in Rhode Island.[65] None of these individuals were ill. The specificity of the MIF IgM assay can be affected by the presence of rheumatoid factor in the serum. A study from the Netherlands reported that with increasing age of the patient there appears to be an increased probability of false positives due to rheumatoid factor.[95] These sera should be routinely absorbed before MIF IgM testing.

There are also some questions about the specificity of the MIF test in general. There can be cross-reacting antibody to the chlamydial genus LPS antigen. Although this antibody should give a different pattern of fluorescence in the MIF assay than the species-specific MOMP, it can be difficult to differentiate one from the other. Although there is less than 10% DNA homology between the three *Chlamydia* species, the MOMP gene appears to be highly conserved, with 67% to 72% for nucleotide sequences and 63% to 76% for amino acid sequences.[52] It is not known whether this may cause cross-reactions in the MIF test, but the MOMP does not appear to be immunodominant in the antibody response to *C. pneumoniae*.[93, 96] This may be more of a problem in adolescents and adults, who can have coexisting or previous genital *C. trachomatis* infection. We have observed that many of the adolescents and adults we evaluate for *C. pneumoniae* infection have MIF antibody to *C. trachomatis* at similar titers. A recent report by Moss and colleagues from England found that antibodies to *C. pneumoniae* and *C. psittaci* accounted for up to half of all chlamydial IgG–positive persons attending a sexually transmitted disease clinic.[97] The initial serologic studies that suggested that *C. trachomatis* was a cause of community-acquired pneumonia and pharyngitis in adults were probably detecting antibody to *C. pneumoniae*.[60, 61]

TREATMENT

To date there have been few published data describing the response of *C. pneumoniae* infection to antibiotic therapy. In vitro susceptibilities indicate that tetracyclines and erythromycin as well as several new macrolides (azithromycin and clarithromycin) and quinolones (ofloxacin) are active[96, 98, 99] (see Table 3). Like *C. psittaci*, *C. pneumoniae* is highly resistant to sulfonamides.[96]

The optimum dose and duration of therapy are uncertain. Anecdotal data suggest that prolonged therapy (i.e., at least 2 weeks) may be desirable since recrudescent symptoms have been described following 2-week courses of erythromycin and even after 30 days of tetracycline or doxycycline.[77] The dose and duration of therapy recommended for treating *M. pneumoniae*, 1 g of erythromycin per day for 10 days, do not appear to be adequate inasmuch as Grayston et al. reported a number of clinical failures.[48] There are no published studies of treatment of *C. pneumoniae* infection that have used cultures and assessed microbiologic efficacy. Studies examining the efficacy of clarithromycin and azithromycin are currently being conducted. Results of the multicenter pediatric pneumonia treatment study[22] found that erythromycin suspension, 40 mg/kg/day divided in two doses for 10 days, successfully eradicated *C. pneumoniae* from 86% of the positive children whereas clarithromycin suspension at 15 mg/kg/day divided in two doses for 10 days eradicated the organism from 79% of the positive children (see Table 4). All of these children improved clinically despite persistence of the organism. Persistence was not related to the development of antibiotic resistance since all of the isolates remained susceptible to erythromycin and clarithromycin during and after treatment.

Preliminary data from an open study evaluating azithromycin for the treatment of bronchitis and pneumonia in adults found that 1.5 g of the drug given over a 5-day period had 75% efficacy in eliminating *C. pneumoniae* from the nasopharynx. Despite persistence of the organism, these patients also improved clinically.[100] We are currently recommending for adults either doxycycline, 100 mg/day divided in two doses for 21 days, or erythromycin, 500 mg/day divided in 4 doses also for 21 days. For children under 8 years of age, we recommend erythromycin suspension, 50 mg/kg/day divided in 4 doses for 21 days. These regimens will clearly raise problems with compliance, but until more data are available about the efficacy of the newer macrolides, these seem to be the regimens that work best.

CHLAMYDIA PSITTACI

Human infection with *C. psittaci* was probably first described by Juergensen in 1874 or Ritter in 1876. Ritter described seven cases of an unusual pneumonia that appeared to be caused by parrots and finches that were caged in the study of his brother's home in Switzerland. Following these reports there were several outbreaks of a similar disease in Europe that established the association with an exposure to birds. The term *psittacosis* was coined by Morange in 1892 from the Greek word for parrots, *psittakos*.[101]

ORGANISM

Chlamydia psittaci is now known to be a very diverse species that affects nonpsittacine birds and many mammalian species as well. There is only 10% DNA homology between *C. psittaci* and *C. trachomatis*. *Chlamydia psittaci* can also be differentiated from *C. trachomatis* by lack of glycogen in the inclusions, inclusion morphology, and resistance to sulfonamides (see Table 5).

The diversity of *C. psittaci* is probably a reflection of this wide host range. Strains of *C. psittaci* analyzed by restriction endonuclease analysis demonstrated at least five biovars.[101] The avian biovar appears to contain at least four serovars as determined by monoclonal antibody staining. Two of these serovars, psittacine and turkey, are of major importance in the avian population of the United States. They are each associated with important host preferences and disease characteristics.

Strains of the turkey serovar have all been associated either with serious disease in birds or human beings or with major epizootics in turkeys and often result in disease in humans. The psittacine serovar has also been associated with serious disease in humans; however, human involvement is usually limited to sporadic cases following exposure to pet birds or pigeons.

EPIDEMIOLOGY

According to the most recent report from the Centers for Disease Control (CDC), 1,136 cases and 8 deaths from psittacosis were reported in the United States from 1975 to 1984.[102] Seventy percent of these reported cases were the result of exposure to pet caged birds. Those at highest risk of acquiring psittacosis included bird owners or fanciers, pet shop employees, or pigeon fanciers. Since

1984 there have been several major outbreaks of psittacosis in turkey processing plants where approximately 300 individuals contracted the infection.[103, 104] Workers exposed to turkey viscera were at the highest risk of infection.

Inhalation of infectious aerosols derived from feces, fecal dust, and secretions of *C. psittaci*–infected animals is believed to be the primary route of infection. The source birds can be asymptomatically infected or can show signs of infection such as anorexia, ruffled feathers, depression, and watery green droppings. Psittacosis is frequently a systemic infection in birds. The turkey strains can induce severe pericarditis. The gastrointestinal tract is also frequently infected. The psittacine serovar appears to much less virulent in both turkeys and pigeons and psittacine birds.[101]

Psittacosis is uncommon in children, but it can occur. In one large series of 135 patients from Australia seen over a 15-year period, the youngest patient was 17 years of age.[105] Children may be less likely exposed to birds because bird keeping is often an adult hobby. An outbreak of psittacosis involving two adolescents has been reported from a small village in Scotland. The source of the infection appeared to be the local pet shop, which had taken delivery of four lovebirds, two of whom died shortly after arrival.[106] Another report describes a family outbreak in which three members of a family of nine persons contracted severe pneumonia.[107] A newly purchased cockatiel appeared to be the primary source, but person-to-person transmission was likely to have taken place between 19-years-old twin brothers who shared a bedroom, one of whom had no direct contact with the bird. A retrospective review of the records of the Public Health Laboratory at Leeds, England, for cases with a fourfold rise in chlamydia complement fixation titers identified 219 patients over a 14-year period from 1965 to 1989.[108] The ages ranged from 9 months to 87 years; only five (2.2%) of the patients were younger than 10 years of age, but only 34 cases were believed to be psittacosis on review. All had antecedent avian exposures, but the ages of the patients were not specified.

CLINICAL MANIFESTATIONS

The mean incubation period is 15 days after exposure (range, 5 to 21 days). The onset is usually abrupt, with complaints of fever, cough, and headache. The fever is high and frequently associated with rigors and sweats. The headache can be so severe that meningitis may be considered a possibility; 33% of the patients in the Australian series had lumbar punctures.[105] The cough is usually nonproductive. Rales may be heard on auscultation. Chest x-ray findings are usually abnormal with variable infiltrates. Pleural effusions may also be present.

The WBC count is usually not elevated, although there may be a mild leukocytosis. Almost 50% of the patients in the Australian series had abnormal liver function test results, including elevated aspartate aminotransferase, alkaline phosphatase, and bilirubin levels.[105]

DIAGNOSIS AND TREATMENT

Because of the varying clinical findings, the diagnosis of psittacosis can be difficult. A history of exposure to birds is very important. However, as many as 20% of patients with psittacosis may not have a history of contact with birds.[101, 102] In the Australian series, 85% of their patients had a history of recent bird contact; 71% of these described a very strong bird contact history.[105] Exposure to poultry was found in only 5 patients. Pneumonia caused by *C. psittaci* can also have a similar clinical appearance and should be suspected if there is evidence of person-to-person spread, which is unusual with psittacosis, and secondary cases tend to be very severe. Other infections that can produce the syndrome of pneumonia with high fever, unusually severe headache, and myalgia include *M. pneumoniae* infection, tularemia, tuberculosis, fungal infections, legionnaires' disease, and of course, bacterial infection. The diagnosis of psittacosis in humans is primarily based on clinical findings, epidemiology, and serology. Culture of *C. psittaci* is not available outside of research laboratories. A recent report by Oldach et al.[109] suggests that direct fluorescent antibody staining of sputum or the use of chlamydial EIAs can be used for the rapid diagnosis of psittacosis. They describe two patients in whom these methods were used successfully. Both patients were culture-positive and had reliable histories of avian exposure. One raced pigeons, four of which had died 6 weeks before the onset of illness, and the other had a pet cockatiel that died 2 weeks earlier. These cases also emphasize the importance of a history of avian exposure.

The CDC[103] differentiates three classes of cases of psittacosis based on laboratory findings or exposures.

1. Confirmed case: clinical specimen yielding *C. psittaci* or compatible clinical illness and a fourfold rise in complement fixation antibody titer.
2. Presumptive case: compatible clinical illness and single serum

sample titer of 1:32 or higher or a stable antibody titer of 1:32 or higher in two samples.

3. Suspect case: a case that does not meet the criteria in nos. 1 or 2 but was associated with another case or avian chlamydiosis.

The complement fixation test is a genus-specific test; thus infection caused by *C. pneumoniae* can give titers of 1:32 or greater. Early treatment with tetracycline may also suppress the antibody response.

The recommended treatment for psittacosis in humans is 500 mg of tetracycline every 6 hours orally for 7 to 10 days. Erythromycin, 2 g/day for 7 to 10 days, can also be used.

Immunity following an initial infection does not appear to be long-term. Reinfection and clinical disease can develop within 2 months of treatment. There are two well-documented cases of reinfection. A pet shop employee had two episodes of psittacosis 11 months apart. Each episode met the CDC-confirmed case definition.[110]

Q FEVER (COXIELLA BURNETII)

Q fever, caused by the rickettsial organism *Coxiella burnetii*, is a zoonotic infection endemic worldwide in a variety of vertebrates and invertebrates. *Coxiella burnetii* is resistant to desiccation and environmental degradation and is extremely infectious by small-particle aerosol.[111] Cattle, sheep, goats, parturient cats, and ticks are the primary reservoirs. Q fever is usually subclinical in animals, although the organism can be excreted in milk, urine, and feces. *Coxiella burnetii* can be found in especially high numbers in amniotic fluid, placenta, and fetal membranes in late gestation, which makes parturient animals especially infectious. It is thought that highly infectious aerosols are generated during delivery. Persons with Q fever usually have severe headache, high fever (≥104°F), shaking chills, general malaise, myalgia, chest pain, and sometimes pneumonia and hepatitis. Q fever usually occurs sporadically, but large outbreaks have occurred, particularly among workers in abattoirs and research laboratories.[111] As a cause of atypical pneumonia, *Coxiella burnetii* is relatively uncommon, even in adults. However, cases have been reported in children. As with psittacosis, the epidemiologic history is very important for making the diagnosis.

Richardus et al.[112] reported infection with *C. burnetii* in 18 children less than 3 years of age in the Netherlands over a 16-month period. The major manifestations of the disease were fever, often relapsing, and malaise; all required hospitalization. Four children had pneumonia, their ages ranging from 7 months to 3 years. Most of the children had not been outside the Netherlands before the onset of their disease. A possible source was identified in 8 (44%) children and included exposure to goats, sheep, wool, cattle, and in 1 case, mother's milk. The 4 children with pneumonia had cough and abnormal chest examinations, with crepitant rales heard on auscultation. Chest radiographs revealed lobar consolidation or diffuse infiltrates. One child had a large pleural effusion. Additional symptoms were anorexia, diarrhea, and vomiting. Two of the children had skin manifestations, an erythematous macular rash, and vasculitis. Ruiz-Contreras et al. recently reported 13 children, 2 to 14 years of age, with Q fever from Spain.[113] Although 4 of these children were coughing, only 1 had pneumonia radiographically. This child also had a *M. pneumoniae* complement fixation titer of 1:512. Concomitant symptoms included headache, vomiting, and abdominal pain. Eleven children had hepatomegaly or splenomegaly. Six of these children had identified epidemiologic risk factors, including contact with sheep, residence in a rural area, or ingestion of raw milk. A survey of 323 hospitalized patients with Q fever in France found the mean age to be 45.5 years; however, there were 4 children under 9 years of age and 8 children between 10 and 19 years of age.[114] Pneumonia was present in approximately half of the total group of patients, but no details were given on the children. A likely epidemiologic risk factor(s) was identified in approximately half of the patients; exposure to sheep or placentas from ewes or goats was most frequent. An outbreak of Q fever has been reported from a secondary school in England where the source appeared to be goats.[115] Another source of Q fever, parturient cats, has been associated with several outbreaks in Canada and one in the United States.[116, 117] These outbreaks occurred in urban as well as rural settings.

Q fever should be diagnosed serologically. Cultivation of *C. burnetii* is very hazardous and not recommended for routine diagnosis.[111] There are a number of methods available for the detection of specific anti–*C. burnetii* antibody. The methods used most commonly are the complement fixation and indirect fluorescent antibody (IFA) tests. Complement fixation titers do not peak until 12 weeks, whereas IFA titers reach their maximum levels 4 to 8 weeks after the onset of disease. The IFA test is believed to be more sensitive and allows for detection of IgM antibodies, which can help to distinguish acute infection from earlier illness. Both complement fixation and IFA antibodies may persist for a year or more.

Coxiella burnetii displays an antigenetic phase variation (phase I and II) analogous to the smooth-to-rough variation that occurs with some species of enteric bacteria. Antibodies to phase II are prominent in patients with acute, self-limited Q fever, whereas phase I antibodies are more prominent in patients with chronic infection. The ratio of phase II to phase I antibodies in acute Q fever is usually greater than 1.[111]

Most acute cases of Q fever will resolve without specific treatment, but the potential for development of chronic infection makes treatment advisable. There are no controlled studies of the treatment of Q fever in children. Experience with adults suggests that tetracyclines are the treatment of choice. In adults and children 8 years of age and older, tetracycline, 25 mg/kg/day in four divided doses for 2 weeks, or in adults, doxycycline, twice daily, also for 2 weeks, is recommended.[111] In younger children chloramphenicol is an alternative, but its efficacy has not been proved. Erythromycin, clindamycin, and cephalosporins are not active against *C. burnetii*.[118] Quinolones have been shown to be active in vitro but are also contraindicated in children.[118]

LEGIONNAIRES' DISEASE

Legionnaires' disease is an acute illness characterized by pneumonia or a febrile, nonpneumonic systemic illness. The etiologic agents, *Legionella* spp., are fastidious, gram-negative bacilli. Legionnaires' disease was first recognized as a clinical entity when it was found to be responsible for the notorious epidemic of pneumonia that occurred among participants at the American Legion Convention at the Bellevue-Stratford Hotel in Philadelphia in 1976.[119] Over 200 people were affected, and 34 died. The genus *Legionella* comprises 30 species and multiple serogroups. The 1976 epidemic was caused by *Legionella pneumophila,* which is estimated to cause 90% to 95% of all cases of legionnaires' disease in individuals without underlying disease.

Legionella is ubiquitous in the environment, especially in water. It can be found in lake water, ponds, bath water, hot water tanks, and air-conditioning cooling towers.

Infection with *Legionella* occurs sporadically and in outbreaks. The latter have frequently occurred in hospitals and are associated with environmental sources. In most cases where thorough investigations have been done, the reservoirs most commonly identified have been potable water distribution systems, air-conditioning cooling towers, or both.[120] Most of these outbreaks have mainly affected adults. Individuals who are at highest risk of acquiring legionnaires' disease after exposure usually have a defect in their pulmonary defense mechanisms that can be secondary to general anesthesia, steroids, cigarette smoking, chronic lung disease, or immunodeficiency.

By 5 years of age, 20% to 50% of normal children will have anti-*Legionella* antibody titers of 1:64 or greater, which suggests that subclinical exposure in early childhood occurs frequently.[121, 122] Yet several serologic studies have found that fewer than 4% of normal children with community-acquired pneumonia will have a fourfold rise in antibody to *Legionella*.[123] The incidence of *Legionella* infection in children is unknown, and the diagnosis is probably rarely considered.

To date there have been fewer than 20 cases of culture-documented legionnaires' disease reported in children. Two thirds have occurred in children with underlying disease, including severe combined immunodeficiency, malignancies, SLE, asthma treated by corticosteroids, and chronic granulomatous disease.[124–129] Most were evidently hospital acquired. In many cases the diagnosis was made only at autopsy. Five cases of pneumonia due to *Legionella* have been reported in neonates, most of whom were premature and undergoing assisted ventilation; 3 died.[130] In several cases, including children and neonates, the diagnosis was made at autopsy.

Clinically, *Legionella* pneumonia cannot be readily differentiated from other severe bacterial pneumonias. Frequent symptoms and signs include rapid onset, fever, cough, pleuritic chest pain, dyspnea, abdominal pain, diarrhea, and headache; respiratory failure is frequent. Laboratory findings include an elevated WBC count with a shift to the left. Chest radiographs usually reveal lobar consolidation, pleural effusions, and rarely, cavitation.

The most specific method for the diagnosis of legionnaires' disease is isolation of the organism from sputum or other respiratory tract specimen, e.g., BAL fluid. *Legionella* may also be detected directly in these specimens with immunofluorescence staining. Other nonculture methods available are detection of *L. pneumophila* antigenuria and *Legionella* rRNA probes.[120]

Serology appears to be of use in epidemiologic studies but is not very helpful for the acute diagnosis of sporadic cases. The method used is an IFA test. Little is known about the immune response to *Legionella* in children. In adults, approximately 25% of patients with culture-documented disease fail to seroconvert against the homologous serotype. It may take up to 3 months (median, 2 weeks) for a patient to seroconvert. Since the background seropositivity rate in healthy individuals, including young children, may reach 25%, only a fourfold rise in titer to *Legionella* should be considered significant.[120]

There are no prospective studies of treatment of legionnaires' disease in adults, and even fewer data are available regarding treatment in children. Erythromycin has been the drug of choice and is used intravenously at 15 mg/kg per dose four times daily for 18 to 21 days or longer if there is severe immunosuppression. Part of the course can be given orally. Some experts recommend the addition of rifampin, 15 mg/kg/day, in patients with serious illness or those who fail to respond to monotherapy. Some normal, healthy individuals with legionnaires' disease will improve without treatment, which may make it difficult to assess the efficacy of any regimen. Relapses have occurred when intravenous erythromycin was changed to the oral route or after a short course of treatment. *Legionella pneumophila* can survive intracellularly in alveolar macrophages, which may be a major reason for antibiotic failure since erythromycin does not penetrate phagocytic cells very well.[131] Alternate therapies include tetracycline and sulfamethoxazole-trimethoprim, neither of which has been extensively evaluated. Recent clinical and laboratory evidence suggests that some quinolones (ciprofloxacin and ofloxacin) and new macrolides (azithromycin and clarithromycin) may be more effective than erythromycin.

SUMMARY

The major agents responsible for atypical pneumonia in children include a wide variety of organisms, one *Mycoplasma* species, two *Chlamydia* species, a rickettsia, and one fastidious bacterium. *Mycoplasma pneumoniae* and *C. pneumoniae* together may be responsible for over 40% of these infections. Recognition of the role that these agents play in pneumonia is important since many of the diagnostic methods used to detect these organisms are not available in most hospital microbiology laboratories. If you don't look, you won't find. Epidemiologic factors can provide valuable clues, especially with the less frequently encountered infections, since it is almost impossible to make a clinical diagnosis on which to base treatment. A reliable history of avian exposure should suggest psittacosis, exposure to sheep or pregnant cats suggests Q fever, and children with underlying malignancy or immunodeficiency or those receiving systemic steroids may have legionnaires' disease.

None of these organisms are susceptible to β-lactam antibiotics. Sometimes the diagnosis is not considered until after the child has failed to respond to a penicillin or a cephalosporin and routine bacteriology is negative. In view of the role played by *M. pneumoniae* and *C. pneumoniae*, a macrolide may be the first-line antibiotic for atypical pneumonia in children.

REFERENCES

1. Osler W: *The Principles and Practice of Medicine*, ed 4. New York, Appleton, 1901, p 108.
2. Broughton RA: Infections due to *Mycoplasma pneumoniae* in childhood. *Pediatr Infect Dis J* 5:71–85, 1986.
3. Clyde WA: Clinical overview of typical *Mycoplasma pneumoniae* infections. *Clin Infect Dis* 17(suppl):32–36, 1993.
4. Foy HM: Infections caused by *Mycoplasma pneumoniae* and possible carrier state in different populations of patients. *Clin Infect Dis* 17(suppl):37–46, 1993.
5. Smith W, Andrewes CH, Laidlaw PP: A virus isolated from influenza patients. *Lancet* 2:66–68, 1933.
6. Loda FA, Clyde WA, Glezea WP, et al: Studies on the role of viruses, bacteria and *M. pneumoniae* as causes of lower respiratory tract infections in children. *J Pediatr* 72:161–176, 1968.
7. Glezen WP, Loda FA, Clyde WA, et al: Epidemiologic patterns of acute lower respiratory tract disease in a pediatric group practice. *J Pediatr* 78:397–406, 1971.
8. Mufson MA, Krause HE, Mocega HE, et al: Viruses, *Mycoplasma pneumoniae* and bacteria associated with lower respiratory tract disease among infants. *Am J Epidemiol* 91:192–202, 1970.
9. Maletzky AJ, Cooney MK, Luce R, et al: Epidemiology of viral and mycoplasmal agents associated with childhood lower respiratory illness in a civilian population. *J Pediatr* 78:407–414, 1971.
10. Foy HM, Cooney MK, McMahan R, et al: Viral and mycoplasmal pneumonia in a prepaid medical care group during an eight year period. *Am J Epidemiol* 97:93–102, 1973.
11. Glezen WP, Denny FW: Epidemiology of acute lower respiratory disease in children. *N Engl J Med* 288:498–505, 1973.
12. Hu PC, Cole RM, Huang YS, et al: *Mycoplasma pneumoniae* infection: Role of a surface protein in the attachment organelle. *Science* 216:313–315, 1982.
13. Collier AM, Clyde WA: Appearance of *Mycoplasma pneumoniae* in lungs of experimentally infected hamsters and sputum from patients with natural disease. *Am Rev Respir Dis* 110:756–773, 1974.
14. Foy HM, Kenny GE, McMahan R, et al: *Mycoplasma pneumoniae* pneumonia in an urban area. *JAMA* 214:1666–1672, 1970.
15. Mirza AA, Ahmad OAS, Ifere AS, et al: Prevalence of *Mycoplasma*

pneumoniae in children with pneumonia in Zaiia, Nigeria. *Ann Trop Pediatr* 11:51–55, 1991.
16. Saikku P, Ruutu P, Leinonen M, et al: *Mycoplasma pneumoniae* and *Chlamydia trachomatis* in acute lower respiratory infections in Filipino children. *Am J Trop Med Hyg* 49:88–92, 1993.
17. Mogabgab WJ: *Mycoplasma pneumoniae* and adenovirus respiratory illness in military and university personnel, 1959–1966. *Am Rev Respir Dis* 7:345–358, 1968.
18. Chanock RM, Fox HH, James WD, et al: Epidemiology of *M. pneumoniae* infection in military recruits. *Ann N Y Acad Med* 143:484–496, 1967.
19. Fernald GW, Clyde WA: Epidemic pneumonia in university students. *J Adolesc Health Care* 10:520–526, 1989.
20. Broome CV, LaVenture M, Kaye HS, et al: An explosive outbreak of *Mycoplasma pneumoniae* infection in a summer camp. *Pediatrics* 66:884–888, 1980.
21. Nagayama Y, Sakurai N, Yamamoto K, et al: Isolation of *Mycoplasma pneumoniae* from children with lower-respiratory-tract infections. *J Infect Dis* 157:911–917, 1988.
22. Hammerschlag MR, Roblin PM, Cassell G, et al: Role of infection with *Chlamydia pneumoniae* among children with community acquired pneumonia in the USA (abstract 1377). Presented at the Interscience Conference on Antimicrobial Agents and Chemotherapy, New Orleans, 1993, p 371.
23. Stadel BV, Foy HM, Nuckolls JW, et al: *Mycoplasma pneumoniae* infection followed by *Haemophilus influenzae* pneumonia and bacteremia. *Am Rev Respir Dis* 112:131–133, 1975.
24. Nagayama Y, Sakurai N, Yamamato K: Clinical observations with pleuropneumonia due to *Mycoplasma pneumoniae. Pediatr Pulmonol* 8:182–187, 1990.
25. Fernald GW, Collier AM, Clyde WA: Respiratory infections due to *Mycoplasma pneumoniae* in infants and children. *Pediatrics* 55:327–335, 1975.
26. Lind K, Bentzon MW: Ten and a half years seroepidemiology of *Mycoplasma pneumoniae* infection in Denmark. *Epidemiol Infect* 107:189–199, 1991.
27. Foy HM, Grayston JT, Kenny GE, et al: Epidemiology of *Mycoplasma pneumoniae* infection in families. *JAMA* 197:859–866, 1966.
28. Biberfeld G, Sterner G: A study of *Mycoplasma pneumoniae* infections in families. *Scand J Infect Dis* 1:39–46, 1969.
29. Cherry JD: Anemia and mucocutaneous lesions due to *Mycoplasma pneumoniae* infections. *Clin Infect Dis* 17(suppl):47–51, 1993.
30. Loo VG, Richardson S, Quinn P: Isolation of *Mycoplasma pneumoniae* from pleural fluid. *Diagn Microbiol Infect Dis* 14:443–445, 1991.
31. Miller ST, Hammerschlag MR, Chirgwin K, et al: The role of *Chlamy-*

dia pneumoniae (sp. TWAR) in acute chest syndrome of sickle cell disease. *J Pediatr* 118:30–33, 1991.

32. Kai M, Kamiya S, Yabe H, et al: Rapid detection of *Mycoplasma pneumoniae* in clinical samples by polymerase chain reaction. *J Med Microbiol* 38:166–170, 1993.
33. Kleemola SRM, Karjalainen JE, Raty RKH: Rapid diagnosis of *Mycoplasma pneumoniae* infection. Clinical evaluation of a commercial probe test. *J Infect Dis* 162:70–75, 1990.
34. Kleemola M, Heiskanen-Kosma T, Nohynek, et al: Diagnostic efficacy of a *Mycoplasma pneumoniae* hybridization test in nasopharyngeal aspirates in children. *Pediatr Infect Dis J* 12:344–345, 1993.
35. Garrow DH: A rapid test for the presence of increased cold agglutinins. *BMJ* 2:206–208, 1958.
36. Griffin JP: Rapid screening for cold agglutinins in pneumonia. *Ann Intern Med* 70:701–705, 1969.
37. Rasch JR, Mogabgab WJ: Therapeutic effect of erythromycin on *Mycoplasma pneumoniae* pneumonia. *Antimicrob Agents Chemother* 5:693–699, 1965.
38. Shames JM, George RB, Holliday WB, et al: Comparison of antibiotics in the treatment of mycoplasmal pneumonia. *Arch Intern Med* 125:680–684, 1970.
39. Smith CB, Friedwell WT, Chanock RM: Shedding of *Mycoplasma pneumoniae* after tetracycline and erythromycin. *N Engl J Med* 276:1172–1175, 1967.
40. McCracken GH: Current status of antibiotic treatment for *Mycoplasma pneumoniae* infections. *Pediatr Infect Dis J* 5:167–171, 1986.
41. Rodvold KA, Piscitelli SC: New oral macrolides and fluoroquinolone antibiotics: An overview of pharmacokinetics, interactions and safety. *Clin Infect Dis* 17(suppl):192–199, 1993.
42. Cassell GH, Crnec J, Waites KB, et al: Efficacy of clarithromycin against *Mycoplasma pneumoniae*. *J Antimicrob Chemother* 27(suppl A):47–59, 1991.
43. Bebear C, Dupon M, Renandin, et al: Potential improvements in therapeutic options for mycoplasmal respiratory infections. *Clin Infect Dis* 17(suppl):202–207, 1993.
44. Anderson G, Esmond TS, Coles S, et al: A comparative safety and efficacy study of clarithromycin and erythromycin stearate in community acquired pneumonia. *J Antimicrob Chemother* 27(suppl A):117–124, 1991.
45. Chien SM, Pichotta P, Siepman N, et al: Treatment of community acquired pneumonia. A multicenter, double-blind randomized study comparing clarithromycin with erythromycin. *Chest* 103:697–701, 1993.
46. Schonwald S, Skerk V, Petricevic I, et al: Comparison of three-day and five-day courses of azithromycin in the treatment of atypical pneumonia. *Eur J Clin Microbiol Infect Dis* 10:877–880, 1991.

47. Block S, Hedrick J, Hammerschlag MR, et al: Unpublished data, 1993.
48. Grayston JT, Kuo CC, Wang SP, et al: A new *Chlamydia psittaci* strain, TWAR, isolated in acute respiratory tract infections. *N Engl J Med* 315:161–168, 1986.
49. Grayston JT, Campbell LA, Kuo C-C, et al: A new respiratory tract pathogen: *Chlamydia pneumoniae* strain TWAR. *J Infect Dis* 161:618–625, 1990.
50. Saikku P, Wang S-P, Kleemola M, et al: An epidemic of mild pneumonia due to an unusual strain of *Chlamydia psittaci. J Infect Dis* 151:832–839, 1985.
51. Chi EY, Kuo C-C, Grayston JT: Unique ultrastructure in the elementary body of *Chlamydia* sp. strain TWAR. *J Bacteriol* 169:3757–3763, 1987.
52. Carter MW, Al-Mahdawi SAH, Treharne JD, et al: Nucleotid sequence and taxonomic value of the major outer membrane protein gene of *Chlamydia pneumoniae* 106–207. *J Gen Microbiol* 137:465–475, 1991.
53. Popov VL, Shatkin AA, Pankratova VN, et al: Ultrastructure of *Chlamydia pneumoniae* in tissue culture. *FEMS Microbiol Lett* 84:129–134, 1991.
54. Campbell LA, Kuo C-C, Grayston JT: Characterization of the new *Chlamydia* agent, TWAR, as a unique organism by restriction endonuclease analysis and DNA-DNA hybridization. *J Clin Microbiol* 25:1911–1916, 1987.
55. Hyman CL, Augenbraun MH, Roblin PM, et al: Asymptomatic respiratory tract infection with *Chlamydia pneumoniae* TWAR. *J Clin Microbiol* 29:2082–2083, 1991.
56. Falsey AR, Walsh EE: Transmission of *Chlamydia pneumoniae. J Infect Dis* 168:393–396, 1993.
57. Kleemola M, Saikku P, Visakorpi R, et al: Epidemics of pneumonia caused by TWAR, a new *Chlamydia* organism, in military trainees in Finland. *J Infect Dis* 157:230–360, 1988.
58. Ekman M-R, Grayston JT, Visakorpi R, et al: An epidemic of infections due to *Chlamydia pneumoniae* in military conscripts. *Clin Infect Dis* 17:420–425, 1993.
59. Yamazaki T, Nakada H, Sakuri N, et al: Transmission of *Chlamydia pneumoniae* in young children in a Japanese family. *J Infect Dis* 162:1390–1392, 1990.
60. Komaroff AL, Aronson MD, Schachter J: *Chlamydia trachomatis* infection in adults with community-acquired pneumonia. *JAMA* 245:1319–1322, 1981.
61. Komaroff AL, Aronson MD, Pass TM, et al: Serologic evidence of chlamydial and mycoplasmal pharyngitis in adults. *Science* 222:927–929, 1983.
62. Kanamoto Y, Ouchi K, Mizui M, et al: Prevalence of antibody to *Chlamydia pneumoniae* TWAR in Japan. *J Clin Microbiol* 29:816–818, 1991.

63. Montes M, Cilla G, Alcorta M, et al: High prevalence of *Chlamydia pneumoniae* infection in children and young adults in Spain. *Pediatr Infect Dis J* 11:972–973, 1992.
64. Freidank HM, Braula D: Prevalence of antibodies to *Chlamydia pneumoniae* TWAR in a group of German medical students. *J Infect* 27:89–93, 1993.
65. Kern DG, Neill MA, Schachter J: A seroepidemiologic study of *Chlamydia pneumoniae* in Rhode Island. *Chest* 104:208–213, 1993.
66. Fryden A, Kihlstrom E, Maller R, et al: A clinical and epidemiological study of "ornithosis" caused by *Chlamydia psittaci* and *Chlamydia pneumoniae* (strain TWAR). *Scand J Infect Dis* 21:681–691, 1989.
67. Bruu A-L, Haukenes G, Aasen S, et al: *Chlamydia pneumoniae* infections in Norway 1981–87 earlier diagnosed as ornithosis. *Scand J Infect Dis* 23:299–304, 1991.
68. Pether JVS, Noah ND, Lan YK, et al: An outbreak of psittacosis in a boys' boarding school. *J Hyg Camb* 92:337–343, 1984.
69. Pether JVS, Wang S-P, Grayston JT: *Chlamydia pneumoniae,* strain TWAR, as the cause of an outbreak in a boys' school previously called psittacosis. *Epidemiol Infect* 103:395–400, 1989.
70. Saikku P, Ruutu P, Leinonen M, et al: Acute lower-respiratory-tract infection associated with chlamydial TWAR antibody in Filipino children. *J Infect Dis* 158:1095–1097, 1988.
71. Chirgwin K, Roblin PM, Gelling B, et al: Infection with *Chlamydia pneumoniae* in Brooklyn. *J Infect Dis* 163:757–761, 1991.
72. Marrie TJ, Grayston JT, Wang SP, et al: Pneumonia associated with the TWAR strain of *Chlamydia. Ann Intern Med* 106:507–511, 1987.
73. Thom DH, Grayston JT, Wang S-P, et al: *Chlamydia pneumoniae* strain TWAR. *Mycoplasma pneumoniae* and viral infections in acute respiratory disease in a university student health clinic population. *Am J Epidemiol* 132:248–256, 1990.
74. Grayston JT, Diwan VK, Cooney M, et al: Community and hospital acquired pneumonia associated with *Chlamydia* TWAR infection demonstrated serologically. *Arch Intern Med* 149:169–173, 1989.
75. Shermer-Avni Y, Goonen R, Liebermann D: Inhibition of ciliary-motion of bronchus cells by *C. pneumoniae,* in Mardh PA, La Placa M, Ward M: *Proceedings of the European Society for Chlamydia Research.* Uppsala, Sweden, Uppsala University Center for STD Research, 1992, p 169.
76. Grayston JT, Mordhorst C, Bruu A-L, et al: Country wide epidemic of *Chlamydia pneumoniae,* strain TWAR in Scandinavia, 1981–1983. *J Infect Dis* 159:1111–1114, 1989.
77. Hammerschlag MR, Chirgwin K, Roblin PM, et al: Persistent infection with *Chlamydia pneumoniae* following acute respiratory illness. *Clin Infect Dis* 14:178–182, 1992.
78. Berdal BP, Scheel O, Ogaard AR, et al: Spread of subclinical *Chlamy-*

dia pneumoniae infection in a closed community. *Scand J Infect Dis* 24:431–436, 1992.
79. Gnarpe J, Gnarpe H, Sundelof B: Endemic prevalence of *Chlamydia pneumoniae* in subjectively healthy adults. *Scand J Infect Dis* 23:387–388, 1991.
80. Emre U, Roblin PM, Gelling M, et al: Association of *Chlamydia pneumoniae* and reactive airway disease in children. *Arch Pediatr Adolesc Med* 148:727–732, 1994.
81. Augenbraun MH, Roblin PM, Mandel LJ, et al: *Chlamydia pneumoniae* pneumonia with pleural effusion: Diagnosis by culture. *Am J Med* 91:43:437–438, 1991.
82. Rumback MJ, Baselski V, Belenchia JM, et al: Case report: Acute postoperative respiratory failure caused by *Chlamydia pneumoniae* and diagnosed by bronchoalveolar lavage. *Am J Med Sci* 305:390–393, 1993.
83. Augenbraun MH, Roblin PM, Chirgwin K, et al: Isolation of *Chlamydia pneumonice* from the lungs of patients infected with the human immunodeficiency virus. *J Clin Microbiol* 29:401–402, 1991.
84. Gaydos CA, Fowler CL, Gill VJ, et al: Detection of *Chlamydia pneumoniae* by polymerase chain reaction–enzyme immunoassay in an immunocompromised population. *Clin Infect Dis* 17:718–723, 1993.
85. Hahn DL, Dodge RW, Galubjatnikov R: Association of *Chlamydia pneumoniae* (strain TWAR) infection with wheezing, asthmatic bronchitis and adult-onset asthma. *JAMA* 266:225–230, 1991.
86. Kuo CC, Grayston JT: Factors affecting viability and growth in HeLa 229 cells of *Chlamydia* sp. strain TWAR. *J Clin Microbiol* 26:812–815, 1988.
87. Cles LD, Stamm WE: Use of HL cells for improved isolation and passage of *Chlamydia pneumoniae*. *J Clin Microbiol* 28:934–940, 1990.
88. Roblin PM, Dumornay W, Hammerschlag MR: Use of HEp-2 cells for improved isolation and passage of *Chlamydia pneumoniae*. *J Clin Microbiol* 30:1968–1971, 1992.
89. Campbell LA, Melgosa MP, Hamilton DJ: Detection of *Chlamydia pneumoniae* by polymerase chain reaction. *J Clin Microbiol* 30:434–439, 1992.
90. Gaydos CA, Quinn TC, Eiden JJ: Identification of *Chlamydia pneumoniae* by DNA amplification of the 16srRNA gene. *J Clin Microbiol* 30:796–800, 1992.
91. Gaydos CA, Roblin PM, Hammerschlag MR, et al: Diagnostic utility of PCR-EIA, culture and serology for detection of *Chlamydia pneumoniae* in symptomatic and asymptomatic patients. *J Clin Microbiol* 32:903–905, 1994.
92. Grayston JT, Aldous MB, Easton A, et al: Evidence that *Chlamydia pneumoniae* causes pneumonia and bronchitis. *J Infect Dis* 168:1231–1235, 1993.
93. Roblin PM, Dumornay W, Hammerschlag MR, et al: Unpublished data, 1993.

94. Hyman CL, Roblin PM, Schachter J, et al: Prevalence of *Chlamydia pneumoniae* infection in asymptomatic health care workers. Presented at the 32nd Interscience Conference on Antimicrobial Agents and Chemotherapy, Anaheim, Calif, Oct 12, 1992.
95. Verkooyen RP, Hazenberg MA, Van Haaren GH, et al: Age-related interference with *Chlamydia pneumoniae* microimmunofluorescence serology due to circulating rheumatoid factor. *J Clin Microbiol* 30:1287–1290, 1992.
96. Chirgwin K, Roblin PM, Hammerschlag MR: In vitro susceptibilities of *Chlamydia pneumoniae* (*Chlamydia* sp. strain TWAR). *Antimicrob Agents Chemother* 33:1634–1635, 1989.
97. Moss TR, Darougar S, Woodland RM, et al: Antibodies to *Chlamydia* species in patients attending a genitourinary clinic and the impact of antibodies to *C. pneumoniae* and *C. psittaci* on the sensitivity and specificity of *C. trachomatis* serology tests. *Sex Transm Dis* 20:61–65, 1993.
98. Hammerschlag MR, Hyman CL, Roblin PM: In vitro activity of five quinolones against *Chlamydia pneumoniae. Antimicrob Agents Chemother* 36:682–682, 1992.
99. Hammerschlag MR, Qumei K, Roblin PM: In vitro activity of azithromycin, clarithromycin, L-ofloxacin and other antibiotics against *Chlamydia pneumoniae. Antimicrob Agents Chemother* 36:1573–1574, 1992.
100. Roblin P, DuMornay W, Emre V, et al: Serologic response to *Chlamydia pneumoniae* infection in children. Presented at the 34th Interscience Conference on Antimicrobial Agents and Chemotherapy, Orlando, 1994.
101. Williams LP: Review of the epidemiology of chlamydiosis in the United States. *J Am Vet Med Assoc* 195:1518–1521, 1989.
102. Centers for Disease Control: *Psittacosis surveillance 1975–1984*. Atlanta, Centers for Disease Control, 1987, pp 1–60.
103. Centers for Disease Control: Psittacosis at a turkey processing plant–North Carolina, 1989. *MMWR* 39:460–469, 1990.
104. Hedberg K, White KE, Forfang JC, et al: An outbreak of psittacosis in Minnesota turkey industry workers: Implications for modes of transmission and control. *Am J Epidemiol* 130:569–577, 1989.
105. Yung AP, Grayston ML: Psittacosis—a review of 135 cases. *Med J Aust* 148:228–233, 1988.
106. Morrison WM, Hutchinson RB, Thomason J, et al: An outbreak of psittacosis. *J Infect* 22:71–75, 1991.
107. Bourke SJ, Carrington D, Frew CE, et al: Serologic cross-reactivity among chlamydial strains in a family outbreak of psittacosis. *J Infect* 19:41–45, 1989.
108. Crosse BA: Psittacosis: A clinical review. *J Infect* 21:251–259, 1990.
109. Oldach DW, Gaydos CA, Mundey LM, et al: Rapid diagnosis of *Chlamydia psittaci* pneumonia. *Clin Infect Dis* 17:338–343, 1993.

110. Cartwright KAV, Caul EO, Lamb RW: Symptomatic *Chlamydia psittaci* reinfection. *Lancet* 1:1004, 1988.
111. Sawyer LA, Fishbein DB, McDade JE: Q fever: Current concepts. *Rev Infect Dis* 9:935–946, 1987.
112. Richardus JH, Dumas AM, Huisman AM, et al: Q fever in infancy, a review of 18 cases. *Pediatr Infect Dis* 4:969–973, 1985.
113. Ruiz-Contreras J, Montero RG, Amador JTR, et al: Q fever in children. *Am J Dis Child* 147:300–302, 1993.
114. Dupont HT, Raoult D, Broqui P, et al: Epidemiologic features and clinical presentation of acute Q fever in hospitalized patients: 323 French cases. *Am J Med* 93:427–434, 1992.
115. Jorm LR, Lightfoot NF, Morgan KL: An epidemiological study of an outbreak of Q fever in a secondary school. *Epidemiol Infect* 104:467–477, 1990.
116. Langley JM, Marrie TJ, Covert A, et al: Poker players' pneumonia; an urban outbreak of Q fever following exposure to a parturient cat. *N Engl J Med* 319:354–356, 1988.
117. Pinsky RL, Fishbein, Green CR, et al: An outbreak of cat-associated Q fever in the United States. *J Infect Dis* 164:202–204, 1991.
118. Yearman MR, Mitscher LA, Baca OG: In vitro susceptibilities of *Coxiella burnetii* to antibiotics including several quinolones. *Antimicrob Agents Chemother* 31:1079–1084, 1989.
119. McDade JE, Shepard CC, Frazer DW, et al: Legionnaires' disease isolation of a bacterium and demonstration of its role in other respiratory diseases. *N Engl J Med* 297:1197–1203, 1977.
120. Edelstein PH: Legionnaires' disease, Pontiac fever, and related illnesses, in Feigin RD, Cherry JD: *Textbook of Pediatric Infectious Diseases*. Philadelphia, WB Saunders, 1992, pp 1141–1148.
121. Foy HM, Broome CV, Hayes PS, et al: Legionnaires' disease in a prepaid medical-care group in Seattle 1963–75. *Lancet* 1:767–770, 1979.
122. Anderson R, Lauer B, Fraser D, et al: Infections with *Legionella pneumophila* in children. *J Infect Dis* 143:386–390, 1981.
123. Orenstein WA, Overturf GD, Leedom J, et al: The frequency of *Legionella* infection prospectively determined in children hospitalized with pneumonia. *J Pediatr* 99:403–406, 1981.
124. Cutz E, Thorner PS, Rao P, et al: Disseminated *Legionella pneumophila* infection in an infant with severe combined immunodeficiency. *J Pediatr* 100:760–762, 1982.
125. Beyer P, Kahn D, Horback J, et al: Unusual progression of a *Legionnella pneumophila* infection in a young child. *Eur J Pediatr* 141:173–175, 1984.
126. Joly JR, Dery P, Gauvreau L, et al: Legionnaires' disease caused by *Legionella dumoffii* in distilled water. *Can Med Assoc J* 135:1274–1277, 1986.
127. Ephros M, Englehard D, Maayan H, et al: *Legionnella gormanii* pneu-

monia in a child with chronic granulomatous disease. *Pediatr Infect Dis J* 8:726–727, 1989.
128. Brady MT: Nosocomial legionnaires disease in a children's hospital. *J Pediatr* 115:46–50, 1989.
129. Carlson NC, Kuskie MR, Dobyns EL, et al: Legionellosis in children: An expanding spectrum. *Pediatr Infect Dis J* 9:133–137, 1990.
130. Holmberg RE, Pavia AT, Montgomery D, et al: Nosocomial legionella pneumonia in the neonate. *Pediatrics* 92:450–452, 1993.
131. Horowitz MA, Silverstein SC: Legionnaires' disease bacteria (*Legionella pneumophila*) multiplies intracellularly in human monocytes. *J Clin Invest* 66:441–450, 1980.

Brain Abscess and Other Intracranial Suppurative Complications

Charles Reece Woods, Jr., M.D.
Assistant Professor of Pediatrics, Bowman Gray School of Medicine, Wake Forest University, Winston-Salem, North Carolina

Intracranial suppurative infections include brain abscess, subdural empyema, cranial epidural abscess, and suppurative thrombophlebitis of the intracranial venous system. These infectious complications often occur in specific clinical settings. The sudden occurrence of seizures, whether focal or generalized, in association with altered mental status or meningeal signs should raise suspicion of an intracranial infection. The development of neurologic symptoms in children with sinusitis, otitis media, or congenital heart disease, especially when associated with new or increasing fever, should bring to mind the possibility of an infectious intracranial complication. The persistence of fever and/or the development of new neurologic findings in children receiving treatment for bacterial meningitis or paranasal sinus infections can also be manifestations of intracranial suppurative complications. Because current therapies often permit cure of these infections with good neurologic outcomes, intracranial suppurative processes should be part of the common knowledge of physicians involved in the care of children. This chapter discusses brain abscess in children beyond the neonatal period, neonatal brain abscess, tuberculous mass lesions of the central nervous system (CNS), subdural empyema, cranial epidural abscess, and suppurative thrombophlebitis of the intracranial venous system.

BRAIN ABSCESS BEYOND THE NEONATAL PERIOD

About 25% of all brain abscesses occur in children less than 15 years of age.[1] In the era before the use of *Haemophilus influenzae* type b (Hib) vaccines in the United States, 1 child with brain abscess was seen for every 40 cases of bacterial meningitis.[2] The incidence of brain abscess relative to bacterial meningitis is likely increased now as a result of the dramatic vaccine-related decline in Hib disease in the past few years. A male:female ratio of about 1.7:1 was consistently observed among 12 series of brain abscess in children (459 males in 738 total cases).[1,3–13] Brain abscess in children is rare between 1 month and 2 years of age. In neonates it is usually associated with concurrent gram-negative bacillary meningitis (see the section Neonatal Brain Abscess).[14,15]

PATHOGENESIS

Brain abscesses may become established by (1) spread of infection from a contiguous extracranial site, (2) hematogenous spread from a remote site of infection, or (3) primary inoculation of microbes into the brain parenchyma during a penetrating traumatic injury.[16] Before the 1960s, ear infections were by far the leading cause of brain abscess in children worldwide.[1,4,5,17–19] Over the past three decades, congenital cyanotic heart disease (CCHD) has become the most common predisposing risk factor for brain abscess in childhood (Table 1).[1,7–9,19–21] Sinus and ear infections combined are the next most frequent cause of brain abscess in this era and almost equal CCHD as a predisposing factor in children from developing countries.[6,11–13] The predisposing cause remains unknown in about one in seven children with brain abscess. In children beyond the neonatal period in developed nations, brain abscess is rarely a complication of bacterial meningitis, although a brain abscess may lead to meningitis if it ruptures into either a ventricle or the subarachnoid space.[2,16] Both the location of the abscess within the brain and the causative organism(s) usually reflect the mechanism by which parenchymal infection was established (Table 2).[16] Abscesses occur most commonly in the frontal and temporal lobes, followed by the parietal lobe, the cerebellum, and the occipital lobes. Abscesses within the sella, brain stem, basal ganglia, and thalamic structures are rare in children.[1,3,8,10,11]

Contiguous spread of infection from an extracranial site such as the middle ear or paranasal sinuses occurs by either direct extension through areas of associated osteomyelitis or through retrograde thrombophlebitis of emissary veins that connect the extracranial and dural venous circulations. Otogenic infections may also spread through pre-existing channels in the structures of the inner ear or between suture lines in the temporal bone. Initiation of a brain abscess requires compromise of an area of brain parenchyma,[22] but the precise mechanism(s) by which this occurs in continguously spreading infection is unclear. Tissue injury may result from thrombophlebitis and venous stasis. The factors that determine which manifestation of intracranial extension (meningitis,

TABLE 1.
Conditions Predisposing to Brain Abscess in Children

Predisposing Condition	Western Countries: Mid-1940s to 1960*	Western Countries: 1960s to Present†	Developing Nations: 1960s to Present‡
Congenital cyanotic heart disease	14.5%	35.5%	25.8%
Ear, nose, throat infection	43.9	23.1	23.9
Ear infection§	36.2	9.3	21.6
Sinusitis§	7.6	12.6	6.1
Head trauma	9.0	6.6	7.6
Neurosurgery	—¶	3.3	1.7
Ventricular shunt	—	2.6	2.2
Pulmonary infection	3.6	0.7	2.0
Dental infection	0.5	0.7	0.8
Bacterial meningitis‖	1.4	2.2	13.5
Tuberculosis	—	1.5	—
Other	11.3	9.5	4.8
Unknown	15.6	14.3	24.2

*n = 221; references 1, 4, 5, 17–19; includes a few cases from the early and mid 1960s.
†n = 273; references 1, 7–9, 19–21; includes a few cases from the late 1950s.
‡n = 356; references 6, 11–13; includes a few cases from the United States (references 6, 11). Percentages total more than 100% because two factors were reported for 23 cases (reference 11).
§Abscesses of otogenic and sinusitis origins were not separated in all series: n = 196, 151, and 231, respectively, across the columns of the table.
¶Not reported in these series.
‖Many cases of brain abscess associated with bacterial meningitis were in young infants.

brain abscess, epidural abscess, or subdural empyema) will occur in an individual patient also remain unknown.[16]

A microinfarct is believed to be the mechanism of injury that precedes brain abscess of hematogenous origin. In patients with CCHD this may result from hyperviscosity secondary to cyanosis or from microemboli that, by way of the right-to-left intracardiac shunt, bypass the normal filtering process of the pulmonary capillary bed and gain access to the cerebral arterial circulation. The infarcted area is susceptible to seeding during subsequent bactere-

TABLE 2.
Relationship of Predisposing Condition to Site of Brain Abscess and Microbial Isolates*

Predisposing Condition	Site of Abscess	Usual Microbial Isolate(s)
Contiguous site		
Otitis media or mastoiditis	Temporal lobe or cerebellum	Streptococci (anaerobic or aerobic), *Staphylococcus aureus*, *Bacteroides fragilis*, *Proteus* spp., and other Enterobacteriaceae, *Haemophilus* spp., *Pseudomonas aeruginosa*
Frontoethmoidal sinusitis	Frontal lobe	Predominantly streptococci; also *Bacteroides*, Enterobacteriaceae, *S. aureus*, *Haemophilus* spp.
Sphenoidal sinusitis	Frontal or temporal lobe	Same as frontoethmoidal sinusitis
Dental infection	Frontal lobe	Mixed *Fusobacterium* spp., *Bacteroides* spp., streptococci

Primary infection		
Penetrating cranial trauma or postsurgical infection	Related to the site of the wound or surgery	*S. aureus*, streptococci (including pneumococci), Enterobacteriaceae, *Clostridium* spp.
Distant infection site		
Congenital cyanotic heart disease (CCHD)	Middle cerebral artery distribution common, can occur at any site; multiple abscesses common	Viridans, anaerobic, and microaerophilic streptococci, *Haemophilus* spp.
Lung abscess, other pulmonary infections	Same as in CCHD	*Fusobacterium*, *Actinomyces*, and *Bacteroides* spp., streptococci, *Nocardia* spp.
Bacterial endocarditis	Same as in CCHD	*S. aureus*, streptococci
Compromised hosts	Same as in CCHD	*Toxoplasma gondii*, *Nocardia* spp., fungi, Enterobacteriaceae

*Adapted from Wispelwey B, Dacey RG, Scheld WM: Brain abscess, in Scheld WM, Whitley RJ, Durack DT: *Infections of the Central Nervous System*. New York, Raven, 1991, p 459. Used by permission.

mia. Septic emboli may arise from valvular vegetations in patients with endocarditis or other intrathoracic infections such as lung abscess.[16, 23]

Contiguous Spread

In the preantibiotic era, intracranial complications occurred in 3% to 6% of patients with otogenic infections, and brain abscess represented about 15% of these complications.[14, 24] The frequency of intracranial complications of otogenic infections has decreased markedly in developed countries in recent years, and this decline likely reflects the ready availability of antimicrobial agents, follow-up care, and surgical intervention. Chronic otitis media and/or mastoiditis lead to intracranial extension four to eight times more frequently than acute otitis media.[16] Acute mastoiditis can lead to intracranial suppuration, and this may rarely occur without the external signs of swelling over the mastoid bone or abnormal appearance of the tympanic membrane.[25] Most brain abscesses related to the middle ear complex occur as solitary lesions. More than half develop in the temporal lobe, and 20% to 30% occur in the cerebellum. Greater than 80% of cerebellar abscesses arise from an otitic focus.[16]

The majority of patients with brain abscess secondary to sinusitis are in the 10- to 30-year-old age range. The frontal lobe is almost exclusively involved (Fig 1). The rare occurrence of sinusitis-related brain abscess in children under age 10 years reflects the developmental absence of the frontal sinuses during early childhood. The frontal sinuses begin to develop by a child's sixth birthday and are not completed until late adolescence.[26] Brain abscess occurs more commonly in association with frontal and/or ethmoidal than maxillary sinusitis. Ethmoidal sinusitis may cause brain abscess indirectly as a complication of orbital cellulitis. Sphenoidal sinusitis has been associated with pituitary abscess[27] and cavernous sinus thrombosis,[28] which in turn can lead to brain abscess. Isolated sphenoid sinusitis often leads to intracranial complications with-subsequent long-term morbidities. Early surgical intervention is warranted when isolated sphenoid sinusitis is recognized.

Dental infections cause brain abscess infrequently despite their relatively common occurrence. Meningitis, subdural empyema, and cavernous sinus thrombosis are much more frequent complications of dental infection than brain abscess. Most intracranial complications of dental infection appear to occur after a recent tooth extraction or other dental manipulation. Brain abscess occurs

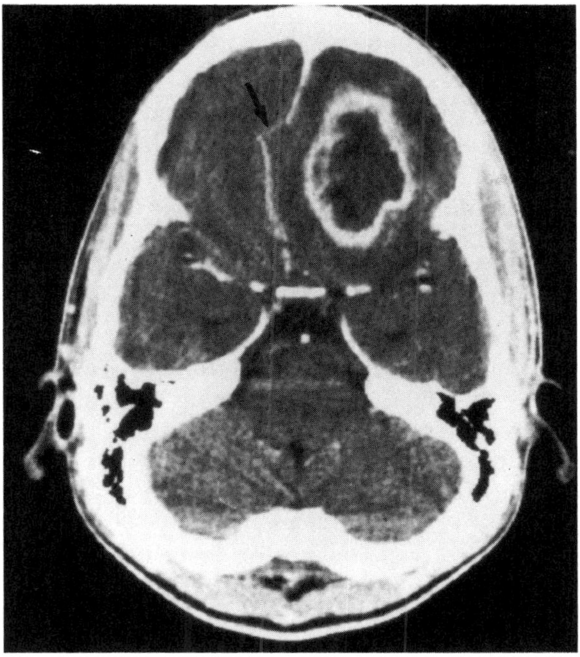

FIGURE 1.

Contrast-enhanced computed tomographic scan of the brain of a 13-year-old boy. A left frontal lobe brain abscess, which shows the characteristic ring-enhancing lesion with a hypodense center and surrounding hypodense areas consistent with parenchymal edema, is present. Midline shift from a mass effect is present *(arrow)*. At the initial evaluation he had periorbital edema and proptosis, but neurologic findings were normal. Sinusitis and orbital cellulitis were also present, and he recovered without sequelae.

more often following acute rather than chronic dental infection. The frontal lobe is most commonly but not exclusively involved.[16]

Brain abscess following cavernous sinus thrombosis is well recognized but rare. Cavernous sinus thrombosis may result from sphenoidal sinusitis or infections of the soft tissues of the face or scalp. Two thirds of brain abscesses associated with face or scalp infections are caused by *Staphylococcus aureus*.[29] Carbuncles and other infections of the soft tissues of the neck can lead to cerebellar abscess.

Hematogenous Spread

Brain abscesses that result from hematogenous spread of infection occur most commonly in the distribution of the middle cerebral artery (predominantly the parietal and temporal lobes) but can be seen in any region of the brain. These abscesses usually have their initial location at the gray matter–white matter junction of the cerebral cortex and are often poorly encapsulated. Multiple or multiloculated abscesses result more often from hematogenous than contiguous spread of infection.[1, 16]

Congenital cyanotic heart disease is by far the most common predisposing factor for hematogenously derived brain abscess in children.[1, 8, 9, 19–21] The male-to-female ratio is nearly equal among children with CCHD and brain abscess.[30, 31] Children with low arterial oxygen saturations (<81%) are more likely for brain abscess to develop than those with higher saturations.[32] The tetralogy of Fallot accounts for over 60% of CCHD-related brain abscess among children in five recent series,[6, 12, 13, 21, 31] but this predominance over other cyanotic congenital cardiac anomalies probably reflects its greater frequency of occurrence rather than a specific increased risk of brain abscess. Any cardiac abnormality with a component of right-to-left shunting of blood can predispose to brain abscess. The majority of abscesses related to CCHD are solitary, but multiple abscesses arise quite often. For reasons that are unclear, brain abscesss in patients with CCHD are rare in those under 2 years of age.[30, 31] Many children with CCHD now undergo corrective surgery in the first few years of life, and it is possible that this will lead to a reduction in CCHD-associated brain abscess in future series of patients with brain abscess.

Evidence of associated endocarditis is usually lacking at the time brain abscesses are detected in children with CCHD.[2] Brain abscess seldom results from the persistent bacteremia of subacute endocarditis, but it is a relatively common complication of acute bacterial endocarditis. This may reflect a greater intensity of bacteremia (in colony-forming units per milliliter) seen in acute vs. subacute endocarditis, greater virulence of the most common causative organism (*S. aureus* vs. viridans streptococci), and/or an increased likelihood of septic emboli during acute vs. subacute endocarditis.[16]

Brain abscess can result from hematogenous spread of chronic pyogenic lung infections, including lung abscess and bronchiectasis. Brain abscess is uncommon in children with cystic fibrosis (CF), and the few cases reported have occurred in patients at least 17 years of age.[33] Organisms isolated from the brain abscesses of patients with CF differed from those cultured from their sputa. Chronic sinusitis is common in patients with CF, but most patients with CF and brain abscess had multiple abscesses in parenchymal sites remote from the sinuses, thus suggesting a hematogenous rather than contiguous origin. Brain abscess may also be associated with skin, wound, and pelvic infections, osteomyelitis, intra-abdominal septic processes, thrombophlebitis, and infections of peripheral arteriovenous shunts.[2, 16]

Patients with hereditary hemorrhagic telangiectasia (Osler-Weber-Rendu disease) or other syndromes with arteriovenous shunts that permit access of venous blood to the cerebral arterial circulation have an increased lifetime risk of development of a brain abscess,[34] but brain abscesses in these patients generally occur in the third to fifth decades of life. The procedure of esophageal dilatation has also been associated with brain abscess formation, although the pathogenesis of this infection is unknown.[35]

Cranial Penetration

Brain abscess is a much less common complication of neurosurgical procedures or head trauma than is meningitis. Transsphenoidal surgery, given its inherently nonsterile operative field, may carry a slightly higher risk of brain abscess than other surgical procedures. Brain abscess following placement of ventricular shunts for relief of hydrocephalus is uncommon (see Table 1). Causative organisms that must be considered include staphylococci and enteric flora. The latter may cause ascending infection when the distal portion of the shunt is placed within the peritoneum.[36] The risk of brain abscess following penetrating cranial injuries appears to correlate with the severity of injury to the underlying brain. Retained fragments of bone are an important risk factor. Cranial penetration by lawn darts and pencil tips and cranial trauma from dog bites have led to brain abscesses in children.[16, 37] Brain abscess has also occurred following use of halo devices for cervical immobilization. Such abscesses may occur several months to a few years after removal of the halo device.[16] Congenital malformations such as dermal sinuses and encephalocoeles are also risk factors for brain abscess formation. Dermal sinus–associated abscesses usually occur in the posterior fossa. Rupture of encephalocoeles may allow direct access of microorganisms into brain tissue.[2]

PATHOLOGY

Once organisms establish infection in the brain parenchyma, the host mounts an acute inflammatory cellular response that initially consists of neutrophils. The mechanism by which neutrophils are recruited into the CNS is unknown. Astrocytes, which undoubtedly have contact with the invading microbes, appear to be capable of producing interleukin-8, a potent chemoattractant for neutrophils, after stimulation with lipopolysaccharide or other proinflammatory cytokines in vitro.[38] Other chemoattractant factors may also be involved. Microglia, the resident macrophages of the brain, may also play roles in recruitment of inflammatory cells and/or early containment of the infection.[39]

Histologic studies from experimental models have defined four distinct stages of brain abscess evolution.[40] The first stage, early cerebritis, begins with the arrival of neutrophils. Over a period of about 3 days the center of the lesion becomes necrotic and is surrounded by a perivascular inflammatory response. The adjacent white matter may become profoundly edematous. In the second stage, late cerebritis, a well-formed necrotic center develops, which usually requires about 7 days. Fibroblasts appear during this time, and an associated marked increase in neovascularity occurs at the periphery of the necrotic zone. The newly formed capillaries usually lack tight junctions and leak proteinaceous fluid. A reactive astrocyte response surrounds the lesion, and edema of the adjacent white matter persists.[16, 41]

The third stage is early capsule formation, which occurs on days 10 to 13. Fibroblasts form a well-developed layer around the necrotic center, which may decrease slightly in size. A region of persisting cerebritis and neovascularity lies outside the developing capsule, and the reactive astrocyte response increases. These processes continue into the final stage of late capsule formation. The capsule continues to thicken, and by the end of the third week, an abundance of reactive collagen is present.[16] Capsules may become more than 1 cm thick in chronic abscesses.[2] Capsule formation is often more complete on the cortical side of the abscess than on the ventricular side, which may explain in part why brain abscesses rupture more often into the ventricles than the subarachnoid space.[16, 40, 41]

This sequence and pace are not followed precisely by all brain abscesses, but the descriptive progression from cerebritis to capsule formation correlates well with findings on computed tomography (CT) scans and magnetic resonance imaging (MRI) of brain abscesses. This distinction between stages can help guide clinical management (see later). The histologic course of a brain abscess is influenced by the predisposing condition, microbial virulence factors, and the host immune response. Less extensive capsules develop in brain abscesses that arise from hematogenous spread than in those resulting from contiguous spread.[16] Animal models of brain abscess show that abscesses caused by *Bacteroides fragilis* enlarge quickly and have delayed capsule formation with an increased likelihood of early ventricular rupture.[42] Experimental abscesses caused by *S. aureus* are larger and take longer to reach a stable size than those caused by α-hemolytic streptococci.[43] Separation of the stages of experimental abscesses caused by *S. aureus* is also not as distinct as described earlier. In immunocompromised hosts, the early inflammatory response and its associated edema may be decreased, and the increase in size of the abscess cavity usually seen during the second stage may be delayed in comparison with immunocompetent hosts.[16]

MICROBIOLOGY

Brain abscesses can be caused by a wide range of microorganisms, including most bacteria and certain fungi and parasites. In an individual patient, the causative organisms usually depend on the predisposing factor for brain abscess and the immunologic status of the host (see Table 2). The organisms and their frequencies of isolation from brain abscesses in children are similar to those in adults.[8, 11, 13, 20, 21] The most significant exception occurs during the neonatal period, when gram-negative enteric organisms predominate.[11]

One third of brain abscesses in children are of polymicrobial origin (two or more organisms).[8, 9, 11, 20] Purulent material from brain abscesses in the past have been reported to be sterile in about 25% of cases. However, many of these cases likely represented inadequate culture methods, especially for anaerobic bacteria, rather than the absence of viable microbes.[2, 8, 20] Microbial isolation rates have ranged from 90% to 100% in recent years.[8, 11, 44] Anaerobes are present in about one third of cases. Anaerobes are often found in mixed culture with aerobes but may be the only type of organisms isolated.[8, 11, 20, 21]

The aerobic bacteria cultured most frequently from brain abscesses are streptococci. These include α-hemolytic and nonhemolytic streptococci (viridans streptococci), group A and occasionally other β-hemolytic streptococci, and enterococci.[23] Strains of the *Streptococcus milleri* group of α-hemolytic streptococci are the most common streptococci isolated from brain abscesses. These organisms also cause focal suppurative disease outside the brain, but no specific virulence factors have been identified.[16] α-Hemolytic streptococci are the most common microbes isolated from brain abscesses associated with CCHD.

Staphylococcus aureus is the most common cause of brain abscess following trauma[16] and can be a cause of brain abscess resulting from sinus or ear disease and acute endocarditis. Coagulase-negative staphylococci should be considered true pathogens when isolated from patients with intracranial foreign bodies such as ventricular shunts.[23] Pneumococci were much more common causes of brain abscess in the past than in recent years.[2, 16]

Many aerobic gram-negative organisms can cause brain abscess, and these are often found in mixed culture.[16] *Proteus* species are the most common of this group and are particularly associated with otogenic and neonatal brain abscesses.[15, 45] *Escherichia coli*, *Klebsiella-Enterobacter* species, and *Pseudomonas* species are also common gram-negative aerobic isolates. The latter are commonly associated with chronic middle ear disease in children. *Salmonella* species occasionally cause brain abscesses in children.[46] Brucellosis is only rarely complicated by brain abscess. *Eikenella corrodens* has been reported as a cause of brain abscess in association with dental, sinus, and ear infections.[16]

Haemophilus species are occasionally isolated from brain abscesses associated with sinus or ear infections and CCHD. *Haemophilus aphrophilus* is a common cause of brain abscess related to CCHD in some series.[23] This organism requires an atmosphere with enriched carbon dioxide and decreased oxygen tensions for cultivation. *Haemophilus influenzae* type b, despite its historical status as the most common cause of bacterial meningitis in childhood, only rarely causes brain abscess.[2, 16] Isolation of *Pasteurella multocida* and *Moraxella catarrhalis* from brain abscesses has been reported.[11]

Bacteroides species, including *B. fragilis*, are the most common anaerobic isolates from brain abscesses. Many other anaerobic genera have been isolated, including anaerobic streptococci (peptostreptococci), *Clostridium*, *Fusobacterium*, and *Actinomyces*.[16, 20, 44] *Propionibacterium acnes* can cause brain abscess following trauma or neurosurgical procedures.[47]

Listeria monocytogenes and *Nocardia asteroides* have also been isolated from brain abscesses, primarily in immunocompromised hosts. *Nocardia asteroides* can invade and survive intracellularly within murine astrocytes, which may explain in part its ability to cause brain abscesses.[48] Brain abscess caused by *Bacillus cereus* has been reported in an immunocompromised child.[49] *Mycobacterium tuberculosis* may also cause brain abscess (see later).

The vast majority of fungal brain abscesses occur in immunocompromised hosts but are uncommon even in such children. *Candida* species, *Aspergillus* species, *Cryptococcus neoformans*, and

Xylhypha bantianum (formerly *Cladosporium trichoides*) are the most common fungal isolates from brain abscesses. Many other fungi have also been reported as causes of brain abscess.[2, 16, 23]

Toxoplasma gondii has become a leading cause of brain abscess in immunosuppressed patients, especially those with the acquired immunodeficiency syndrome (AIDS).[2, 16] *Entamoeba histolytica* is the most common cause of amebic brain abscess, and these usually occur in association with abscesses in extracranial sites, primarily the liver. Brain abscess may occur when helminths such as *Strongyloides stercoralis* migrate to the brain and transport with them bacteria with which they were colonized during passage in the gastrointestinal tract.[16]

CLINICAL MANIFESTATIONS

Clinical manifestations of brain abscess vary greatly among individual patients and are influenced by the causative organism(s), immunologic status of the host, predisposing factor(s) for brain abscess, location of the abscess(es), and presence or absence of associated meningitis or ventricular rupture. The progression of neurologic symptoms can be fulminant or insidious. Most brain abscesses are recognized within 2 weeks of the onset of symptoms, but many patients can have symptoms for weeks to months before diagnosis. The prominent clinical manifestations of brain abscess are often those of an expanding intracerebral mass rather than an acute inflammatory response. Symptoms and laboratory findings compatible with infection are more common in patients with acute clinical courses, but rupture of a chronic abscess into the ventricular system can be an acute and catastrophic event (see later).[2, 16, 23]

The frequencies of specific symptoms and signs of brain abscess among children reported in 13 pediatric series are listed in Table 3. Headache is the most common symptom, occurs in about two thirds of children, and results from increased intracranial pressure (ICP). Fever and vomiting occur in slightly more than half of the children. Altered mental status, which may range from mild lethargy to coma, is present in almost half of the children, and this may be manifested as irritability in infants. Lethargy and subtle mental status changes such as confusion were probably underreported in several of the aforementioned series. Various combinations of fever, vomiting, headache, malaise, and even lethargy are relatively nonspecific in infants and young children, and headache is often difficult to document in these age groups.[2, 16, 23] Intracranial infections, including brain abscess, are part of the differential diagnosis, however, and become likely when these symptoms are

TABLE 3.
Signs and Symptoms of Children With Brain Abscess: Compilation From 13 Series of Pediatric Patients Encountered From 1945 to 1990

Manifestation	Percent	n*	References
Headache	65	691	3,5,7–9,11,13,17–19
Fever	55	634	1,3,5,7–9,11–13,17,21
Vomiting	53	709	1,3,5,7–9,11–13,17,19
Papilledema	48	382	1,3,5,7,8,11,12,17
Focal neurologic deficit	47	750	1,3,5,7–9,11–13,17–19,21
Mental status changes†	43	552	1,3,5,7,9,11,13,17,19
Meningeal signs	36	422	1,3,5,7,9,11,17,19
Seizure	34	645	1,3,5,7–9,11–13,17,18

*Total cases for which the presence or absence of the manifestation could be determined. The specific manifestations described varied among the series.
†Mental status changes range from drowsiness, lethargy, or confusion to a comatose state in these series.

associated with any focal neurologic finding. Young infants may have a bulging anterior fontanelle as an early manifestation of increased ICP.

Focal neurologic signs, which are present in about half of patients, depend on the site(s) of the lesion(s). Hemiplegia, hemianopia, and cranial nerve palsies are common. Frontal lobe abscesses may exhibit few focal signs for weeks, whereas abscesses that involve regions of the cerebral cortex concerned with motor, sensory, speech, or visual functions usually cause recognizable neurologic deficits early in their courses. Signs of meningeal irritation are less common and suggest associated meningitis and/or rupture of an abscess into the ventricular system. Seizures are more often generalized than focal in nature. Papilledema is present in almost half of the children in whom it is sought but is less common when symptoms have been present for only a few days. The classic triad of fever, headache, and a focal neurologic deficit occurs in fewer than half of patients with brain abscess.[11, 16]

Frontal Lobe Abscess

Frontal lobe abscesses (see Fig 1) often become apparent only when sufficient size is achieved to create a mass effect with its subsequent focal neurologic signs. Disturbed behavior may be seen and, in the absence of evidence of systemic inflammation, can be misdiagnosed as a primary psychiatric disorder. Forced grasping and sucking may be prominent findings, and hemiparesis may develop over time. A mass effect may occur suddenly and cause depressed consciousness and signs of temporal lobe herniation.[2]

Temporal Lobe Abscess

Temporal lobe abscesses are commonly associated with epidural and subdural space infections and may have concurrent thrombophlebitis of the lateral venous sinus or cortical veins (Fig 2). Clinical manifestations include fluent or nonfluent dysphasia when the dominant hemisphere is involved, as well as a contralateral upper quadrant visual field defect or complete homonymous hemianopia. Anterior extension of the abscess process can impinge on motor

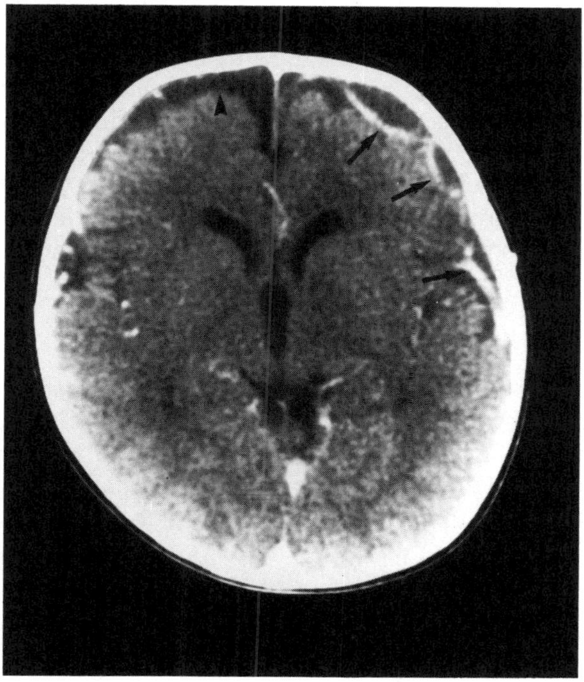

FIGURE 2.

Computed tomographic scan of the brain of a 4-month-old male with pneumococcal meningitis. A multilobular extra-axial fluid collection with an enhancing medial rim, which is characteristic of subdural empyema, is present over the left frontal lobe *(arrows)*. Subdural effusion is evident over the right frontal lobe *(arrowhead)*.

function and predominantly affects the face and arm. Ipsilateral third nerve palsy and upper brain stem dysfunction may result from herniation of the mesial temporal lobe through the incisura of the tentorium. Prognosis is poor once herniation begins.[2]

Parietal Lobe Abscess

These remain relatively clinically silent until encroachment on the sensorimotor cortex occurs. Posterior and inferior extensions may cause inferior quadrant visual field defects or homonymous hemianopia. Dysphasia may develop if the dominant hemisphere is involved. Involvement of the nondominant hemisphere may lead to dyspraxia and contralateral spatial neglect.

Cerebellar Abscess

Most cerebellar abscesses occur in the hemispheres, and neurologic manifestations are consequently lateralized and ipsilateral to the involved hemisphere. Ataxia and tremor are the most common findings. Dizziness and nystagmus may be present. The latter will be most prominent on gaze toward the side of the lesion. Swelling within the posterior fossa can impair outflow of cerebrospinal fluid (CSF) from the fourth ventricle, which leads to a diffuse increase in ICP. Vomiting is a prominent symptom, and papilledema is present in about half of such cases. Sudden death may result from downward herniation of cerebellar tissues through the foramen magnum. Upward herniation through the incisura of the tentorium can occur and clinically mimics downward herniation of supratentorial lesions.[2]

Brain Stem Abscess

Brain stem abscesses are rare and were seldom diagnosed premortem in the pre–CT scan era. Otogenic and hematogenous sources have been reported. Patients may have multiple cranial nerve palsies and signs of involvement of ascending and descending sensory and motor tracts. In children these lesions are often clinically confused with primary brain stem gliomas. Vomiting, papilledema, and herniation can occur as a result of increased pressure within the posterior fossa.[2]

DIAGNOSIS

Laboratory findings in children with brain abscesses are frequently nonspecific. The peripheral white blood cell (WBC) count and erythrocyte sedimentation rate (ESR) are elevated in most cases but normal in a significant minority.[2, 5, 8, 11, 16] There are no data available regarding C-reactive protein in patients with brain abscess. Blood cultures are seldom positive for microbes present in the brain abscess except when acute endocarditis is the predisposing factor. Blood cultures were positive in 9% of cases in a recent series; all blood isolates also were recovered from cultures of the brain abscess.[11] Although blood culture has a low yield when a brain abscess is known to be present, it remains an essential part of the evaluation of children with acute or chronic inflammatory symptoms of unknown cause, especially in children with congenital heart disease who are at risk for bacterial endocarditis. Examination of the urine is rarely helpful once the diagnosis of brain abscess is known. Serum electrolytes should be examined for the presence of hyponatremia, which may result from the syndrome of inappropriate antidiuretic hormone secretion.[2, 16, 23]

Cerebrospinal fluid findings range from normal WBC counts and chemistries to a marked pleocytosis with an elevated protein concentration and hypoglycorrhachia. About 15% of children with brain abscess have normal CSF findings.[5, 6, 8, 11, 18] Others have marked pleocytosis with WBC counts as high as 6,000/mm^3.[3, 5, 8] Pleocytosis with greater than 1,000 WBCs/mm^3 is usually associated with neutrophil predominance, whereas lesser CSF WBC counts usually have mononuclear cell predominance.[8, 18] Higher counts with neutrophil predominance may indicate rupture of an abscess into the ventricular system. Cultures of CSF are rarely positive for the causative organisms unless the abscess has ruptured into a ventricle.[2, 8, 11, 16]

Intracranial pressure is elevated in most patients with brain abscess, and clinical deterioration and/or death from downward herniation in children following lumbar puncture has been reported in many series. Because the information gained from evaluation of the CSF is of minimal diagnostic or therapeutic usefulness in most cases of brain abscess, a CT scan or MRI study of the brain should be performed before lumbar puncture is attempted when a brain abscess or other focal CNS lesion is suspected.[1, 2, 11, 13, 16, 19, 23]

Imaging Studies

Before the advent of CT and MRI technologies, skull radiography, electroencephalography (EEG), arteriography, and ventriculography were the main tools available for diagnosis and localization of brain abscesses. Skull radiographic findings are usually normal, but the presence of a collection of air within a cavity is pathognomonic for brain abscess. The EEG is abnormal in most children with brain abscesses and may lateralize to the side of the lesion, but more precise localization is seldom achieved.[1, 5, 8, 11] Arteriograms, which are abnormal in most patients, and ventriculograms are unnecessary in this era.[16] The technetium 99 radionuclide brain scan is very sensitive for the detection of brain abscess in children[1, 6, 8] and is the procedure of choice if CT scanning and MRI are unavailable or their results are normal when there is high suspicion of a brain abscess.[16]

The introduction of CT scanning has had a major positive impact on the diagnosis, management, and outcome of brain abscess. The characteristic features of a brain abscess on CT are a mass with a hypodense center, a uniform ring of enhancement around the center (after a contrast agent is administered), and a hypodense region of parenchymal edema outside the ring. These features are strongly suggestive of but not pathognomonic for brain abscess. Hydrocephalus and/or mass effects with midline shifts may be seen, and ependymal enhancement may occur if ventriculitis is present.[16, 50]

The CT scan appearance correlates with the histopathologic stage of the brain abscess. During the cerebritis stages, precontrast images show an area of low density with ring enhancement appearing 10 minutes after contrast infusion; the enhancement persists 60 minutes after contrast infusion. Diffusion of contrast into the center of the lesion may be seen. Frank abscess with capsule development appears as a low-density lesion with a faint ring before contrast infusion and shows ring enhancement that decays within 60 minutes after administering contrast. The contrast agent does not diffuse into the center.[16]

Experience with MRI in brain abscess in pediatric patients is emerging. Magnetic resonance imaging appears to be more sensitive than CT in detecting the early cerebritis phase and delineating the extent of surrounding edema. As the frank abscess develops, the central portion becomes hypointense on T1-weighted images and hyperintense on T2-weighted images. The capsule appears hyperintense on T1-weighted images and hypointense on T2-weighted images. After administration of the MRI contrast agent gadolinium, the abscess capsule demonstrates increased signal intensity.[51] The three regions of a brain abscess—the central abscess cavity, the capsular rim, and the surrounding cerebral edema—are differentiated more accurately on gadolinium-enhanced MRI than on contrast-enhanced CT. Magnetic resonance imaging may also be more accurate in differentiating brain abscess from other CNS lesions with a similar appearance on CT.[7, 11, 16]

Unenhanced MRI scans can show a resolution of abnormal rim (capsule) signals within 2 months of therapy, whereas CT enhancement may persist for more than 9 months after successful therapy. This may make MRI more useful for follow-up studies. Other advantages of MRI are its lack of radiation exposure and the absence of bone artifact, which improves sensitivity for posterior fossa lesions. Gadolinium also does not have the potential for toxicity that is associated with iodine-based CT contrast agents.[16] The longer time period required for performance of an MRI, with its inherent requirement for a longer period of sedation, is a disadvantage of MRI for some pediatric patients. Computed tomography probably remains the procedure of choice for rapid diagnosis in patients with progressing signs of increased ICP.

Differential Diagnosis

Other infections that can have manifestations similar to brain abscess include meningitis, viral encephalitis, subdural empyema, epidural abscess, cranial osteomyelitis, mycotic aneurysms (especially in the setting of infective endocarditis), neurocysticercosis, echinococcosis, and tuberculoma. The symptomatic and radiologic features of brain abscess sometimes overlap those of cerebrovascular diseases (migraine headache, intracerebral or subarachnoid hemorrhage, cerebral venous sinus thrombosis, or cerebral infarct) and primary or metastatic tumors of the CNS. Chronic subdural hematomas in children, which can result from child abuse, can also mimic brain abscess.[16, 23]

TREATMENT

Initial Approach

Appropriate management of the predisposing condition(s) of a patient with a brain abscess is critical for a good outcome. Surgical drainage of associated extracranial head and neck infections is often required. Brain abscesses generally require a combined surgical plus medical approach for optimal outcome. Antibiotic therapy should be instituted immediately once the presence of a brain abscess is discovered. Close monitoring of the mental status and neurologic examination are required. Patients with signs of increased ICP often require invasive monitoring of their ICP in an intensive care setting. Anticonvulsant therapy is required when seizures have occurred.

The major surgical techniques currently in use are aspiration and excision. Excision provides definitive therapy, but neither method has been conclusively shown to be superior to the other.[11, 16] Since the introduction of CT scanning, aspiration has been used more often than excision in pediatric patients.[9, 11, 13] Aspiration has been advocated over excision as the initial procedure of choice because of its potential for less injury to brain tissue. Neurologic sequelae have been fewer following aspiration than excision in some series.[11,12] Mortality rates are comparably low for both procedures. Aspiration has a very low associated morbidity and can be accomplished with stereotactic CT guidance, which allows accurate (within 1 mm) access to almost any intracranial point. Specimens sufficient for histologic and etiologic diagnosis are obtained in over 90% of cases. Aspiration guided by CT has been used successfully in patients with multiple abscesses, multiloculated lesions, and deep-seated lesions, including brain stem abscesses.[16]

Excision may be required when there is clinical deterioration from a mass effect or lack of improvement after aspiration plus antimicrobial therapy. Excision may also be required when the causative organism(s) are resistant to available therapies or the effective agents penetrate poorly into brain tissue. Fungal brain abscesses will often require excision. Patients undergoing aspiration in the past had higher mortality rates than those whose abscesses were excised, but this probably reflected a case selection bias in that aspiration was reserved for patients too ill to undergo excision.[1,11,18,52] The duration of antimicrobial therapy necessary for microbial eradication appears to be shorter following excision than aspiration[12] (10 to 28 days with a mean of 17 days vs. 21 to 42 days with a mean of 28 days in a recent pediatric series).[11] Ultimately, the procedure used and the timing of the intervention must be individualized in each case. Factors that influence this decision include the clinical course and immunologic status of the patient and the number, size, location(s), and apparent stage, based on CT scan or MRI appearance, of the abscess(es).[12,16,23]

Antimicrobial therapy alone has been used increasingly in the past two decades and may be adequate for some lesions. Several reports have demonstrated success of this approach in children.[50,53–55] A number of the patients in these reports had cerebritis rather than frank abscess. Greater success has been achieved with lesions less than 4 cm in diameter than with those that are larger.[11,54] Before consideration of medical therapy without surgical intervention, the following minimum criteria should be met: (1) a high degree of certainty regarding the causative organism(s) should exist and be based on positive culture results from CSF, blood, or the primary site of infection, and (2) clinical signs of increased ICP must be absent. Lesions that are in the stages of cerebritis are more reasonable candidates for medical therapy alone than are those that have progressed to the stage of frank abscess. Medical therapy alone may be necessary in some patients who have multiple abscesses or abscesses for which any surgical approach might cause damage to vital brain structures. The decision to treat with antimicrobial agents without surgical intervention should be made in consultation with a neurosurgeon since urgent intervention may be required should signs of increased ICP develop.[54, 55]

The appropriate duration of antimicrobial therapy is unknown. The traditional recommendation for pediatric patients has been a 6- to 8-week course.[23] This is believed by many experts to be longer than necessary, and shorter courses of 7 to 10 days following excision or 3 to 4 weeks following aspiration have been suggested.[11] Other authorities recommend 4 to 6 weeks.[16] Successful therapy usually results in progressive decreases in abscess size, mass effect, edema, and the degree of ring enhancement on serial CNS imaging studies within the first 4 weeks of therapy.[54] It is not necessary to continue antimicrobial therapy to the point of complete resolution of the abscess(es) on imaging studies, which for CT scan does not occur for an average of 3 to 4 months (range, 1 to 11 months).[16, 50] Magnetic resonance imaging may provide evidence of resolution earlier in the course than CT and will likely prove to be the modality of choice for monitoring therapeutic efficacy.

Antimicrobial Regimens

No controlled trials of antimicrobial regimens for brain abscess have been performed. The standard empirical regimen for brain abscesses until recently has been a combination of penicillin G and chloramphenicol.[2, 16] Penicillin remains bactericidal for most nonenterococcal streptococci and most anaerobes other than *B. fragilis*. Penicillin penetrates well into abscess cavities but may be inactivated by bacterial or leukocytic products in the purulent material. Chloramphenicol is bactericidal against most bacteria encountered in abscesses other than *S. aureus* and Enterobacteriaceae, but it is also associated with an increased risk of aplastic anemia and requires close monitoring of serum drug concentrations. Chloramphenicol attains higher concentrations in brain abscesses than in serum, but this agent has been noted to antagonize the effects of penicillin in experimental models of meningitis.[2, 11, 16, 23]

The clinical settings in which penicillin-chloramphenicol might not be adequate are those in which *S. aureus*, various gram-negative enteric organisms, and *Pseudomonas* species are likely causative organisms (see Table 2). When *S. aureus* infection is a potential cause, a semisynthetic penicillin such as nafcillin is required. Vancomycin, which penetrates well into brain abscess fluid, should be used if methicillin resistance is suspected. Third-generation cephalosporins have activity superior to that of chloramphenicol against most Enterobacteriaceae and are effective against most pneumococcal and *Haemophilus* strains. Ceftazidime also has added activity against *P. aeruginosa*.[11] These agents are highly effective in bacterial meningitis in childhood and are appropriate components of empirical antimicrobial regimens for brain abscess in many settings.

Other agents that are useful for the treatment of brain abscess include metronidazole and trimethoprim-sulfamethoxazole. Metronidazole has been used effectively in several series of brain abscess.[11] This agent is highly active against obligate anaerobes but not aerobic bacteria. Because early animal data suggested a carcinogenic potential, general use of metronidazole in pediatric patients was once limited. This fear has not been substantiated in subsequent wide clinical use. Trimethoprim-sulfamethoxazole is effective against a broad range of organisms and may assume a more important role in abscess management in future years, especially against organisms multiply resistant to β-lactam antibiotics. Excellent concentrations in brain tissue and pus are achieved in most patients treated with this combination drug.

Aminoglycosides do not penetrate well into abscesses and have decreased activity in the acidic pH and anaerobic conditions encountered in purulent material. These drugs may be useful adjuncts, however, for the prevention of emergence of resistance to the β-lactam agents used to treat gram-negative organisms such as *Serratia* and *Enterobacter* species, which may possess inducible chromosomal β-lactamases. Direct instillation of antibiotics into abscess cavities is of uncertain efficacy when compared with intravenous administration alone. Diffusion of directly instilled β-lactam antibiotics into surrounding brain tissue may cause seizures.[11, 23]

The choice of empirical antimicrobial therapy for brain abscess must take into consideration the likely predisposing factor(s) and immunologic status of the patient. Recent recommendations[11, 56] are listed in Table 4. The combination of metronidazole and a third-generation cephalosporin is a reasonable substitute for chloramphenicol. Coverage for anaerobes is essential, with the possible exception of ventriculoperitoneal shunt–related brain abscess.

The purulent material from brain abscesses should be cultured for aerobic and anaerobic bacteria, mycobacteria, and fungi and should be sent for routine histopathology and Gram, acid-fast, and

TABLE 4.
Suggested Initial Empirical Antimicrobial Regimens for Brain Abscess in Children According to Predisposing Condition*

Underlying Condition	Antimicrobial Regimen
Congenital cyanotic heart disease†	Penicillin + chloramphenicol
Sinusitis or head trauma	Nafcillin‡ + chloramphenicol
Otitis/mastoiditis	Nafcillin‡ + ceftazidime + metronidazole
Ventricular shunt infection	Vancomycin + ceftazidime
Meningitis	Third-generation cephalosporin ± aminoglycoside
Unknown	Nafcillin‡ + third-generation cephalosporin + metronidazole
Immunocompromised host	Nafcillin‡ + ceftazidime + metronidazole with consideration of amphotericin B

*Adapted from Sáez-Llorens XJ, Umaña MA, Odio CM, et al: *Pediatr Infect Dis J* 8:455, 1989. Used by permission.
†Children with brain abscess and congenital cyanotic heart disease who have recently undergone corrective heart surgery should probably be treated similarly to children with ventriculoperitoneal shunt–related infections.
‡Vancomycin should be substituted for nafcillin or other semisynthetic antistaphylococcal penicillins if a gram-positive organism with significant potential for resistance to these agents is suspected. A vancomycin dosage of up to 60 mg/kg/day given intravenously is indicated for intracranial infections. Peak concentrations should be monitored to ensure efficacy.[23]

fungal stains. The Gram-stained smear should be carefully reviewed for the presence of multiple types of microbes. This may provide the only evidence of anaerobes and may be helpful in interpreting subsequent culture results. Once culture results are known, the antimicrobial regimen may be tailored to the organism(s) identified, although this should be done with caution if multiple morphologies are evident on Gram stain but only a single organism is present in culture.

Corticosteroids

The use of corticosteroids in the management of children with brain abscess remains controversial.[23] These agents may be necessary and lifesaving in the setting of increased ICP and rapid neurologic deterioration. Although steroids may decrease antibiotic entry into the CNS, there is no evidence that these agents delay sterilization of brain abscesses.[13] Ring enhancement on CT may increase after withdrawal of corticosteroids, but this does not by itself indicate a worsening clinical situation.[50] Patients ill enough to require corticosteroids often require monitoring of ICP as well as other methods for controlling increased ICP such as mannitol infusion and hyperventilation.[23]

PROGNOSIS

Significant improvement in mortality and morbidity rates associated with brain abscess in children and adults has occurred in the past 10 to 15 years. This change is largely attributed to advances in imaging modalities and the subsequent improvement in diagnosis and management of brain abscesses.[11, 16] Mortality rates among pediatric patients with brain abscess in the United States in recent years have dropped to 5% to 14% from 25% to 30% or greater before the early 1960s.* Mortality rates after the advent of CT scanners in the mid-1970s ranged from 0% to 6% in several pediatric series.[6, 9, 10] Mental status at the time of initial evaluation is a significant prognostic factor. There were no deaths among 22 children in a recent series who were alert or only drowsy when first seen vs. 15 deaths among 20 who were comatose (no response to pain).[1] Mortality rates appear to be increased in patients with CCHD as a predisposing condition.[23, 31] This may reflect the increased likelihood of multiple abscesses in these patients or abscess locations that were not amenable to surgical intervention in the pre-CT era.

The proportion of survivors without any neurologic sequelae is 56% to 59% in recent pediatric series from developed countries.[7–9, 21] Seizures are the most common neurologic sequela and occur in 10% to 30% of survivors.[5, 7–11, 19, 58] The onset of seizures related to a brain abscess may not occur for several years after the abscess is diagnosed, and the risk development of a seizure disorder may increase with increasing abscess size. Children may have less than adults for development of epilepsy as a sequela of brain abscess. Abscesses in the frontal and temporal lobes carry a greater risk of seizure than abscesses in other sites.[58] Intellectual impairment as a result of brain abscess is more common in children under the age of 5 years. Behavioral changes and learning disabilities

*References 1, 3, 5, 7–10, 13, 18, 19, 50, 57.

may also result from brain abscess during early childhood.[10] Focal deficits persist in about 15% of patients and include hemiparesis, ataxia, spasticity, cranial nerve palsies, optic atrophy, and visual field deficits. Hydrocephalus also may develop.[6–11, 23]

RUPTURE OF A BRAIN ABSCESS INTO THE VENTRICULAR SYSTEM

Rupture of an abscess into a ventricle is usually a catastrophic clinical event. Mortality exceeds 50%, and residual neurologic deficit in survivors, including hydrocephalus, is the rule. Rupture often occurs before diagnosis of the underlying brain abscess. The sudden deposit of purulent material into the ventricular system, essentially forming a ventricular empyema, rapidly leads to high fever, shock, meningeal signs, and often an altered sensorium. If the patient survives to undergo CSF evaluation, extreme pleocytosis of 50,000 to 100,000 WBCs/mm^3 and profound hypoglycorrhachia are usually present. Organisms are often demonstrable on Gram stains of CSF, and cultures are usually positive. Successful treatment requires prompt surgical drainage in addition to antimicrobial and supportive therapies. The possibility of rupture into the ventricular system must be kept in mind during the management of patients with brain abscess.[2]

BRAIN ABSCESS IN NEONATES

Brain abscesses in neonates are commonly associated with gram-negative bacillary meningitis and may become very large before causing clinical signs.[2, 15] Multiple abscesses are often present, and the frontal lobes are frequently involved. The incidence of brain abscess in neonates has reportedly increased,[15] but this may reflect improvement in diagnosis with modern imaging techniques in neonates who were previously thought to have meningitis alone. Undetected brain abscesses in neonates may partially explain the high mortality observed in early series of neonatal gram-negative bacillary meningitis.[16]

The vast majority of brain abscesses complicating meningitis in neonates are caused by either *Proteus mirabilis* or *Citrobacter diversus. Proteus mirabilis* accounted for 27 of 30 neonatal brain abscesses observed over a 12-year period in one recent series.[15] This contrast sharply with its relatively low incidence of 4% or less as a cause of neonatal meningitis.[16] Greater than 70% of cases of neonatal meningitis caused by *C. diversus* have associated brain abscess(es).[59] *Escherichia coli* and *Klebsiella pneumoniae*, the two most common causes of gram-negative bacillary meningitis in neonates,[60] seldom cause brain abscess.[61] *Enterobacter sakazakii* may also have an increased propensity to cause brain abscess.[62] *Salmonella* strains, with or without concurrent meningitis,[46] and other gram-negative enteric bacteria such as *Serratia marcescens* occasionally cause brain abscess in neonates.[61] *Haemophilus influenzae* type b, pneumococci, and meningococci have been reported as rare causes of brain abscess in neonates.[11] Group B *Streptococcus*, the most common cause of neonatal meningitis, rarely causes brain abscess.

The increased propensity for *C. diversus* and *P. mirabilis* to cause brain abscess is not understood. Autopsies of two infants with *C. diversus* brain abscess found evidence of intraparenchymal necrotizing vasculitis with subsequent hemorrhagic necrosis of subcortical white matter.[63] This suggests that brain abscesses caused by *C. diversus* are established after penetration of the endothelial blood-brain barrier. Findings in a neonatal rat model of *C. diversus* meningitis suggest that these bacteria reach the brain parenchyma after destruction of the ependymal cell lining of the ventricles.[64] A 32-kDa outer-membrane protein appears to be a marker for *C. diversus* strains that cause CNS infection.[65] Strains that express this protein do not have an increased ability to invade human umbilical vein endothelial or HEp-2 epithelial cells in vitro, which may indicate that it has a CNS-specific role in the pathogenesis of *C. diversus* infection.[66]

The presence of a brain abscess should be considered (along with hydrocephalus and other intracranial suppurative processes) in neonates with meningitis of any cause whose CSF cultures are persistently positive or neonates who have clinical evidence of a bacterial infection in association with an enlarging head circumference, other signs of increased ICP, or focal neurologic findings. Head CT or MRI should be considered in these neonates and in those whose CSF cultures yield *Citrobacter* or *Proteus* species.[59] Management considerations for brain abscess in neonates are similar to those in older infants and children. Aspiration is often therapeutic and should be considered even when the causative organism is known from cultures of blood or CSF. Decompression may help to prevent rupture of an abscess into the ventricular system. Ultrasonography has been successfully used to guide needle aspiration in neonates.[67] Antimicrobial regimens should be continued for 4 to 6 weeks. Mortality rates of neonatal brain abscess in the current era are unknown but may still exceed 30%. Most survivors of neonatal brain abscess caused by *C. diversus* and *P. mirabilis*, and probably most other causes, suffer mental retardation.[15, 68]

TUBERCULOMA AND TUBERCULOUS BRAIN ABSCESS

Invasion of the CNS by *M. tuberculosis* leads to the formation of tubercles (caseating granulomas), as in other tissue sites. Tuberculous meningitis results when a tubercle ruptures into the subarachnoid or ventricular space. Tuberculomas result from enlargement of tubercles that are confined within the parenchyma or walled off within the meninges. Tuberculomas are the most common intracranial mass lesions caused by *M. tuberculosis* and, like tuberculous meningitis, occur most often in young children. These two conditions seldom coexist in a patient, however. Tuberculomas are surrounded by a dense fibrous capsule and range in size from less than 1 cm to several centimeters in diameter. Lesions may occur throughout the brain, and infratentorial tuberculomas develop in children more commonly than in adults. Multiple tuberculomas may be present. Tuberculomas are often asymptomatic unless they induce seizures or enlarge enough to create mass effects. Fever is rarely present. The CSF may show an elevated protein concentration but is often entirely normal. Computed tomography or MRI often reveals a ring-enhancing lesion with surrounding edema that is not distinct from pyogenic brain abscess. Current antituberculosis chemotherapies without surgery are usually curative, although biopsy may be necessary to make the diagnosis. Resolution may be evident on CT scan as early as 12 weeks after initiation of therapy. Corticosteroids should be used if signs of increased ICP are present. Tuberculomas are not highly destructive of surrounding brain tissue, and patients usually recover without neurologic sequelae after appropriate therapy.[51, 69]

Tuberculous brain abscess, which develops when the caseous core of a tuberculoma liquefies, is extremely rare.[70] Patients with tuberculous brain abscess usually show systemic signs of inflammation. The classic triad of fever, headache, and a focal neurologic deficit is commonly seen. These lesions are also difficult to distinguish from pyogenic brain abscess by CT scan.[69] The majority of pediatric patients reported with tuberculous brain abscess have done well following surgical excision and antituberculosis chemotherapy.[70]

SUBDURAL EMPYEMA

Subdural empyema is the second most common intracranial suppurative process in children.[2, 71] Subdural empyema may occur at any age but is seen predominantly in children under 3 years or over 12 years of age. The peak incidence throughout life is in the second decade.[72] In younger children subdural empyema usually occurs as a complication of bacterial meningitis. It develops in about 2% of cases of bacterial meningitis in infants[73, 74] and is thought to result from spread of infection from the subarachnoid space into an initially sterile sympathetic subdural fluid collection (subdural effusion). In older children and adolescents, subdural empyema usually results from contiguous spread of infection from chronic sinusitis or mastoiditis. Subdural empyema is an infrequent complication of intracranial surgery and is rarely hematogenous in origin. Osteomyelitis of the adjacent calvarium and thrombophlebitis of contiguous cortical veins and dural venous sinuses are often associated with infection of the subdural space. Unlike the epidural space, the subdural space is not limited by the tight adhesion of the dura at the suture lines of the skull. This allows a subdural empyema to extend widely over one or both hemispheres. Interhemispheric accumulation of purulent material occurs in about one fourth of cases.[2, 73, 75, 76]

Subdural empyema associated with primary bacterial meningitis can be caused by any of the common meningitis pathogens of childhood. *Haemophilus influenzae* type b was the most common causative organism in the pre–Hib vaccine era but will likely be supplanted by pneumococci in the 1990s. Persistent fever with the onset of new neurologic findings during treatment for bacterial meningitis suggests the development of a subdural empyema or other intracranial suppurative process. A bulging anterior fontanelle, lethargy, enlarging head circumference, and vomiting are common findings in infants. Transillumination of the skull may reveal the location of the empyema in young infants.[2]

Fluid obtained from empyema associated with primary meningitis is often turbid rather than grossly purulent. The distinction between subdural effusion and empyema is important since the former process is common in children with bacterial meningitis and usually resolves spontaneously whereas the latter requires drainage. Subdural empyema and effusion both have increased white cell counts and protein concentrations, but empyema is distinguished from effusion by the neutrophilic predominance of the cell count (effusions generally have mononuclear cell predominance) and low glucose concentration (usually normal in effusions). The subdural fluid usually has a greater white cell count with greater predominance of neutrophils and higher protein and lower glucose concentrations than concurrent samples of CSF. Gram stains and cultures of subdural empyemas may be negative when obtained several days after initiation of antibiotics for the meningitis.[74, 75, 77]

The manifestations of subdural empyema in older children are similar to those of brain abscess. The clinical course may be rapid or insidious. The symptoms and signs of the primary source of infection may predominate. As the empyema progresses, high fever, increasingly severe headache, signs of meningeal irritation, vomiting, and altered mental status generally develop. Focal neurologic deficits vary according to the location of the empyema and are referable to the cortical regions that lie beneath it. Hemiparesis or hemiplegia occur in about two thirds of cases and ocular palsies in about one quarter. Focal or generalized seizures occur in about half of the patients.[71] Progressive enlargement of the empyema can cause a mass effect that may lead to herniation. If the process develops slowly, papilledema may be seen. Antimicrobial therapy directed at the primary source of infection before suspicion of the subdural empyema may attenuate the acute inflammatory signs and symptoms and sometimes delays diagnosis. Postoperative empyema often follows an indolent course and may not become evident for weeks to months after surgery.[76]

Laboratory findings in older children are also similar to those of brain abscess. Peripheral leukocytosis with a left shift is present in most cases. The CSF findings are usually more suggestive of a parameningeal focus than bacterial meningitis. White blood cell counts in the CSF range from a few hundred to seldom more than 1,000 cells/mm^3. The CSF protein concentration is often mildly to moderately elevated, the glucose concentration is usually normal, cultures are generally sterile, and the opening pressure is usually elevated. Cultures of the empyema material are usually positive unless the patient has received prior antibiotic therapy.[2, 75] The causative organism(s) of subdural empyema in these children are the same as those isolated from brain abscesses associated with the primary site of infection (see Table 2). Anaerobes are frequently isolated from subdural empyemas associated with ear or sinus infections.[20]

The distinction between empyema and other intracranial suppurative processes usually cannot be made on clinical grounds alone. The differential diagnosis of subdural empyema also includes meningitis, meningoencephalitis, and subdural hematoma.[72] Central nervous system imaging studies are the diagnostic procedures of choice. As with brain abscess, lumbar puncture should be undertaken with caution, if at all, in a patient with focal neurologic signs or signs of increased ICP until the safety of the procedure is determined by a CNS imaging study.[72, 78]

On CT scan an empyema usually appears as a hypodense extra-axial fluid collection (density equal to or slightly greater than that of CSF) with contrast enhancement of the medial rim. Extensive mass effect manifested by ventricular compression, sulcal effacement, and a midline shift is usually present and may overshadow the inciting empyema. Diffuse empyemas appear crescentic in shape and may become multilobular over time (see Fig 2). More confined lesions may appear lentiform in shape. These appearances are not distinct from those seen with epidural abscesses. The presence of subjacent gyral enhancement indicates meningitis, cerebritis, and/or venous thrombosis. Spindle-shaped collections associated with thick, irregular enhancement of the falx are seen in interhemispheric subdural empyema.[72]

Magnetic resonance imaging is becoming the procedure of choice for patients with extra-axial fluid collections. Because of its lack of bone artifact, MRI is more sensitive than CT for small extra-axial fluid collections. It allows more definitive separation of the collection from cerebritis, cerebral edema, and venous thrombosis. Purulent collections, because of their higher protein concentration, appear hyperintense to CSF on MRI, which permits differentiation of sterile collections (subdural effusion, cystic hygroma) from empyema. Subdural effusion is seldom associated with underlying parenchymal abnormality. Magnetic resonance imaging is more specific than CT in differentiating subdural empyema from epidural abscess. A hypodense medial rim, which represents the inflamed, displaced dura, is seen on unenhanced MRI of epidural but not subdural empyema.[72] The presence of rim enhancement on either modality generally allows empyema to be distinguished from hematoma. Lack of rim enhancement on CT does not rule out the presence of empyema.[76]

Drainage of the subdural empyema is essential. In infants a diagnostic paracentesis (to differentiate empyema from effusion) coupled with antibiotic therapy is usually sufficient, but repeated subdural taps may be required. The fluid in subdural empyemas secondary to sinus or ear infections and trauma is usually grossly purulent and thick and requires a more definitive initial drainage procedure. This may be accomplished by craniotomy or through burr holes. There is no consensus as to the preferred procedure. Factors that should be considered in determining the surgical approach include the location and extent of the empyema and the level of consciousness of the patient.[2, 71, 72]

The choice of antimicrobial agents depends on the primary source of infection. Patients with subdural empyema secondary to meningitis who are receiving appropriate antibiotic therapy at the time of diagnosis may continue to receive the same therapy. Third-generation cephalosporins such as ceftriaxone or cefotaxime currently provide adequate empirical coverage in this setting, although this may change in the near future if multidrug-resistant pneumococci become more common. Empirical antimicrobial therapy for subdural empyema caused by other primary infections is the same as for brain abscess (see Table 4). Definitive data are not available, but antimicrobial therapy should probably be continued for 3 weeks after drainage.[56] Serial CNS imaging studies can be helpful in gauging the adequacy of therapy. As with brain abscess, fluid collections and enhancement may persist for weeks to months after resolution of all other clinical features and, alone, do not indicate a need for more prolonged therapy.[51, 76, 77] Duration of therapy greater than 4 weeks is seldom required after appropriate drainage. The ESR and other laboratory tests are not helpful in determining the length of therapy.[56]

Subdural empyemas were uniformly fatal in the preantibiotic era. Mortality rates fell to 30% to 40% in the 1950s. In recent years mortality rates less than 10% have been achieved. Infants with subdural empyemas caused by Hib usually recover fully. Long-term neurologic sequelae following empyema secondary to meningitis are more likely a consequence of the subarachnoid than subdural space infection.[74, 75, 77] Permanent neurologic sequelae following subdural empyema of nonmeningitis origin usually represent persistence of the focal neurologic findings present at the time of diagnosis. Persistence or resolution of the initial findings depends on the degree of brain injury from associated parenchymal abscess or infarction from increased ICP or venous thrombosis. Long-term follow-up CNS imaging studies often demonstrate atrophy of the cortex subjacent to the empyema.[72]

CRANIAL EPIDURAL ABSCESS

Cranial epidural abscesses occur almost exclusively in older children and adults. The vast majority are associated with infections of the sinuses or middle ears.[71, 75] Trauma, neurosurgical procedures, orbital cellulitis, fetal scalp monitoring, and rhinocerebral mucormycosis may also lead to cranial epidural abscess. Because the dura adheres tightly to the inner aspect of the cranium, especially at the suture lines, epidural abscesses rarely become large enough to exert significant pressure on the underlying brain. However, epidural abscesses often serve as foci for subdural spread of infection. Subdural empyema, meningitis, and/or brain abscess are frequently associated with cranial epidural abscess. Osteomyelitis of the overlying diploic bone is often present and may lead to cellulitis of the scalp or face.[2, 79]

Local pain, tenderness, and fever are often the only signs early in the course. Focal neurologic findings are unusual. Vomiting and alterations in mental status are unusual with uncomplicated epidural abscess unless a mass effect develops. Seizures occur in a few patients. When the apex of the petrous temporal bone is involved in the primary process, Gradenigo syndrome (unilateral facial pain and lateral rectus weakness resulting from involvement of cranial nerves V and VI, respectively) may be seen. Because the uncomplicated epidural abscess grows slowly, it is often the striking symptoms and signs of further intracranial extension of infection that first indicate an intracranial suppurative process. Posttraumatic and postoperative epidural abscesses may not become apparent for months to years following the event.[2, 71, 79]

The diagnosis can be established with either CT or MRI. Contrast CT reveals medial rim enhancement that is usually thicker and more irregular than in subdural empyema. The intracranial fluid collection may be lentiform or crescentic in shape when it overlies a cerebral convexity. Epidural collections may also occur in the interhemispheric fissure. Findings on MRI are similar, and this modality may distinguish epidural from subdural abscess more readily than CT, as noted earlier. In addition, MRI offers greater sensitivity for small loculations associated with sinusitis early in the course because of its lack of bone artifact and high degree of contrast between purulent collections and normal CSF. These properties make MRI especially useful for evaluating epidural fluid collections that occur following trauma or surgical procedures.[51, 79]

Surgical drainage of cranial epidural abscess is required in addition to antimicrobial therapy.[2, 56, 79] Causative organisms are the same as those of subdural empyema and brain abscess and likewise vary depending on the primary site of infection (see Table 2). Empirical antibiotic regimens are also selected as for subdural empyema and brain abscess (see Table 4). Other associated intracranial sites of infection must be excluded when this diagnosis is made. As for subdural empyema, antimicrobial therapy should generally be continued for 3 weeks after surgical drainage. Serial CNS imaging studies can be helpful in evaluating the effectiveness of therapy. Longer courses of therapy (4 to 6 weeks) should be given when associated osteomyelitis of the skull is present.[56] The combination of medical and surgical management of uncomplicated cranial epidural abscess is highly successful, and recent series report no fatalities or long-term neurologic sequelae. The outcome of complicated cranial epidural abscess depends on the associated sites of infection.[75, 79]

SUPPURATIVE THROMBOPHLEBITIS OF THE INTRACRANIAL VENOUS SYSTEM

Syndromes of intracranial suppurative thrombophlebitis are rare in children, but prompt recognition and intervention can be lifesaving. These occur primarily in the dural venous sinus system. Septic thrombosis of cortical veins within the subarachnoid space was believed in the past to be the cause of many of the focal neurologic deficits and seizures that occurred in patients with bacterial meningitis, but this finding is present in fewer than 0.3% of children under 16 years of age with bacterial meningitis.[80] Septic thrombosis of the dural venous sinus system may be divided into three categories: lateral sinus (including sigmoid sinus) thrombosis, sagittal sinus thrombosis, and cavernous sinus thrombosis.[81]

Lateral sinus thrombosis is the most common of these in children and results almost exclusively from contiguous spread of infection from the middle ear/mastoid air spaces. This may occur following acute or chronic otitis media. Headache, which may be generalized or unilateral and occipitofrontal, and vomiting are the most common complaints. Diplopia and vertigo occasionally occur. Otologic findings are almost universally abnormal. Fever, papilledema, sixth nerve palsy, and nuchal ridigity are also common findings. Ipsilateral periorbital soft tissue swelling may be seen. Peripheral leukocytosis is common but not always present. Cerebrospinal fluid is usually normal but shows evidence of a parameningeal infection in about one third of cases. Intracranial pressure is usually elevated. Cultures of CSF rarely yield the causative organism(s).[81] Diagnosis is best made by angiography, and MRI angiography is an appropriate alternative to carotid angiography (Fig 3).[82] Causative organisms and therefore empirical antimicrobial regimens are the same as for brain abscess associated with otogenic infections (see Tables 2 and 4, respectively). Radical mastoidectomy is usually required for cure. Antibiotics should be continued for 2 to 3 weeks after surgery. The mortality rate has been 12% or less in the antibiotic era. Chronic sequelae such as otitic hydrocephalus, dysfunctions of cranial nerves VII or VIII, or decreased visual acuity occur in 13% of patients.[81]

Septic cavernous sinus thrombosis is usually associated with

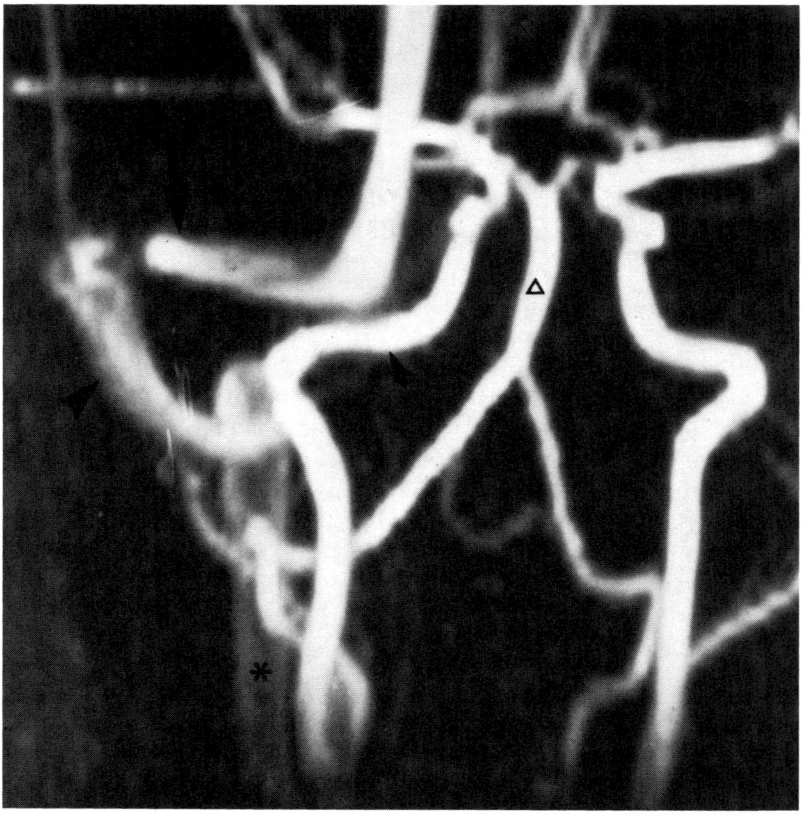

FIGURE 3.

Magnetic resonance imaging flow angiogram of a 10-year-old boy with septic thrombosis of the left lateral venous sinus. The right lateral venous sinus is normal in appearance (*large arrow*). The thrombotic left lateral venous sinus, which has no blood flow, is not seen. This process was associated with acute otitis media with bilateral purulent otorrhea. *Arrowhead* = sigmoid sinus; *star* = internal jugular vein; *small arrow* = internal carotid artery; *triangle* = basilar artery.

sphenoidal or ethomoidal sinusitis or infections of the soft tissues of the face. Dental and ear infections may also lead to this process. Fever, signs suggestive of an intraorbital process (ptosis, proptosis, chemosis, and palsies of cranial nerves III, IV, and VI), and headache are common. Headache may be chronic, especially when sphenoidal sinusitis is the underlying cause. Orbital findings result from occlusion of the ophthalmic vein, which drains into the cavernous sinus. Concurrent orbital cellulitis may be present, especially when the ethmoidal sinus is the primary site of infection. Most patients have CSF findings consistent with meningitis or a parameningeal infection. Angiography can help to establish the diagnosis. Antibiotic coverage for *S. aureus*, streptococci, and anaerobes should be instituted when cavernous sinus thrombosis is suspected. Surgical drainage of infected paranasal sinuses, especially the sphenoidal sinus, may result in rapid clinical improvement. Antibiotics should be continued for 2 or more weeks, depending on the clinical course, primary site of infection, and the presence of associated complications such as brain abscess. Mortality remains about 30% (data primarily from adults), and residual focal deficits are common among survivors. Residual pituitary insufficiency may be seen.[29, 81]

Septic thrombosis of the superior sagittal sinus is exceedingly rare in childhood. The most common predisposing cause is bacterial meningitis, but paranasal sinusitis, lateral venous sinus thrombosis, pulmonary infections, tonsillitis, and dental infections have been reported as causes of superior sagittal sinus thrombosis. The symptoms, signs, and laboratory findings of this process are similar to those of other intracranial suppurative infections, but the course is usually fulminant. Intracranial pressure rises rapidly because of loss of the CSF reabsorptive function of the sagittal venous sinus. Craniotomy may hasten deterioration. Thrombosis of the entire sinus, which is the usual event associated with bacterial meningitis, has a mortality rate in excess of 70%, and survivors usually have significant neurologic sequelae. Patients with paranasal sinusitis may have thrombosis only of the anterior segment of the sagittal venous sinus and may recover with minimal sequelae. Appropriate antibiotic regimens vary depending on the primary site of infection.[81]

The benefit of anticoagulation therapy for septic thrombosis of dural venous sinuses is unclear and must be weighed against the risk of subsequent intracranial hemorrhage. Early use in cavernous sinus thrombosis may help prevent the spread of thrombosis to other dural venous sinuses.[29]

REFERENCES

1. Nielsen H: Cerebral abscess in children. *Neuropediatrics* 14:76–80, 1983.
2. Dodge PR, Pomeroy SL: Parameningeal infections (including brain abscess, epidural abscess, subdural empyema), in Feigin RD, Cherry JD: *Textbook of Pediatric Infectious Diseases*, ed 3. Philadelphia, WB Saunders, 1992, pp 455–462.

3. Nestadt A, Lowry RB, Turner E: Diagnosis of brain abscess in infants and children. *Lancet* 2:449–453, 1960.
4. Arseni C, Horvath L, Dumitrescu L: Cerebral abscesses in children. *Acta Neurochir* 14:197–224, 1966.
5. Eberhard SJ: Diagnosis of brain abscess in infants and children. A retrospective study of twenty-six cases. *N C Med J* 30:303–313, 1969.
6. Idriss ZH, Gutman LT, Kronfol NM: Brain abscesses in infants and children. *Clin Pediatr (Phila)* 17:738–746, 1978.
7. Hirsch JF, Roux FX, Sainte-Rose C, et al: Brain abscess in childhood. *Child Brain* 10:251–265, 1983.
8. Jadavji T, Humphreys RP, Prober CG: Brain abscesses in infants and children. *Pediatr Infect Dis J* 4:394–398, 1985.
9. Moss SD, McLone DG, Arditi M, et al: Pediatric cerebral abscess. *Pediatr Neurosci* 14:291–296, 1988.
10. Buonaguro A, Colangelo M, Daniele B, et al: Neurological and behavioral sequelae in children operated on for brain abscess. *Child Nerv Syst* 5:153–155, 1989.
11. Sáez-Llorens XJ, Umaña MA, Odio CM, et al: Brain abscess in infants and children. *Pediatr Infect Dis J* 8:449–458, 1989.
12. Wong TT, Lee LS, Wang HS, et al: Brain abscesses in children—a cooperative study of 83 cases. *Child Nerv Syst* 5:19–24, 1989.
13. Tekkök IH, Erbengi A: Management of brain abscess in children: Review of 130 cases over a period of 21 years. *Child Nerv Syst* 8:411–416, 1992.
14. Spires JR, Smith RJH, Catlin FI: Brain abscesses in the young. *Otolaryngol Head Neck Surg* 93:468–474, 1985.
15. Renier D, Flandin C, Hirsch E, et al: Brain abscesses in neonates. A study of 30 cases. *J Neurosurg* 69:877–882, 1988.
16. Wispelwey B, Dacey RG, Scheld WM: Brain abscess, in Scheld WM, Whitley RJ, Durack DT: *Infections of the Central Nervous System*. New York, Raven, 1991, pp 457–486.
17. McGreal DA: Brain abscess in children. *Can Med Assoc J* 86:261–268, 1962.
18. Wright RL, Ballantine HT: Management of brain abscesses in children and adolescents. *Am J Dis Child* 114:113–122, 1967.
19. Fischer EG, McLennan JE, Suzuki Y: Cerebral abscess in children. *Am J Dis Child* 135:746–749, 1981.
20. Brook I: Bacteriology of intracranial abscess in children. *J Neurosurg* 54:484–488, 1981.
21. Theophilo F, Markakis E, Theophilo L, et al: Brain abscess in childhood. *Child Nerv Syst* 1:324–328, 1985.
22. Molinari GF, Smith L, Goldstein MN, et al: Brain abscess from septic cerebral embolism: An experimental model. *Neurology* 23:1205–1210, 1973.
23. Patrick CC, Kaplan SL: Current concepts in the pathogenesis and management of brain abscesses in children. *Pediatr Clin North Am* 35:625–636, 1988.
24. Gower D, McGuirt WF: Intracranial complications of acute and

chronic infectious ear disease: A problem still with us. *Laryngoscope* 93:1028–1033, 1983.
25. Ogle JW, Lauer BA: Acute mastoiditis. *Am J Dis Child* 140:1178–1182, 1986.
26. Wald ER: Sinusitis in children. *N Engl J Med* 326:319–323, 1992.
27. Nelson DA, Holloway WJ, Kara-Eneff SC, et al: Neurological syndromes produced by sphenoid sinus abscess. *Neurology* 17:981–987, 1967.
28. Lew D, Southwick FS, Montgomery WW, et al: Sphenoid sinusitis. A review of 30 cases. *N Engl J Med* 309:1149–1154, 1983.
29. DiNubile MJ: Septic thrombosis of the cavernous sinus. *Arch Neurol* 45:567–572, 1988.
30. Clark DB: Brain abscess and congenital heart disease. *Clin Neurosurg* 14:274–287, 1967.
31. Kagawa M, Takeshita M, Yato S, et al: Brain abscess in congenital cyanotic heart disease. *J Neurosurg* 58:913–917, 1983.
32. Fischbein CA, Rosenthal A, Fischer EG, et al: Risk factors for brain abscess in patients with congenital heart disease. *Am J Cardiol* 34:97–102, 1974.
33. Kline MW: Brain abscess in a patient with cystic fibrosis. *Pediatr Infect Dis J* 4:72–73, 1985.
34. Gelfand MS, Stephens DS, Howell EI, et al: Brain abscess: Association with pulmonary arteriovenous fistula and hereditary hemorrhagic telangiectasia: Report of three cases. *Am J Med* 85:718–720, 1988.
35. Leahy WR, Toyka KV, FischBeck KH: Cerebral abscess in children secondary to esophageal dilatation. *Pediatrics* 59:300–301, 1977.
36. Gower DJ, Horton D, Pollay M: Shunt-related brain abscess and ascending shunt infection. *J Child Neurol* 5:318–320, 1990.
37. Foy P, Sharr M: Cerebral abscess in children after pencil-tip injuries. *Lancet* 2:662–663, 1980.
38. Nitta T, Allegretta M, Okumura K, et al: Neoplastic and reactive human astrocytes express interleukin-8 gene. *Neurosurg Rev* 15:204–207, 1992.
39. Chao CC, Hu S, Close K, et al: Cytokine release from microglia: Differential inhibition by pentoxifylline and dexamethasone. *J Infect Dis* 166:847–853, 1992.
40. Kurzydlowski H, Wollenschlager C, Venezio FR, et al: Reevaluation of an experimental streptococcal canine brain abscess model. *J Neurosurg* 67:717–720, 1987.
41. Waggener JD: Pathophysiology of bacterial meningitis and cerebral abscesses: An anatomical interpretation. *Adv Neurol* 6:1–17, 1974.
42. Britt RH, Enzmann DR, Placone RC, et al: Experimental anaerobic brain abscess. Computerized tomographic and neuropathological correlations. *J Neurosurg* 60:1148–1159, 1984.
43. Enzmann DR, Britt RR, Obana WG, et al: Experimental *Staphylococcus aureus* brain abscess. *AJNR Am J Neuroradiol* 7:395–402, 1986.
44. DeLouvois J: Bacteriological examination of pus from abscesses of the central nervous system. *J Clin Pathol* 33:66–71, 1980.

45. DeLouvois J: The bacteriology and chemotherapy of brain abscess. *J Antimicrob Chemother* 4:395–413, 1978.
46. Wessalowski R, Thomas L, Kivit J, et al: Multiple brain abscesses caused by *Salmonella enteritidis* in a neonate: Successful treatment with ciprofloxacin. *Pediatr Infect Dis J* 12:683–688, 1993.
47. Berenson CS, Bia FJ: *Propionibacterium acnes* causes postoperative brain abscesses unassociated with foreign bodies: Case reports. *Neurosurgery* 25:130–134, 1989.
48. Beaman L, Beaman BL: Interactions of *Nocardia asteroides* with murine glia cells in culture. *Infect Immun* 61:343–347, 1993.
49. Jenson HB, Levy SR, Duncan C, et al: Treatment of multiple brain abscesses caused by *Bacillus cereus*. *Pediatr Infect Dis J* 8:795–798, 1989.
50. Whelan MA, Hilal SK: Computed tomography as a guide in the diagnosis and follow-up of brain abscesses. *Radiology* 135:663–671, 1980.
51. Smith RR: Neuroradiology of intracranial infection. *Pediatr Neurosurg* 18:92–104, 1992.
52. Matson DD, Salam M: Brain abscess in congenital heart disease. *Pediatrics* 27:772–789, 1961.
53. Berg B, Franklin G, Cuneo R, et al: Nonsurgical cure of brain abscess: Early diagnosis and follow-up with computerized tomography. *Ann Neurol* 3:474–478, 1978.
54. Rennels MB, Woodward CL, Robinson WL, et al: Medical cure of apparent brain abscesses. *Pediatrics* 72:220–224, 1983.
55. Keren G, Tyrell DL: Nonsurgical treatment of brain abscesses: Report of two cases. *Pediatr Infect Dis J* 3:331–334, 1984.
56. Wiedermann BL: Subdural, epidural, and subgaleal infections, in Kaplan SL: *Current Therapy in Pediatric Infectious Disease,* ed 3. St Louis, Mosby, 1993, pp 152–153.
57. Rosenblum ML, Hoff JT, Norman D, et al: Decreased mortality from brain abscesses since advent of computerized tomography. *J Neurosurg* 49:658–668, 1978.
58. Koszewski W: Epilepsy following brain abscess. The evaluation of possible risk factors with emphasis on new concept of epileptic focus formation. *Acta Neurochir* 113:110–117, 1991.
59. Kline MW: *Citrobacter* meningitis and brain abscess in infancy: Epidemiology, pathogenesis, and treatment. *J Pediatr* 113:430–434, 1988.
60. Kaplan SL, Patrick CC: Cefotaxime and aminoglycoside treatment of meningitis caused by gram-negative enteric organisms. *Pediatr Infect Dis J* 9:810–814, 1990.
61. McCracken GH, Threlkeld N, Mize S, et al: Moxalactam therapy for neonatal meningitis due to gram-negative enteric bacilli. *JAMA* 252:1427–1432, 1984.
62. Willis J, Robinson JE: *Enterobacter sakazakii* meningitis in neonates. *Pediatr Infect Dis J* 7:196–199, 1988.
63. Foreman SD, Smith EE, Ryan NJ, et al: Neonatal *Citrobacter* meningitis: Pathogenesis of cerebral abscess formation. *Ann Neurol* 16:655–659, 1984.

64. Kline MW, Kaplan SL, Hawkins EP, et al: Pathogenesis of brain abscess formation in an infant rat model of *Citrobacter diversus* bacteremia and meningitis. *J Infect Dis* 157:106–112, 1988.
65. Kline MW, Mason EO, Kaplan SL: Characterization of *Citrobacter diversus* strains causing neonatal meningitis. *J Infect Dis* 157:101–105, 1988.
66. Woods CR, Mason EO, Kaplan SL: Interaction of *Citrobacter diversus* strains with HEp-2 epithelial and human umbilical vein endothelial cells. *J Infect Dis* 166:1035–1044, 1992.
67. Obana WG, Cogen PH, Callen PW, et al: Ultrasound-guided aspiration of a neonatal brain abscess. *Child Nerv Syst* 7:272–274, 1991.
68. Graham DR, Band JD: *Citrobacter diversus* brain abscess and meningitis in neonates. *JAMA* 245:1923–1925, 1981.
69. Zuger A, Lowy FD: Tuberculosis of the central nervous system, in Scheld WM, Whitley RJ, Durack DT: *Infections of the Central Nervous System*. New York, Raven, 1991, pp 425–456.
70. Henrickson M, Weisse ME: Tuberculous brain abscess in a three-year-old South Pacific Islander. *Pediatr Infect Dis J* 11:488–491, 1992.
71. Yogev R: Suppurative intracranial complications of upper respiratory tract infections. *Pediatr Infect Dis J* 6:324–327, 1987.
72. Helfgott DC, Weingarten K, Hartman BJ: Subdural empyema, in Scheld WM, Whitley RJ, Durack DT: *Infections of the Central Nervous System*. New York, Raven, 1991, pp 487–498.
73. Farmer TW, Wise GR: Subdural empyema in infants, children and adults. *Neurology* 23:254–261, 1973.
74. Jacobson PL, Farmer TW: Subdural empyema complicating meningitis in infants: Improved prognosis. *Neurology* 31:190–193, 1981.
75. Smith HP, Hendrick EB: Subdural empyema and epidural abscess in children. *J Neurosurg* 58:392–397, 1983.
76. Zimmerman RD, Leeds NE, Danziger A: Subdural empyema: CT findings. *Radiology* 150:417–422, 1984.
77. Curless RG: Subdural empyema in infant meningitis: Diagnosis, therapy, and prognosis. *Child Nerv Syst* 1:211–214, 1985.
78. Krauss WE, McCormick PC: Infections of the dural spaces. *Neurosurg Clin North Am* 3:421–433, 1992.
79. Gellin BG, Weingarten K, Gamache FW, et al: Epidural abscess, in Scheld WM, Whitley RJ, Durack DT: *Infections of the Central Nervous System*. New York, Raven, 1991, pp 499–514.
80. DiNubile MJ, Broom WH, Southwick FS: Septic cortical thrombophlebitis. *J Infect Dis* 161:1216–1220, 1990.
81. Southwick FS, Richardson EP, Swartz MN: Septic thrombosis of the dural venous sinuses. *Medicine (Baltimore)* 65:82–106, 1986.
82. Medlock MD, Olivero WC, Hanigan WC, et al: Children with cerebral venous thrombosis diagnosed with magnetic resonance imaging and magnetic resonance angiography. *Neurosurgery* 31:870–876, 1992.

Botulism

Norman D. Ferrari III, M.D.
Associate Professor of Pediatrics and Internal Medicine, Chief, General Pediatrics and Adolescent Medicine, Associate Dean, Ambulatory Services, West Virginia University School of Medicine, Morgantown, West Virginia

Martin E. Weisse, M.D.
Assistant Professor of Pediatrics, Sections of General Pediatrics and Adolescent Medicine, and Infectious Diseases, West Virginia University School of Medicine, Morgantown, West Virginia

Botulism is a neuroparalytic disease caused by the most potent toxin known to man. The lethal dose of toxin is 1×10^{-9} mg/kg.[1] There are three forms of the disease. Wound botulism occurs when traumatized tissue is infected with toxin-producing strains of *Clostridium botulinum*. Food-borne botulism follows ingestion of preformed toxin from contaminated foodstuff. The most common form of the disease is infantile botulism. This form of illness develops in infants less than 1 year of age whose gastrointestinal tract is colonized by toxin-producing *C. botulinum*. The toxin is produced and absorbed in vivo.

In 1991 there were 114 cases of botulism reported to the Centers for Disease Control in the United States. Of these, 81 (71%) were infantile botulism, 27 (23%) were foodborne botulism, and only 6 (5%) were wound botulism. Since 1960, the peak year for foodborne cases was 1977, when 80 cases were reported from an outbreak in Michigan involving 59 persons who all ate at the same restaurant. The peak year for infantile botulism was in 1984 with 100 cases.[2, 3]

HISTORY

Botulism has been identified as a cause of food poisoning in Europe since the late 18th century, but its folklore goes back considerably further. It has been suggested that botulism killed the leader and captains of Sennacherib's army in 701 B.C. and thus saved Jerusalem (2 Chronicles 32:21). Many outbreaks of botulism in Europe were associated with ingestion of sausage, and Emperor Leo VI of Byzantium (886–911 A.D.) forbade the manufacture of blood sausage, perhaps in response to deaths associated with this food.[4]

Advances in Pediatric Infectious Diseases®, vol. 10

Centuries later, botulism occurred in Europe, particularly in Germany. There was a notable outbreak in Wildbad, Germany, in 1793 that caused the illness of 13 people and the death of 6. This outbreak was caused by eating blunzen, a type of blood sausage that was locally popular. The number of reported cases of sausage poisoning increased rapidly during the ensuing years and prompted a study of this disease by Justinius Kerner (1786–1862), the district medical officer. He collected data on 230 cases of botulism, most of which involved some form of sausage poisoning. He became so well known for his work that botulism became known as "Kerner's disease."[4] Several decades later in Belgium, a music club performed at the funeral of one of its members. After the ceremonies, the amateur musicians gathered at the home of one of their number where they had refreshments, including a portion of raw, salted ham. During the next 2 days, 23 of the 34 members became ill with increasing neuromuscular paralysis; 3 of them died and 10 nearly died. The tragedy came to the attention of a bacteriologist named van Ermengem at the University of Ghent. In his investigations he found that everyone in whom symptoms developed had eaten ham and those with milder symptoms had eaten smaller portions. He isolated an anaerobic, spore-forming bacillus from the ham as well as from the spleen of one of the victims. He was able to reproduce the disease in animals with a cell-free filtrate and postulated the presence of an extracellular toxin. He found that the toxin was heat labile but was resistant to alcohol, proteolytic enzymes, and mild acid. He called the organism *Bacillus botulinus* after *botulus*, the Latin word for sausage.[5] Another outbreak of botulism in Germany in 1904 was caused by canned beans that had not been heated after storage.[6] An organism was isolated that produced a toxin similar to van Ermengem's, but antitoxin did not cross-neutralize, thus indicating that there were at least two types of *B. bolutinus*.[7] It is now known that there are seven distinct toxin types of *C. botulinum*.

Until 1951 all of the reported cases of human botulism were food borne. In that year three cases of wound botulism were reported.[8] Infant botulism, which was not described until 1976,[9] now constitutes the majority of botulism cases.

MICROBIOLOGY

Clostridium botulinum is an ubiquitous gram-positive, spore-forming, obligate anaerobe found globally, with its natural habitat being soil and dust. Spores have been found in close to 20% of soil samples tested in the United States. States with the highest soil concentrations of spores include Colorado, California, Utah, and Pennsylvania.[10] *Clostridium* spores are resistant to heat, light, drying, and radiation, yet specific conditions are necessary for germination. Ideal conditions include neutral pH, temperature of 15 to 45°C, and required amino acids and vitamins. Spores can be found on fresh fruits and vegetables or in various meats and fish. Honey is an important, identified, and avoidable source of spores. Honey should not be given to infants less than 1 year of age since 4% to 25% of honey samples tested contain *Clostridium* spores.[11–13] Conversely, corn syrup is rarely contaminated, with only 0.5% of the samples having spores in close to 1,000 samples.[14]

TOXINS

SEROTYPES

There are seven distinct toxin serotypes (A through G), of which only A, B, E, and F are known to cause disease in man. The first two immunologically distinct toxins were isolated from raw ham[5] and canned beans[6] and were later classified as types A and B.[15] Type C toxin was isolated in the United States from fly larvae[16] and in Australia from carcasses of cattle that had died of bulbar paralysis.[17] The antitoxin prepared from the Bengston strain neutralized the toxins of both the Benston and Seddon strains, but the antitoxin prepared from the Seddon strain did not neutralize the Bengston strain.[18] Type D toxin was also originally recovered from cattle.[19] Toxins C1, C2, and D are immunologically related. Type E was isolated from the intestines of sturgeons in Russia,[20] and type F was implicated in human botulinum poisoning from liver paste in Denmark. Type G was isolated from a soil sample collected in Argentina.

Clostridium botulinum is distinguished from other clostridial species by the production of specific botulinum toxin, and it includes a heterogeneous group of organisms. *Clostridium botulinum* was originally used to designate nonproteolytic strains, whereas proteolytic strains were designated as *Clostridium parabotulinum*. Now all neurotoxin-producing strains are designated as *C. botulinum*. Because of the diversity of colony morphology and biochemical differences, *C. botulinum* has been divided into four groups, I to IV. Group I strains are strongly proteolytic and include all type A strains and some type B and F strains. The spores in this group are all highly heat resistant. Group I strains are found in regions that have relatively little rainfall and where the temperature is moderate. In the United States, type A is found west of the Great Plains and usually in soil of low organic content and neutral to high pH. Type A has been found in soil from Europe, Southeast Asia, Australia, India, and South America. In the United States, type B is localized in the region of the Allegheny range, especially in southeastern Pennsylvania. Group II strains are strongly saccharolytic but nonproteolytic and produce toxin even at temperatures as low as 3 to 4°C. The spores are relatively heat labile. Group E and the other B and F strains are included in this group. Group III strains are nonproteolytic and saccharolytic. The spores are intermediately heat resistant. All type C and D strains belong to this group. Group IV contains only type G strains, which are proteolytic and nonsaccharolytic.

ACTIVATION

Botulinum toxin is produced as a single polypeptide chain (progenitor toxin) without intrinsic activity. Activation requires cleavage, or nicking, of a peptide bond in the single chain to form a two-polypeptide chain held together by at least one disulfide bond. Group I strains, particularly types A and B, produce proteases and may therefore autoactivate toxin. Group II strains include type E and require tryptic activation for toxin activation. For example, type A and B strains usually produce toxin with potencies greater than 1 million mouse median lethal dose units (LD_{50})/mL, whereas type E cultures produce toxin of only 10^2 mouse LD_{50}/mL. Nevertheless, the morbidity (49%) and case fatality rate (19% to 33%) of human type E botulism are comparable to those of type A and B cases.[21]

Botulinum toxin is an oral toxin that is absorbed from all areas of the alimentary tract including the colon. Toxin is absorbed most readily from the small intestine. Toxin absorption is endocytotic like most nutritional proteins.[1] The mechanism of transport to the target cells is unknown.

MECHANISM OF ACTION

Botulinum toxin acts presynaptically by blocking the release of acetylcholine at the neuromuscular junction. Three stages are involved: toxin binding, internalization, and neurotransmitter release.

Botulinum toxin binds rapidly and irreversibly to acceptors at the presynaptic nerve surface.[22, 23] The fact that toxins A and B do not compete for acceptor sites but A and E do compete implies that there is more than one acceptor type[24]; the nature of the acceptor molecules has not yet been ascertained. After binding to the acceptor, the toxin is internalized by an energy-dependent process mediated by the heavy chain of the toxin, a process resembling endocytosis.[25] Intact double-chain toxin is transported into the cytosol and is required for inhibition of neurotransmitter release. Normally, an action potential at the nerve ending triggers an influx of calcium ions, which then promote the exocytosis of acetylcholine from vesicles at active zones on the plasmalemma. The light chain of the toxin acts as a protease and cleaves synaptobrevin, an integral membrane protein of the acetylcholine-containing vesicles, thereby inhibiting acetylcholine release. It is unknown what specific function synaptobrevin plays, but perhaps its cleavage alters the recognition of a complementary binding protein in the cytosol or on the cytoplasmic face of the plasma membrane and impairs neurotransmitter/vesicle fusion.[26, 27]

Type A botulinum neurotoxin and to a lesser extent toxin F[28, 29] have been used therapeutically to replace some surgical treatments for several ophthalmologic and neuromuscular diseases. Examples include various dystonias,[30] cranial nerve palsies,[31, 32] strabismus,[33, 34] torticollis,[35] as well as chronic urinary retention.[36] The spasticity due to cerebral palsy[37] and multiple sclerosis[38] has also been treated with botulinum toxin.

SYMPTOMS, DIAGNOSIS, AND TREATMENT

INFANT BOTULISM

Most patients affected with infantile botulism range from 6 weeks to 9 months of age, with a peak incidence between 2 and 3 months. Several recent reports have described infants 1 week of age,[39, 40] and more than 90% of cases occur in those younger than 6 months old.

As many as 70% of affected infants are breast-fed.[41] Most experts feel that the intestinal environment in a breast-fed infant is more favorable for spore formation. In these infants the predominant microorganism is *Bifidobacterium*, whereas formula-fed infants are more quickly colonized with *Bacteroides* species, coliforms, and enterococci, which inhibit the growth of *Clostridium*.[42]

All peripheral cholinergic synapses are affected, including autonomic parasympathetic and neuromuscular junctions, and this contributes to the clinical symptoms. Autonomic dysfunction occurs first and is manifested as constipation, hypoactive bowel sounds, dry mouth, dilated and sluggish pupils, and neurogenic bladder. Constipation is the most common initial symptom. Next is a descending paralysis (cranial to caudal), usually starting with the cranial nerves. Loss of head control and poor feeding are followed by weak suck and cry, ptosis, decreased ocular movement, drooling, decreased gag reflex, and facial diplegia. Last seen are diminished movement of the extremities and loss of deep tendon reflexes.[43, 44] Before the development of weakness as many as 75% of receptors must be blocked; however, more than 90% of diaphragmatic receptors must be affected before spontaneous respirations cease.[45]

Complications commonly seen with botulism include inappropriate secretion of antidiuretic hormone (SIADH) with seizures, significant hyponatremia, autonomic instability resulting in tachycardia and hypertension, and urinary tract infections from neurogenic bladders resulting from parasympathetic dysfunction. Many infants require intubation as part of their management and may have subsequent atelectasis, pneumonia, sepsis, and subglottic stenosis.[43]

Many different causes should be considered in a hypotonic infant, including systemic infections like sepsis and meningoencephalitis, poliomyelitis, tick paralysis, postinfectious polyradiculoneuropathy (Guillain-Barré syndrome), infantile spinal muscular atrophy (Werdnig-Hoffmann disease), myasthenia gravis, congenital myopathies, and poisoning from heavy metals and organophosphate.[46]

History and electromyelography (EMG) are the primary tools for making the diagnosis of infantile botulism. Nerve conduction velocities are normal. Electromyelograms may be normal initially, and serial evaluations may be necessary to obtain a diagnostic pattern. Brief small-amplitude potentials with a decremental response at low (3 to 10 Hz) repetitive stimulation and an incremental or staircase response are seen at high (20 to 50 Hz) repetitive stimulation.[47] Stool should be examined for *C. botulinum* and toxin to confirm the diagnosis. Serum levels of toxin never reach high enough levels to measure, and cerebrospinal fluid is normal.

Recovery is usually complete with time. Supportive care is the mainstay of all treatment, and infants should be transferred to a center with intensive respiratory care available. Hospitalization has ranged from 2 to 150 days, with a median of 27 days. Nutrition is of paramount importance and requires parenteral or continuous nasojejunal tube feedings. Bolus gastric feedings are not as well tolerated. Intubation is required in as many as 80% of affected infants. Tracheostomy is necessary only for prolonged intubation, an inability to maintain the endotracheal tube, or fear of subglottic stenosis from a tight endotracheal tube. Most fatalities are secondary to avoidable respiratory complications.[43, 48]

Antitoxin is of little use since it will only neutralize toxin not bound irreversibly to receptors. Since most antitoxin is made from horse serum, there is also the risk of serum sickness and anaphylaxis.

Antimicrobials should be used cautiously.[49, 50] Aminoglycosides may enhance neuromuscular blockade. Patients treated with penicillin showed no difference in recovery from those untreated, and some have theorized that treatment may only result in huge release of toxin after lysis of the clostridia.

Cholinesterase inhibitors, like edrophonium and neostigmine, have only a transient benefit because patients rapidly become refractory. Enemas and cathartics have minimal to no usefulness.

FOOD-BORNE BOTULISM

The first reported case of food-borne botulism in the United States was reported in 1920. Between 1976 and 1984 there were 309 reported cases for an average of about 24 cases per year. The case fatality rate is 7.5%. Most cases follow intoxication with type A (60%), type B (30%), or type E (10%) botulinum toxin. Improperly home-canned fruits and vegetables (70%) account for most cases, whereas the rest are from meat and fish (30%). Only a few cases result from commercially prepared foods. Large outbreaks follow mass poisonings at commercial establishments, like the record outbreak in Michigan in 1977. Type E cases are primarily reported from Alaska and are exclusively traced to fish and meat.[4]

These patients are often nauseous and vomiting, findings unique to this form of botulism. Gastrointestinal symptoms occur in 100% of the cases caused by type E toxin. Acute gastritis is followed by blurred vision, diplopia, and photophobia resulting from paralysis of cranial nerves III (oculomotor), IV (trochlear), and VI (abducens). Next comes difficulty swallowing, and neck muscle weakness. Dry mouth results from the paralysis of cranial nerves VII (facial), which innervates the salivary gland, and XII (hypoglossal) to the tongue. If not recognized, the toxin will progress to paralyze the skeletal and respiratory muscles. There is no change in the senses, and patients experience normal hearing and consciousness.[4]

The differential diagnosis for food-borne botulism is similar to infantile botulism but also includes acute alcohol intoxication, basilar artery thrombosis, hypocalcemia, hypermagnesemia, and carbon monoxide poisoning.

The diagnosis is made from clinical symptoms, identification of toxin in the patient's serum, or isolation of the toxin or *Clostridium* in the suspected food. Treatment is supportive care with respiratory support if needed. Unlike infantile botulism, antitoxin may neutralize the large amount of unbound circulating toxin. Some authorities advocate the use of gut lavage with sodium bicarbonate to remove unabsorbed toxin.

WOUND BOTULISM

Wound botulism is the rarest type of botulism. Only 16 cases were reported between 1976 and 1984, for an average of 2 cases per year. This form of the disease carries a case fatality rate of 12.5%. Cases have been related to two toxins: type A (69%) and type B (31%). The most common injuries associated with wound botulism are compound fractures of long bones and severe crush injuries to the extremities. The mean incubation time from injury to neurologic symptoms is about 10 days, with a range of 4 to 14 days.[4] There have also been recent reports linking wound botulism to parenteral drug abuse.[51]

Clinically, bulbar paralysis followed by descending symmetrical motor paralysis is typical. The highest cranial nerves are affected first, and diplopia is often the first symptom, followed by dysphagia and a dry mouth. Should toxin continue to be produced and absorbed, fatal apnea can result from the paralysis of respiratory muscles. The diagnosis is confirmed by obtaining serum toxin levels and isolation of *Clostridium* from the wound. As in infantile botulism, antitoxin is of little use.[4]

REFERENCES

1. Bonventre PF: Absorption of botulinum toxin from the gastrointestinal tract. *Rev Infect Dis* 1:663–667, 1979.
2. Centers for Disease Control: Summary of notifiable diseases, United States. *MMWR* 40:3, 21, 1992.
3. MacDonald K, Cohen M, Blake P: The changing epidemiology of adult botulism in the United States. *Am J Epidemiol* 123:794–799, 1986.
4. Smith LD, Sugiyama H: *Botulism: The Organism, Its Toxins, the Disease,* ed 2. Springfield, Ill, Charles C Thomas, 1988, pp 3–9, 115–133.
5. van Ermengem E: Ueber einen neuen anaeroben Bacillus und seine Beziehugen zum Botulism. *Z Hyg Infekt* 25:1–56, 1897.
6. Landmann G: Ueber die Ursache der Darmstadter Bohnenvergiftung. *Hyg Rundschau* 10:449–452, 1904.
7. Leuchs J: Beitrage zu Kenntnis des Toxins und Antitoxins des *Bacillus botulinus. Z Hyg Infekt* 65:55–84, 1910.

8. Hampton CR: A case of probable botulism due to wound infection. *J Bacteriol* 650:213–215, 1951.
9. Pickett J, Bert B, Chaplin E, et al: Syndrome of botulism in infancy: Clinical and electrophysiologic study. *N Engl J Med* 295:770–772, 1976.
10. Smith L: *Clostridium botulinum:* Characteristics and occurrence. *Rev Infect Dis* 1:637–641, 1979.
11. Midura T, Snowden S, Wood R, et al: Isolation of *Clostridium botulinum* from honey. *J Clin Microbiol* 9:282–283, 1979.
12. Arnon S, Midura T, Damus K, et al: Honey and other environmental risk factors for infant botulism. *J Pediatr* 94:331–336, 1979.
13. Spika JS, Shaffer N, Hargrett-Bean N, et al: Risk factors for infant botulism in the United States. *Am J Dis Child* 143:828–832, 1989.
14. Kautter DA, Lilly T, Solomon HM, et al: *Clostridium botulinum* spores in infant foods: A survey. *J Food Protect* 45:1028–1029, 1982.
15. Meyer KF, Glunnison JB: European strains of *C. botulinum* XXXVI. *J Infect Dis* 45:96–105, 1929.
16. Bengston IA: Preliminary note on a toxin-producing anaerobe isolated from the larvae of *Lucilia caesar*. *Public Health Rep* 37:164–170, 1922.
17. Seddon HR: Bulbar paralysis in cattle due to the action of a toxicogenic bacillus, with a discussion on the relationship of the condition to forage poisoning (botulism). *J Comp Pathol Ther* 35:147–190, 1922.
18. Pfenninger W: Toxico-immunologic and serologic relationship of *B. botulinus*, type C, and *B. parabotulinus*, "Sneddon" SSII. *J Infect Dis* 35:347–352, 1924.
19. Theiler A, Viljoen PR, Green H, et al: Lamsiekte (parabotulism) in cattle in South Africa, in *Union of South Africa Department of Agriculture, 13th and 14th Reports of the Director of Veterinary Education and Research*. 1927, pp 821–1361.
20. Gunnison JB, Cummings JR, Meyer KF: *Clostridium botulinum* type E. *Proc Soc Exp Biol Med* 35:278–280, 1936.
21. Sakaguchi G: *Clostridium botulinum* toxins. *Pharmacol Ther* 19:165–194, 1983.
22. Dolly JO, Williams RS, Black JD, et al: Localization of sites for 125-I labelled neurotoxin at the murine neuromuscular junction and its binding to rat brain synaptosomes. *Toxicon* 20:141–148, 1982.
23. Dolly JO, Black JD, Williams RS, et al: Acceptors for botulinum neurotoxin reside on motor nerve terminals and mediate its internalization. *Nature* 307:457–460, 1984.
24. Hambleton P: *Clostridium botulinum* toxins: A general review of involvement in disease, structure, mode of action and preparation for clinical use. *J Neurol* 239:16–20, 1992.
25. Shone CC, Hambleton P, Melling J: A 60 kDa fragment from the NH2 terminus of the heavy subunit of *Clostridium botulinum* type A neurotoxin forms channels in lipid vesicles. *Eur J Biochem* 167:175–180, 1987.

26. Schiavo G, Fabio B, Poulain B, et al: Tetanus and botulinum B neurotoxins block neurotransmitter release by proteolytic cleavage of synaptobrevin. *Nature* 359:832–835, 1992.
27. Drachman DB, Price DL: Botulism toxin: Mechanism of presynaptic blockade. *Science* 193:1256–1258, 1976.
28. Ludlow CL, Haller M, Rhew K, et al: Therapeutic use of type F botulinum toxin. *N Engl J Med* 326:349–350, 1992.
29. Greene PE, Fahn S: Use of botulinum toxin type F injections to treat torticollis in patients with immunity to botulinum toxin type A. *Mov Disord* 8:479–483, 1993.
30. Marsden CD, Quinn NP: The dystonias: Neurologic disorders affecting 20,000 people in Britain. *BMJ* 300:139–144, 1990.
31. Jankovic J, Brin MF: Therapeutic uses of botulinum toxin. *N Engl J Med* 324:1186–1194, 1991.
32. Hambleton P: Therapeutic application of botulinum toxin. *J Med Microbiol* 39:243–245, 1993.
33. Scott AB: Botulinum toxin injection into extraocular muscles as an alternative to strabismus surgery. *Ophthalmology* 87:1044–1049, 1980.
34. Ing MR: Botulinum alignment for congenital esotropia. *Ophthalmology* 10:318–322, 1993.
35. Anderson TJ, Rivest J, Stell R, et al: Botulinum toxin treatment of spasmodic torticollis. *J R Soc Med* 85:524–529, 1992.
36. Fowler CJ, Betts CD, Christmas TJ, et al: Botulinum toxin in the treatment of chronic urinary retention in women. *Br J Urol* 70:387–389, 1992.
37. Koman LA, Mooney JF, Smith B, et al: Management of cerebral palsy with botulinum A toxin: Preliminary investigation. *J Pediatr Orthop* 13:489–495, 1993.
38. Borg-Stein J, Pine ZM, Miller JR, et al: Botulinum toxin for the treatment of spasticity in multiple sclerosis: New observations. *Am J Phys Med Rehabil* 72:364–368, 1993.
39. Thilo EH, Townsend SF, Deacon J: Infant botulism at one week of age. *Pediatrics* 92:151–153, 1993.
40. Schmidt RD, Schmidt TW: Infant botulism: Case series and review of the literature. *J Emerg Med* 10:713–718, 1992.
41. Thompson JA, Glascow LA, Warpinski JR, et al: Infant botulism: Clinical spectrum and epidemiology. *Pediatrics* 66:936–942, 1980.
42. Hentges D: The intestinal flora and infant botulism. *Rev Infect Dis* 1:668–673, 1979.
43. Schreiner MS, Field E, Ruddy R: Infant botulism: A review of 12 years experience at the Children's Hospital of Philadelphia. *Pediatrics* 87:159–165, 1991.
44. Brown L: Infant botulism. *Pediatr Ann* 13:139–148, 1984.
45. Paton WDM, Waud DR: The margin of safety of neuromuscular transmission. *J Physiol* 191:595, 1967.

46. Brown L: Differential diagnosis of infant botulism. *Rev Infect Dis* 1:625–629, 1979.
47. Gay CT, Marks W, Riley H, et al: Infantile botulism. *South Med J* 81:457–460, 1988.
48. Johnson RO, Clay SA, Arnon SS: Diagnosis and management of infant botulism. *Am J Dis Child* 133:586–593, 1979.
49. Arnon S: Infant botulism. *Annu Rev Med* 31:541–560, 1980.
50. Arnon S, Chin J: The clinical spectrum of infant botulism. *Rev Infect Dis* 1:614–624, 1979.
51. MacDonald K, Rutherford GW, Friedman SM, et al: Botulism and botulism-like illness in chronic drug abusers. *Ann Intern Med* 102:616–618, 1985.

Varicella-Zoster Virus: Prospects for Control*

Anne A. Gershon, M.D.
Department of Pediatrics, Columbia University College of Physicians & Surgeons, New York, New York

BACKGROUND

Varicella (chickenpox) and zoster (shingles) are the two clinical illnesses caused by varicella-zoster virus (VZV). Varicella, the primary infection, usually occurs during childhood and is characterized by a generalized pruritic vesicular exanthem accompanied by fever. Zoster, the secondary infection, usually occurs in adults or immunocompromised patients (including those with acquired immunodeficiency syndrome [AIDS]) and is characterized by a circumscribed, unilateral, painful, vesicular eruption with an associated inflammation of the involved dorsal root or cranial nerve sensory ganglia.

There are about 4 million cases of varicella yearly in the United States. Although most cases are mild, the high frequency of the disease leads to a certain degree of morbidity and mortality. It is estimated that there are about 4,500 hospitalizations yearly as a result of severe varicella or its complications in otherwise healthy children in the United States.[1] About 100 cases of fatal varicella are recorded by the Centers for Disease Control (CDC) yearly, but underreporting of this disease is common. In healthy populations, adults and children less than 1 year of age have the highest rates of hospitalization and death from varicella. A varicella case fatality rate of 6.7 per 100,000 in the population at large has been observed.[2] According to the CDC, for adults aged 30 to 40 years, the case fatality ratio is 25 per 10,000. For children this figure is estimated to be 1 in 10,000.

Zoster is caused by reactivation of latent VZV infection that was acquired during varicella. That zoster results from reactivation of latent virus rather than reintroduction of virus into a partially

*This work was supported in part by Grant AI24021 and Merck Sharpe & Dohme Laboratories.

immune host was long suspected since zoster does not exhibit the seasonal prevalence seen with varicella (late winter and spring), nor does zoster occur frequently in young adults who are exposed to their children when they contract chickenpox. The mode of pathogenesis of zoster by reactivation of latent VZV has now been proved. Molecular studies of VZV isolates from patients with zoster after either natural chickenpox or varicella vaccination have shown that the DNA of viruses causing the primary infection and zoster are similar.[3–5] Reactivation of VZV infection can also occur in the absence of clinical symptoms both after natural infection and after immunization, as can reinfection.[6–11]

During varicella, VZV invades sensory nerves where it establishes latent infection in sensory ganglia, most likely as a result of skin infection but possibly because of viremia. Presumably, latent infection develops in most individuals, but only about 15% will eventually manifest zoster. It is estimated that there are about 400,000 cases of zoster yearly in the United States, mostly in immunocompromised patients and the elderly.

Varicella-zoster virus infection may cause a severe or fatal disease in patients receiving immunosuppressive therapy or those who have decreased cell-mediated immune (CMI) responses. For example, severe, generalized varicella occurred in 30% of leukemic children who acquired chickenpox while receiving chemotherapy and/or radiotherapy, and mortality ranged from 7% to 28% in the preantiviral therapy era.[12, 13] In older immunodeficient patients there is an increased risk of disseminated zoster, and mortality rates may approach those for varicella.[8, 14]

This review will concentrate mainly on new information regarding VZV, including molecular biology, pathogenesis, transmission, congenital infection, diagnostic advances, antiviral therapy, and the use of live vaccine to prevent or modify varicella and zoster.

THE VIRUS

The linear double-stranded DNA genome of VZV consists of approximately 125,000 base pairs. It consists of a 5.8×10^6 dalton, long unique DNA segment U_L flanked by terminal and internal repeats and a 3.4×10^6 dalton, short unique sequence U_S, flanked by internal and terminal repeats.[15–17] The genome, which has been sequenced, exists in a total of four isomers (two majors of 95% and two minors of 5%).[18]

Morphologically, VZV is a typical but rather small herpesvirus. The virion has a diameter of 150 to 200 nm and consists of an inner icosahedral (20-sided) capsid surrounded by a tegument and an envelope composed of two or more membranes. The virus produces approximately 30 structural and nonstructural proteins, including at least five glycoproteins designated I through V, which are analogous to glycoproteins E, B, H, G, and C, respectively, of herpes simplex virus (HSV). Glycoproteins play active roles in invasion and infection of cells, and their recognition by the immune system of the host leads to humoral immunity and CMI to VZV. Immunity to nonstructural viral antigens may also be important in host defense. There is no known antigenic variation of VZV, but minor strain differences have been demonstrated.[19] Varicella-zoster virus DNA shares partial homology with HSV, Epstein-Barr virus (EBV), and certain animal herpesviruses.[20] Varicella-zoster virus shares major antigens with herpesviruses that produce varicella-like disease in various simian species,[21] and it shares minor antigens with HSV.[22, 23]

Varicella-zoster virus is a difficult virus to propagate in vitro since it is highly cell associated and virus yields are low. This peculiarity of VZV has complicated the development and production of a live attenuated vaccine. The virus is able to multiply in human skin in vivo with much greater facility, which accounts for both its high degree of infectivity and person-to-person spread. In vitro, VZV is hypothesized to be inactivated in late endosomes during egress from infected cells.[24, 25] In contrast, this inactivation is hypothesized to not occur in vivo in the human outer layers of the epidermis, where endosomes are not present.

LATENCY

How VZV is maintained in the latent state has been a subject of intense interest for many years. With the development of molecular methods by which virus genes can be studied it has become possible to demonstrate the presence of VZV genes during latent infection in autopsy specimens from patients with a prior history of varicella and no evidence of zoster at death. Varicella-zoster virus DNA was first demonstrated in human trigeminal ganglia by Southern blotting[26] and VZV RNA by in situ hybridization.[27] More recently VZV DNA has been demonstrated in dorsal root ganglia (DRG) by in situ hybridization[28] and polymerase chain reaction (PCR).[29] The exact site of latent infection is still controversial. Some investigators have described VZV transcripts in neurons of trigeminal and thoracic ganglia,[29] and others have reported latent virus in ganglia in satellite cells rather than neurons.[28]

Gene expression in the herpesviruses occurs in a coordinated cascade; immediate early genes activate early genes, which in turn induce expression of late structural genes. Several immediate early and early VZV genes that have mostly regulatory rather than structural viral functions are expressed during VZV latency. These include VZV genes 4 (the HSV-1 equivalent of gene 27), 29, and 62 (the HSV-1 equivalent of ICP4).[28] Since several VZV genes are expressed during latency, there may be some degree of viral multiplication taking place during latent infection.[30] In contrast, during HSV latency only the latency-associated transcript (LAT) gene, which is asymmetrically transcribed from a promoter downstream of HSV ICP0, is expressed; latent HSV is present only in neurons.[28]

TRANSMISSION OF VARICELLA-ZOSTER VIRUS

Historically, transmission of VZV has been believed to occur by way of respiratory droplets, and epidemiologic evidence suggests that transmission can occur before the onset of skin rash.[31–34] Airborne spread of varicella has been documented,[35, 36] but spread by fomites has not. Varicella is most contagious during the onset of rash and for a few days afterward.[37]

Although during infection VZV seems to originate from the respiratory tract, a number of observations are difficult to reconcile with the concept that this is the only source of virus transmission. For example, it is extremely rare to be able to isolate VZV from the pharynx of infected patients. Although Kido et al. used PCR to reveal that VZV DNA is present in the nasopharynx in most children during the early stages of clinical varicella,[38] in the study of Koropchak et al., performed 24 hours after rash onset in 12 patients, only 3% of oropharyngeal samples but 75% of skin vesicles were positive for VZV DNA.[39] In a study by Ozaki et al. of pharyngeal secretions of patients with chickenpox, however, 26% and 90% were positive during the incubation period and after clinical onset, respectively.[40] Although VZV DNA can be demonstrated in the pharynx by PCR, this does not necessarily indicate the presence of infectious virus. Furthermore, in contrast to the throat, VZV can readily be cultured from vesicular skin lesions in both varicella and zoster. Thus it seems likely that the skin is also a source of infectious VZV.

Studies with live attenuated varicella vaccine in leukemic children have demonstrated that varicella can be transmitted from skin lesions. Of over 500 immunized leukemic children in the collaborative study of the National Institute of Allergy and Infectious Disease (NIAID),[9] only those with skin lesions (either maculopapular or vesicular) as a side effect of their vaccination were found to spread vaccine-type virus to varicella-susceptible close contacts.[41] Those with no rash did not transmit the virus to their siblings. In this study there was also a direct relationship between the number of skin lesions present and whether or not the spread of vaccine-type virus occurred. Thus it appears that a major source of infectious VZV is the skin, and it therefore seems likely that transmission from both the respiratory tract and skin occurs.

VARICELLA-ZOSTER VIRUS, PREGNANCY, AND CONGENITAL INFECTION

In 1947, two medical students, LaForet and Lynch, described an infant with multiple congenital anomalies after maternal chickenpox in early pregnancy.[42] The infant had hypoplasia of the entire right lower extremity, talipes equinovarus and absent deep tendon reflexes on the right, cerebral cortical atrophy, cerebellar aplasia, chorioretinitis, right torticollis, insufficiency of the anal and vesical sphincters, and cicatricial cutaneous lesions of the left lower extremity. Since this was only one case and since VZV was not cultured from the infant, the medical community did not seriously consider that a congenital varicella syndrome analogous to the congenital rubella syndrome existed. However, in 1974, Srabstein and his colleagues reported another case, reviewed the scant literature, and concluded that there is such a syndrome typically consisting of some combination of cicatricial skin lesions, ocular abnormalities, limb deformities, mental retardation, and early infant death following maternal varicella in early pregnancy.[43] There have now been 15 reports in the literature of what could be considered the full-blown spectrum of the syndrome and about 35 additional reports of infants with apparently incomplete forms.[44]

At one time it was thought that the syndrome occurred after maternal VZV infection only in the first trimester of pregnancy, but current information indicates that about half of the reported cases developed when the mother had varicella in the second trimester. Of 44 cases, 20 (45%) occurred after maternal varicella in the 7th to 13th weeks, 23 (52%) occurred between weeks 13 and 26, and 1 (2%) occurred in the 28th week.[44] Of the 50 affected infants described in the literature, 45 cases (90%) followed maternal varicella, and 5 (10%) followed maternal zoster (disseminated in 1 instance).[44]

In these 50 infants, scars of the skin, usually cicatricial lesions in a dermatomal distribution, were the most prominent stigmata and were reported in 70%. These scars are thought to be the result of not only varicella in utero but also zoster that occurred before birth. Eye abnormalities including chorioretinitis, microphthalmos, Horner syndrome, cataract, and nystagmus were present in about 70%. Other features include a hypoplastic limb, probably the result of a neuropathy caused by viral invasion of the ganglia and spinal cord, and cortical atrophy and/or mental retardation. Early death has occurred in about one third of affected infants. Half of the infants were also described as premature or had low birth weight for their gestational ages. Of 20 reported infants with a hypoplastic limb, 10 (50%) were described to have had evidence of mental retardation. In 4 infants who died, at autopsy there was apparent dissemination of VZV with varicella-like involvement of the lungs, liver, spleen, adrenals, and/or pancreas.[43–47] The main features of the syndrome are summarized in Table 1.

Seven patients with the congenital varicella syndrome (at least 14%) have contracted clinical zoster in infancy or early childhood,[44] an extremely high incidence of reactivation to a degree usually associated with immunocompromised patients. This is of particular interest since CMI to VZV in two of ten children with the syndrome has been reported to be absent as determined by lymphocyte transformation.[48, 49] Presumably the increased degree of

TABLE 1.
Features of 50 Reported Cases of Congenital Varicella Syndrome Following Maternal Varicella or Zoster in the First (45%) or Second (52%) Trimester of Pregnancy*

Feature	Incidence, %†
Skin scarring	70
Ocular abnormalities	66
cataract, chorioretinitis, Horner syndrome, microphthalmos, nystagmus	
Hypoplastic extremity	40
Low birth weight	50
Cortical atrophy/mental retardation	46
Early death	28

*Adapted from Gershon A: Chickenpox, measles, and mumps, in Remington J, Klein JO: *Infections of the Fetus and Newborn Infant*. Philadelphia, WB Saunders, 1994.
†Of these cases, 90% followed maternal and 10% followed maternal zoster.

reactivation is due to immature CMI when varicella occurs in utero. A higher incidence of zoster is also seen in children whose mothers had varicella during pregnancy but who do not have the congenital varicella syndrome.[50, 51] Attempts to isolate VZV from the skin, cerebrospinal fluid, eye, and other tissues in infants with developmental defects have been negative.[44]

There have now been five reported prospective studies of the incidence of congenital varicella syndrome following maternal varicella.[48, 52–55] If all are considered, there were 3 cases in 171 pregnancies (2%). It is estimated that 2,000 pregnant women in the first or second trimester contract varicella every year in the United States, which would predict an estimated 40 damaged infants yearly.[44] The rarity of the syndrome but its usually serious nature makes counseling of pregnant women extremely difficult. It is hoped that much of this threat of varicella will be relieved when women who are of childbearing age and susceptible to varicella can be immunized before pregnancy.

When onset of the rash of maternal varicella occurs within 5 days before delivery or 2 days after delivery, a severe or fatal infection may develop if the infant contracts varicella. In this situation, protective maternal antibodies to VZV may not have been formed and crossed the placenta. Presumably because of immaturity of CMI, the baby is at risk for the development of severe varicella, much in the way that very young infants are at increased risk of severe HSV infections developing. Hemorrhagic skin lesions and primary viral pneumonia may develop in infants infected with VZV; this can be prevented in over 95% of infants by passive immunization with varicella-zoster immune globulin (VZIG) given as soon as possible after delivery.[44]

LIVE ATTENUATED VARICELLA VACCINE

There is currently a good deal of interest in the use of vaccination to prevent varicella and its complications such as bacterial superinfections and encephalitis, as well as severe or fatal varicella in immunocompromised patients. In addition, it is hoped that with the use of routine immunization there will be better control of nosocomial spread of VZV, fewer cases of the congenital syndrome, and fewer serious cases of varicella in adults.

Live attenuated varicella vaccine was developed in Japan in the early 1970s. It was first licensed there for use in immunocompromised patients, and about 5 years ago it was licensed there for routine use in healthy children.[56, 57] Its routine use in healthy chil-

TABLE 2.
Differences Between Wild Type Varicella-Zoster Virus and the Oka Strain

Decreased pathogenicity for healthy children if administered by injection or inhalation of vaccine-type VZV (A)*[58]
Low level of transmissibility of vaccine-type VZV to others (A)[41]
Modified infection of vaccine-type VZV in contact cases (A)[41]
Decrease in the incidence of zoster after immunization as compared with natural infection (A)
Restriction fragment length polymorphism[3, 60–63]
Lower quantity of the glycoprotein V of VZV in the Oka strain[64]
Temperature sensitivity of the Oka strain in cell culture at 39°C as compared with wild-type VZV[65]

*Differences that indicate or suggest attenuation are indicated by *A*.

dren in the United States has been extremely controversial, where it has remained under consideration for licensure almost 20 years after its development. At this time, however, it seems likely that the Food and Drug Administration (FDA) will approve its routine use in children in 1994 or 1995.

The Oka strain vaccine was derived from a wild-type VZV isolated from a healthy Japanese boy with varicella. It was inoculated into human and guinea pig tissue cultures at 34 and 37°C for over 30 passages. Differences between the Oka strain and wild-type strains of VZV and evidence that Oka is attenuated are shown in Table 2.[10, 56] The molecular basis of the attenuation of VZV has not yet been elucidated. DNA from the vaccine-type and wild-type viruses exhibits significantly different cleavage patterns with *Hpa*I, *Bam*HI, and *Bgl*I enzymes[60, 66] and *Pst*I.[61] A DNA fragment cleaved by *Hpa*I restriction endonuclease that is unique to vaccine-type virus has also been identified.[3] In studies in the United States using *Bgl*I, a novel restriction site in vaccine-type virus, resulted in a different pattern of migration of fragments A to C in comparison with wild-type VZV[60, 66]; this appears to be due to differences between American and Japanese circulating wild-type viruses rather than a marker of attenuation. With *Pst*I, additional cleavage sites are produced from vaccine virus (between the O and L fragments) that are not present in wild-type virus.[61] It is not known whether this is a marker of attenuation or a geographic marker. Other observed differences in vaccine- and wild-type strains include decreased pathogenicity of the vaccine type, differences in temperature sensitivity, and lower quantities of glycoprotein V in the vaccine type.[58, 64, 65]

In the United States, studies of vaccination of leukemic children who had a recognized mortality associated with primary varicella infection of about 10% in the early 1980s and studies of healthy varicella-susceptible adults generally preceded studies in healthy children. The vaccine was found by the Collaborative Varicella Vaccine Study Group to be well tolerated and generate a high degree of protection against both varicella and zoster in these groups.[10, 59] Although the vaccine was originally thought to have its greatest potential use in preventing severe varicella in high-risk patients, today there is even greater interest in vaccinating healthy populations.

In the United States the Oka vaccine produced by Merck Sharpe & Dohme is expected to be licensed for general use. Over 9,000 healthy children have been vaccinated in clinical trials here, and more than 2,000 healthy children between the ages of 1 and 12 years have been immunized with production lots of vaccine. Minor adverse effects in healthy child vaccinees were that 4% had a rash at the injection site, 4% had a mild varicella-like rash, 15% had a brief oral temperature over 102°F, and 24% had temporary discomfort at the injection site. Most of the children with rash had fewer than ten lesions, fewer than half of which were vesicular. Similar mild adverse effects were seen in healthy adolescents and adults, but these groups were given two doses 3 months apart. Children under 12 years of age had a 97% seroconversion rate measured by an enzyme immunoassay using glycoproteins of VZV as antigen.[67] Adolescents (above age 12) and adults had a 82% seroconversion rate after one dose and a 99% seroconversion rate after two doses given 3 months apart.[68] Antibody titers remained positive in over 95% of the children for up to 6 years. Breakthrough cases of varicella occurred in approximately 2% to 3% of the cohort during each year of follow-up but clearly represented a modified form of illness.[68, 69]

A financial analysis for vaccine use in the United States in 1985 revealed that routine use of the vaccine in 1-year-old children would be cost saving if expenses for parental absence from work were considered as well as costs of the illness itself and the price of the vaccine.[70] A more recent cost-benefit analysis has been completed and also reveals that routine use of varicella vaccine would be cost-effective with similar considerations, assuming a cost of about $35 per dose for vaccine.[71] A mathematical model suggests that with more than 90% vaccine coverage in the population, the numbers of cases of varicella in adults will decrease, even if there is waning immunity in as many as 15% of vaccinees.[72] This should dispel fears that with widespread use of the vaccine there will be a risk of increasing the incidence of disease in adults; however, this model assumes almost complete immunization of the population.

When the vaccine is licensed in the United States, it seems likely that most healthy children over the age of 12 months who have not had varicella will be candidates for immunization. It will be recommended that for children over 13 years of age and adults, two doses of vaccine should be given 1 to 2 months apart. Although use of the varicella vaccine has engendered great controversy in the United States for many years, it is predicted to be well received when it becomes available. Postmarketing surveillance to continue to examine its safety and protection as well as to monitor for waning immunity and the incidence of zoster will be important. At present it is clear that immune boosting after re-exposure to VZV is common, but whether this is important in long-term maintenance of immunity to VZV is unknown.

Varicella vaccine will first be licensed in the United States for healthy children. Eventually it is hoped that responses of children with chronic diseases can also be assessed in studies so that it can be determined whether it is safe for these children to be immunized routinely. Such children include those with asthma who are receiving corticosteroids, those with human immunodeficiency virus (HIV) infection, those with rheumatoid arthritis who are receiving aspirin therapy, and those with various forms of cancer who are receiving therapy. The vaccine should not be administered to pregnant women or children with serious intercurrent illnesses or primary or secondary immunodeficiencies, nor should it be used for postexposure prophylaxis.

EFFICACY OF VARICELLA VACCINE

Varicella vaccine does not provide quite the degree of protection against illness that we have come to expect from vaccines. It may be that complete immunity to the herpesviruses cannot ever be achieved for some individuals; this is certainly suggested by the observation that zoster occurs in 15% of persons infected with wild-type VZV. The occurrence of modified breakthrough varicella months to years after VZV immunization was first observed in Japanese studies. In a study of 106 children up to 10 years after immunization, 14 of whom had been receiving steroid therapy when they were immunized, there were 5 cases of breakthrough chickenpox, 4 of which occurred in the first year after vaccination.[73] There were 147 recognized exposures to VZV.

Subclinical reinfection with VZV following immunization is undoubtedly even more common than clinical reinfection. In 38 immunized Japanese children, VZV antibody titers measured by the technique of fluorescent antibody to membrane antigen (FAMA) were 1:4 or greater in 97%. In 29 control children who had experienced natural varicella, FAMA titers were 1:4 or greater in 100%, and both groups had similar geometric mean titers.[73] Since the average VZV antibody titer following immunization is a tenth of that following natural varicella,[74, 75] these results indicate that a boost in antibody titer had occurred in vaccinees, presumably because of subclinical reinfection. Subclinical reinfection with VZV is also extremely common after infection with the wild-type virus if an individual is subsequently re-exposed to the virus.[6, 7, 76]

Experience in the United States in over 9,000 healthy children is that the vaccine's efficacy is on the order of 75% in terms of complete protection from varicella. In other words, no illness will develop in about 85% of children with household exposures to varicella.[69] The remaining 15%, however, will experience a very modified infection with fewer than 25 skin lesions and little or no toxicity.[77, 78] Zoster has not been a significant problem in healthy vaccinees. In 7,000 vaccinees, 6 possible (none proven) cases were observed, calculated to represent 14 per 100,000 person-years; the expected rate after natural varicella for this age group is 20 to 63 per 100,000 person-years.[79]

The efficacy of varicella vaccine has mainly been judged by determining whether vaccinees with household exposures to varicella are protected from illness rather than by double-blind studies. This approach is made possible by the well-recognized clinical attack rate in susceptible individuals that approaches 90% following a household exposure to varicella. Of over 300 healthy immunized children, modified chickenpox has developed in 15% after a household exposure (personal communication, Jo White, M.D., at Merck, 1994). Protection has occurred in 42 of 57 healthy adults (74%) and in 101 of 119 (85%) leukemic children in studies carried out by the NIAID Collaborative Study Group.[10] In the latter two studies, only vaccinees who had a documented immune response to the vaccine were included in the analysis. Importantly, however, the definition of what constitutes breakthrough varicella must be considered. In the aforementioned studies by Merck, the development of even one skin vesicle after household exposure was considered breakthrough varicella. If the definition of "illness" is restricted to healthy child vaccinees in whom more than five vesicles developed, the level of protection after vaccination of healthy children is about 90%. Finally, thus far it appears that two doses of varicella vaccine do not provide significantly more protection than one dose as long as seroconversion has occurred.[9, 76]

In studies of healthy vaccinated children in the United States, the persistence of antibodies for 2 years after vaccination was 94% in one study of 36 immunized toddlers[80] and 100% in 41 children followed for 6 years.[68] This degree of antibody persistence in healthy children is superior to that observed in leukemic children and healthy adults.

In vaccinated leukemic children in the United States, protection has been similar to that observed in healthy children. The overall attack rate of varicella over a period of 11 years has been 10%. Antibody persistence is somewhat lower than in healthy children. Over 85% of leukemic children have persistence of antibodies to VZV (see Table 3). Leukemic children in whom breakthrough varicella has developed have had a more pronounced illness than that seen in healthy children. Those in whom varicella has developed have had an average of 96 vesicles in 39 cases of breakthrough chickenpox in which the number of skin lesions were counted. Nevertheless, for leukemic children, over 45% of whom were still

TABLE 3.
Varicella Vaccine in Leukemic Children*

Year	No.	No. With Varicella (%)	% Seronegative
1	558	23 (4)	5
2	493	11 (2)	12
3	379	18 (5)	21
4	279	5 (2)	23
5–11	215	5 (2)	13

*Long-term follow-up with regard to breakthrough varicella and antibody loss with time. All children were initially seropositive after immunization. Titers were measured by fluorescent antibody to membrane antigen and/or latex agglutination antibody. In the past 10 years, varicella has developed 10% of the cohort.

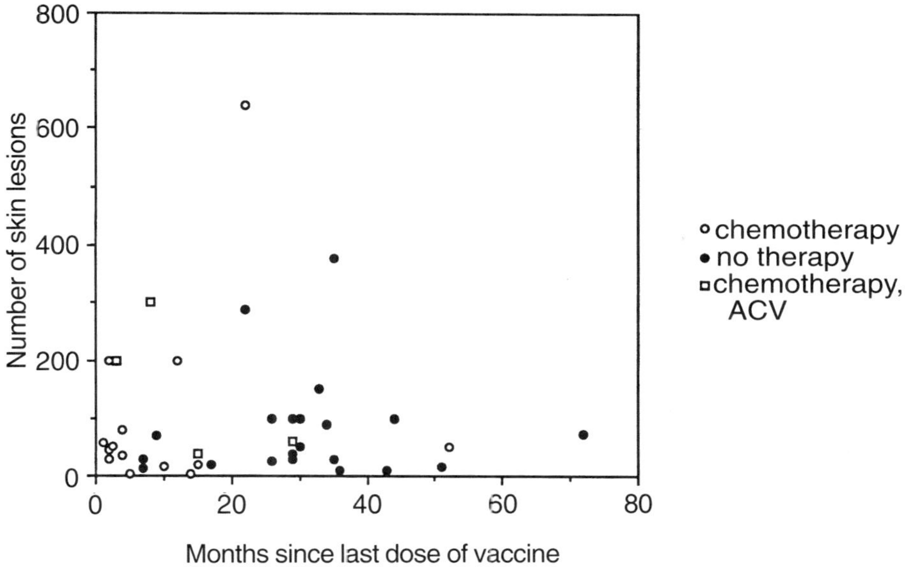

FIGURE 1.

Number of skin lesions in 39 vaccinated leukemic children with subsequent breakthrough varicella months to years later with respect to the time since the last dose of varicella vaccine was given. Note that the severity of illness did not increase with an increasing interval (in months) since immunization. The average number of skin vesicles was 96. Patients still receiving chemotherapy when breakthrough varicella developed are indicated by *open circles or squares.* Four children still receiving chemotherapy (with 40, 60, 200, and 300 vesicles) were treated with acyclovir *(ACV).*

receiving chemotherapy when varicella developed, this degree of illness is clearly modified. In addition, the degree of illness has not increased with time since vaccination (Fig 1).

The most difficult problem in immunizing leukemic children is that a vaccine-associated rash develops in about 50% within 6 weeks after the first dose of vaccine. About 50% of these children will require treatment with the antiviral drug acyclovir which must be given intravenously. For these reasons, the FDA has preferred to distribute the vaccine to these high-risk children under a compassionate use mechanism rather than by licensing the vaccine for them. Once immunity to VZV develops in leukemic vaccinees, protection is similar to that seen in healthy children.

Immune responses to VZV appear to be highly dependent on age. The development of zoster in the elderly because of loss of CMI to VZV has already been mentioned. In addition, in vaccine studies it has been found that young adults do not respond as well immunologically to varicella vaccine as do children, even leukemic children. Adverse effects are slightly increased in degree and incidence, and there is a higher incidence of breakthrough varicella when compared with healthy children.[10] Nevertheless, more than 80% of immunized healthy adults have persistence of antibodies to VZV from 7 to 13 years after immunization (Table 4). Overall, varicella has developed in 9% of the cohort of adults immunized in the NIAID collaborative study. The average number of vesicles in 31 adult vaccinees with breakthrough varicella was 43. The patient with the worst case of breakthrough varicella had about 300 skin lesions and was treated with oral acyclovir.

The severity of varicella in immunized adults did not increase over time (Fig 2). These data suggest that if waning immunity to varicella occurs in immunized adults it is not a significant problem. Since varicella is more likely to be severe in adults than in children, it is preferable for varicella-susceptible adults to be immunized than to take the risk of wild-type varicella developing.

Why the vaccine is less protective in adults than in children is probably related to a lower ability of adults to mount a CMI response to VZV. In CMI studies of leukemic and adult vaccinees using lymphocyte transformation, it was found that CMI responses of adults were extremely low and resembled those of the leukemic children who went on to contract zoster[81] (Fig 3). In contrast, sig-

TABLE 4.
Varicella Vaccine in Healthy Adults*

Year	No.	No. With Varicella (%)	% Seronegative
1	343	8 (2)	34
2	234	8 (3)	33
3	174	2 (1)	40
4	115	5 (4)	10
5	68	4 (6)	30
6	45	2 (4)	10
7–13	40	2 (5)	18

*Long-term follow-up with regard to breakthrough illness and antibody loss with time. Over the past 13 years, breakthrough varicella has developed in 9%.

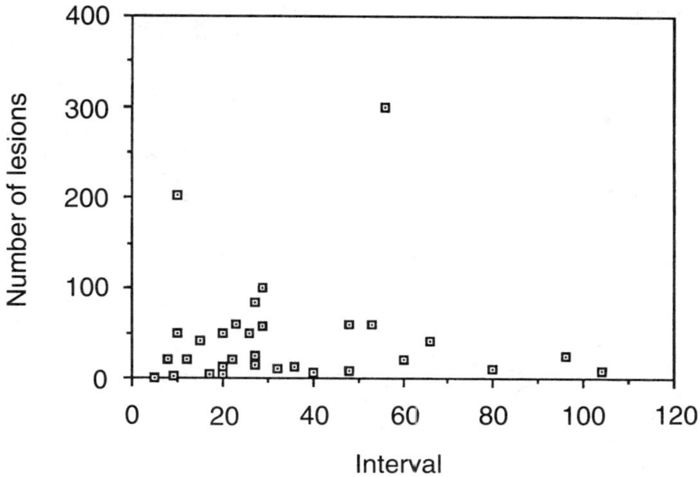

FIGURE 2.
Number of skin lesions in 31 vaccinated adults with breakthrough varicella months to years later with respect to the time since the last dose of varicella vaccine was given. Note that the severity of illness did not increase with an increasing interval (in months) since immunization. The average number of skin vesicles was 43.

nificantly higher CMI responses were present in adult controls who had had varicella many years previously.[76, 81] More recently, CMI responses measured by lymphocyte transformation have been directly compared in vaccinated adults and vaccinated healthy children, and it was found that responses in adults were significantly lower.[82] Interestingly, the poor ability to respond by lymphocyte transformation in adults cannot be ascribed to either a low responder cell frequency of T lymphocytes in adults vs. children or to a deficiency in cytotoxic T cells directed against VZV in adults.[83, 84] It remains unknown why adults respond less well to varicella vaccine than children do.

Differences in the biological behavior between wild-type and vaccine-type VZV are listed in Table 5. There is no question that the vaccine-type virus is attenuated. The number of skin lesions caused by the vaccine-type virus is significantly lower, as is transmissibility and the percentage of persons in whom skin lesions develop. Interestingly, there is some attenuation of disease produced by injection of the virus as compared with the natural route of infection by inhalation (see Table 5). Spread of the vaccine-type virus has occurred only from immunocompromised vaccinees with rash, and only one instance of tertiary spread has been recorded.[41]

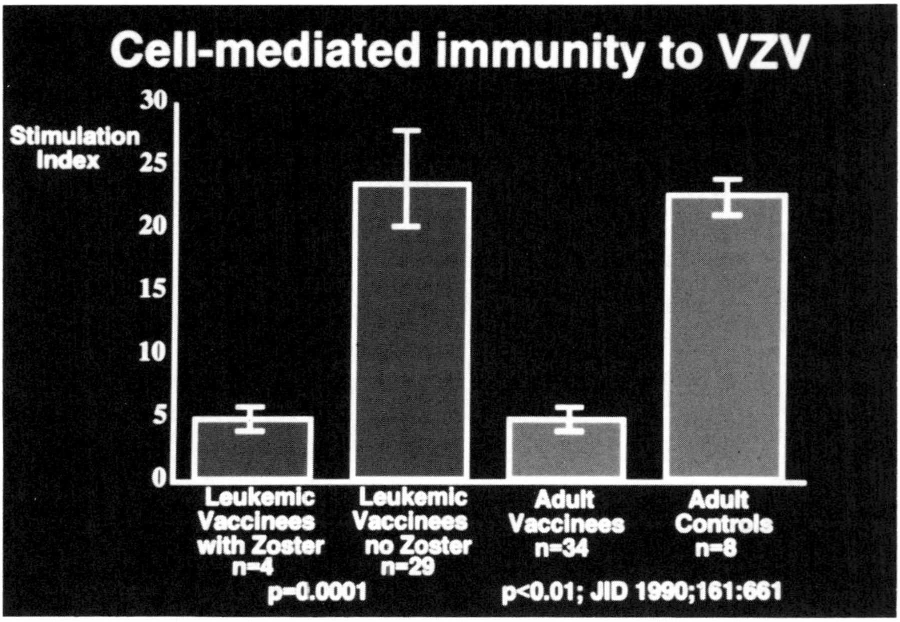

FIGURE 3.
Cell-mediated immunity (CMI) to varicella-zoster virus *(VZV)* measured by lymphocyte stimulation and expressed as a stimulation index in four groups of individuals: leukemic vaccinees in whom zoster subsequently developed, matched leukemic vaccinees in whom zoster did not develop, healthy adult vaccinees, and adults who had natural varicella as children. Note that healthy adult vaccinees had CMI responses similar to leukemic children in whom zoster eventually developed; however, zoster did not develop in any adult. (From Hardy IB, Gershon A, Steinberg S, et al: Incidence of zoster after live attenuated varicella vaccine. Presented at the International Conference on Antimicrobial Agents and Chemotherapy, Chicago, 1991. Used by permission.)

ZOSTER AND VARICELLA VACCINE

An important aspect of immunization of leukemic children in the NIAID study was that it was possible to determine over a period of only a few years whether the incidence of zoster after immunization was higher, lower, or unchanged. As can be seen from the life-table analysis in Figure 4, the incidence of zoster was lower after vaccination than after natural infection in leukemic children. It was possible to prospectively match, according to chemotherapeutic protocol, 96 leukemic vaccinees to 96 leukemic children who had experienced natural varicella. Life-table analysis revealed that the incidence of zoster was significantly lower in vaccinees than in leukemic children who had experienced natural varicella.[59, 85] In the

TABLE 5.
Biological Differences Between Vaccine and Wild-Type Varicella-Zoster Viruses

	Mean/Median No. of Lesions, Otherwise Healthy Children	% With Lesions
Natural infection (80%–90% transmission)	250–500	95
Vaccine, injected (0% transmission from healthy vaccinees)	2–5	7
Vaccine, airborne (14% transmission from immunocompromised patients)	38	73

NIAID collaborative study, the rate of zoster was 2% in vaccinees and 15% in controls. There are several possibilities as to why zoster may be less common after vaccination than after natural infection. One is that the virus is attenuated. Another is that the virus may not have access to sensory nerves if the skin is not infected, as is frequently the case after vaccination; this results in a lower rate of latency than after natural infection with wild-type virus. It is hoped that this projection of a lower incidence of zoster after vaccination than after natural infection will hold true for healthy immunized populations. It is one of the major reasons for routine use of varicella vaccine.

It was observed in Japan that zoster occurred far more frequently in 83 immunized children who had a vaccine-associated rash (16%) than in 249 with no rash after immunization (2%) (Collaborative Study Group of Varicella Vaccine, Ministry of Health and Welfare, Japan, 1974 to 1983). This observation has been confirmed and extended in the NIAID collaborative study.[59] Of 13 vaccinated leukemic children in whom zoster developed, 11 (85%) had a prior history of a VZV-related rash, either vaccine associated (8 children) or breakthrough varicella (3 children). Both children with no history of rash contracted zoster at the injection site of the vaccine. In the 268 leukemic vaccinees who had any type of previous VZV-related rash, the relative risk of subsequent development of zoster was 5.75 when compared with the 280 leukemic vaccinees who had no VZV-associated rash. In the NIAID collaborative study, 2 cases of zoster were due to vaccine-type virus and 2 were caused by wild-type VZV.

It may also be that immunized adults have a lower rate of latent infection since skin rash from vaccine-type or wild-type VZV is unusual after immunization against varicella[81] (Fig 5). This would explain why, despite low CMI responses to VZV, the incidence of zoster in vaccinated adults has been low. Because both a vaccine-associated rash and breakthrough varicella are unusual in healthy vaccinees, it is predicted that the incidence of zoster will be lower in healthy vaccinees than in those who have had natural varicella. Possibly this is due to a low rate of latent infection in vaccinated adults since the virus usually does not reach the skin after vaccination. In the collaborative study, the incidence of any rash developing after vaccination was significantly lower in adult vaccinees than in leukemic vaccinees (see Fig 5). In the collaborative study, of 375 immunized adults only 1 has contracted zoster, and this was caused by the wild-type virus.[86]

Whether breakthrough varicella that occurs after immunization is as contagious to others is important but difficult to determine. Leukemic children with breakthrough varicella can clearly transmit wild-type VZV to close contacts. Virus spread from nonimmunocompromised patients, however, may be less likely to occur. Certainly this has been true for vaccine-associated rashes, in which

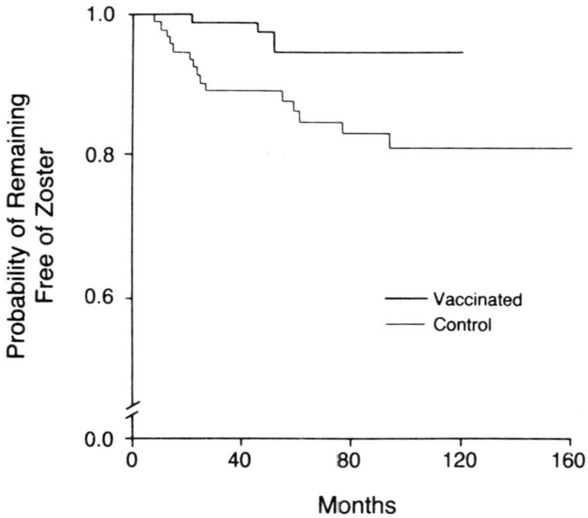

FIGURE 4.
Kaplan-Meier product-limit analysis of the probability of remaining free of zoster in 96 children with leukemia who received varicella vaccine and 96 children with leukemia who had naturally acquired chickenpox before or after the diagnosis of leukemia. (From Hardy IB, Gershon A, Steinberg S, et al: *N Engl J Med* 325:1545–1550, 1991. Used by permission.)

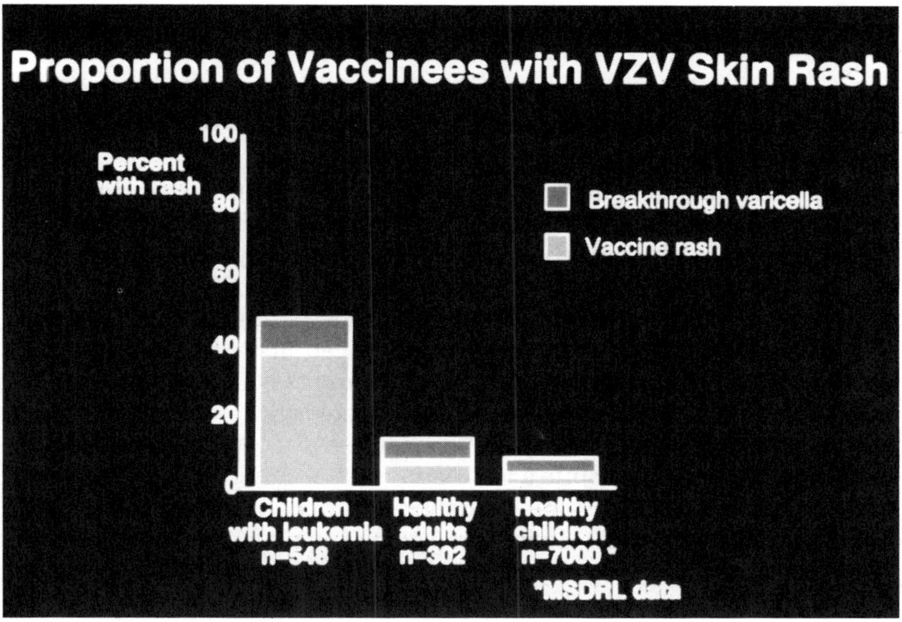

FIGURE 5.
Percentage of vaccinees in whom skin lesions developed because of either a vaccine-associated rash or breakthrough varicella in three groups of individuals: leukemic children, healthy adult vaccinees, and healthy child vaccinees. The incidence of zoster was significantly higher in leukemic vaccinees than in healthy adults or children who were vaccinated. (From Hardy IB, Gershon A, Steinberg S, et al: Incidence of zoster after live attenuated varicella vaccine. Presented at the International Conference on Antimicrobial Agents and Chemotherapy, Chicago, 1991. Used by permission.)

spread from a healthy adult or child with a vaccine-associated rash has not been reported, although spread from leukemic vaccinees with rash to healthy siblings has been 14%.[41] Of interest is the observation that breakthrough varicella with about 50 skin lesions after no recognized exposure to VZV developed approximately 2 years after immunization in one adult vaccinee in the NIAID collaborative study. While she had varicella she cared for her two young children aged 4 and 6 years, in neither of whom did clinical varicella develop. Under ordinary circumstances involving household exposure, one would predict that at least one of the children would have contracted clinical varicella. Thus in healthy populations, spread of wild-type VZV from persons with breakthrough varicella may well be diminished. Obviously more data on this point must be obtained before any firm conclusions can be made.

LONG-TERM CONSIDERATIONS FOR VARICELLA VACCINE USE

The main argument today against the routine use of varicella vaccine in all children is a fear that routine vaccination will lead to an increase in varicella in adults. Theoretically this could be due to a significant degree of waning immunity years after vaccination or to failure to reach all segments of the population with vaccine so that there are pockets of susceptible adults. Although some degree of waning immunity has been observed in adults and leukemic children who were immunized, there is little evidence for waning immunity in healthy child vaccinees.[69, 73] As can be seen from Tables 3 and 4, despite a loss of detectable antibodies in adults and leukemic vaccinees, the incidence of varicella in vaccinees has not increased and has remained constant at about 2% a year. Moreover, the severity of the breakthrough illnesses has not increased with time. Additionally, in a computer modeling study carried out by the CDC, it was found that the incidence of varicella in adults would decrease in a vaccine program in which all children were immunized.[72] This study took the possibility of waning immunity in as many as 15% of vaccinees into account.

THE FUTURE OF VARICELLA VACCINE IN THE UNITED STATES

Immunization is predicted to be recommended for all susceptible children and adults in the United States. It will obviously not be possible to immunize all susceptible persons at once. Priority will be given to infants between 12 and 18 months of age and children approaching puberty. Then, gradually, the rest of the susceptible population will be immunized. A history of prior varicella usually indicates that an individual is immune. Most adults with no history of varicella are also immune when antibody testing is performed. Since administration of vaccine to varicella-immune individuals is not harmful, whether to test adults who believe they are susceptible to varicella or not before immunization must be decided on an individual basis with the cost of the vaccine and the cost of serologic testing kept in mind. With regard to adults who may be susceptible, it has been observed that in tropical climates chickenpox occurs less frequently in younger age groups than in countries with temperate climates,[87] with a higher incidence of varicella in adults. A high rate of varicella in nurses and military recruits who have immigrated from tropical countries to the United Kingdom and the United States has been observed.[62, 87–89]

When varicella vaccine is first licensed in the United States, it will be available only as a monovalent form; several studies of a combined measles-mumps-rubella-varicella (MMRV) vaccine have indicated the utility of this approach.[90–92] There is an excellent response to all four antigens. Advantages of the use of MMRV would be to ensure that virtually all children are vaccinated and that two doses are given. The combination vaccine may also lessen the cost of immunization with the varicella component.

Until more data are available, in the United States it is not recommended that immunocompromised patients other than those with acute lymphoblastic leukemia for more than 1 year in remission be given varicella vaccine. This excludes children about to undergo organ transplantation and those with HIV infection. Eventually, vaccine use in children with these medical problems will be studied in clinical trials under carefully controlled conditions.

Today there is a great deal of interest in determining whether immunization of persons who have already had varicella and are at high risk of the development of zoster will either prevent or modify zoster by boosting CMI responses.

ANTIVIRAL THERAPY

A very effective form of antiviral therapy for VZV infection is the administration of acyclovir intravenously within 3 days of onset of the rash of varicella or zoster.[14, 93, 94] Acyclovir interferes with multiplication of VZV by inhibition of viral DNA replication and also by acting as a DNA chain terminator. There is considerable variability in the sensitivity to acyclovir of VZV isolates that ranges from 0.5 to 10.8 μg/mL of drug.[95] Since only about 20% of orally administered acyclovir is absorbed by the gastrointestinal tract and therapeutic levels may not be achieved for isolates that are less sensitive to acyclovir, intravenous therapy with acyclovir is recommended for patients who are very ill (or highly likely to become so) with VZV infections. Acyclovir is very well tolerated; its main side effects are mild gastrointestinal problems and mild rashes. If given by the intravenous route too rapidly, it can cause renal tubular damage, which is reversible when use of the drug is stopped. Renal complications can be avoided by ensuring that patients receiving acyclovir are well hydrated.

Administration of acyclovir orally within 24 hours of the onset of rash hastens recovery from varicella in otherwise healthy children, but only by about a day, and enthusiasm in the medical community for its routine use is therefore low.[96] The American Academy of Pediatrics has suggested that acyclovir be considered in patients over the age of 13 in whom varicella develops and also for children who have underlying chronic cutaneous and/or pulmonary illnesses.[1] The administration of acyclovir by mouth to adolescents and adults with varicella has a similar efficacy, and the duration of illness is shortened by about a day.[97, 98] There was no efficacy in adults if acyclovir was begun more than 24 hours after the onset of rash.[97]

A number of patients with varicella during pregnancy who were treated with intravenous acyclovir have been reported.[99–107] Although controlled studies have not been performed, the evidence suggests that acyclovir has improved the outcome in this population. Among the 21 treated cases reported, there were nevertheless 3 deaths (14%) caused by varicella, all of which occurred in the third trimester.[106] Whether all pregnant women in whom varicella develops should be treated with acyclovir and whether oral acyclovir during pregnancy has merit are unknown. Congenital abnormalities attributed to the administration of acyclovir to over 600 women, most of whom were in the first trimester of pregnancy, have not been observed.[108, 109]

Successful prophylaxis of varicella in healthy children with oral acyclovir given from 7 to 14 days after exposure has been reported but cannot be recommended. The study included only a small number of patients and was not controlled; there is no information on whether immunity to varicella will be long lasting.[110]

There is currently considerable interest in whether early therapy with acyclovir can prevent damage to sensory neurons and the eventual development of postherpetic neuralgia (PHN),[111] a complication of zoster that occurs particularly in elderly patients and may be both persistent and debilitating. Whether prompt administration of antiviral drugs to elderly patients can prevent PHN will have to await controlled studies.

Resistance of VZV to acyclovir is beginning to be observed, but thus far only in immunocompromised patients. A major mechanism of resistance is loss of the ability of the virus to produce the enzyme thymidine kinase, which phosphorylates acyclovir, a process required for activation. Failure of VZV to produce thymidine kinase results in a resistant virus but also one that is less virulent. The decrease in virulence probably accounts for the low rate of spread of acyclovir-resistant VZV. Spread of thymidine kinase-negative herpesviruses has been observed only from one immunocompromised patient to another. Varicella-zoster virus infections that appear to be clinically resistant to acyclovir can be treated with foscarnet. This antiviral drug inhibits the DNA polymerase of VZV, but at a site different from that of ACV, and therefore viruses that are resistant to acyclovir can be predicted to be sensitive to foscarnet. Foscarnet must be administered intravenously, and unfortunately it is more toxic than acyclovir. Foscarnet is nephrotoxic, and it may also cause hypocalcemia, hypomagnesemia, hypophosphatemia, hypokalemia, anemia, nausea, seizures, neutropenia, and cardiac arrhythmia.[112]

Future antiviral drugs that may soon be licensed for use in the United States include famciclovir, which needs to be given orally only once or twice a day, and valacyclovir, which achieves blood levels that are about four times higher than those achieved by oral acyclovir.

DIAGNOSTIC ADVANCES

Several technological advances for the diagnosis of varicella and zoster have been made recently, and these will have an impact on varicella vaccine and its use. These include the development of simple and inexpensive means to measure antibodies to VZV and use of PCR to diagnose VZV infection and determine whether the illness was caused by wild- or vaccine-type virus without having to first grow the virus in tissue culture.

Rapid diagnosis of varicella or zoster can be accomplished by scraping a suspicious skin lesion, making a smear on a microscope slide, fixing with ethanol, and staining with commercial fluorescein-tagged monoclonal antibody to VZV glycoprotein.[113] With this technique it is possible to diagnose VZV infection within an hour and distinguish between VZV and HSV infection. Should the virus causing the skin infection be found to be HSV, it is even possible to determine whether it is type 1 or type 2 HSV within that time interval.

Polymerase chain reaction has recently been successfully employed for the diagnosis of VZV infection in vesicular fluid, respiratory secretions, and cerebrospinal fluid.[38, 39, 63, 113, 114] Eventually PCR, in which viral DNA is exponentially amplified so that it may be identified by molecular probes, will almost certainly become a standard method for diagnosing VZV infection. In the case of VZV, the infectious virus is much more labile than its DNA, so it is much easier to demonstrate VZV DNA by PCR than the virus itself by isolation techniques. In our laboratory we estimate that for every positive virus culture for VZV there are six positive PCR determinations. It is also possible to distinguish between vaccine-type and wild-type VZV by PCR, also avoiding the step of virus isolation.[63] It is relatively simple to collect the specimens so that even a parent with no medical training can obtain them.[115] Polymerase chain reaction for the diagnosis of VZV is also extremely useful since unlike some of the other herpesviruses, particularly cytomegalovirus, there is no shedding of virus in the absence of disease. Thus demonstration of VZV by PCR is diagnostic of an illness caused by the virus. The current disadvantages of VZV PCR include possible false-positive reactions because of contamination of specimens with amplified DNA (a problem common to PCR in general) and the unavailability of commercially marketed primers. Both of these problems are potentially solvable.

A number of commercially marketed tests for measurement of VZV antibody by enzyme immunosorbent assays (EIAs) are available and have been evaluated.[116–118] These tests are fairly reliable; however, since they may lack sensitivity, some adults with immunity to varicella may be misidentified as being susceptible to chickenpox when so tested. Enzyme immunosorbent assay may also not identify all individuals who have been immunized with live attenuated varicella vaccine.[116, 119] The main advantages of EIA are that it may be automated and kits for its performance are commercially available.

An alternative method to EIA to measure antibodies to VZV is with a commercially marketed latex agglutination (LA) assay.[75, 119] The LA test compares quite favorably with the highly sensitive and specific indirect immunofluorescence FAMA test.[120] The LA test is extremely useful for determining whether past infection with varicella has occurred, presumably indicating immunity to varicella. In approximately 10% to 15% of sera in which VZV antibody cannot be detected by EIA, antibody is detectable by methods such as FAMA and LA. The disadvantages of the FAMA method are that it is cumbersome, requires propagation of fresh virus for each test, and is not routinely available.

The LA test makes use of commercially marketed emulsified latex particles coated with glycoproteins of VZV. Doubling dilutions of test sera are made in 1-cm-diameter flat circles on a wax-coated card supplied by the manufacturer. A standardized drop of latex emulsion is added to each circle, and the card is placed on a mechanical rotator for 10 minutes. Circles are then examined for agglutination (obvious clumping of the latex particles). For screening sera for immunity status, two dilutions of sera are tested at 1:4 and at 1:50. A positive reaction in one or both wells is highly correlated with immunity to varicella. It is strongly recommended that sera that are negative at screening dilutions be retested at dilutions of 1:4 to 1:64 to avoid false-negative results because of prozone phenomena. False-positive reactions may occur in about 5% of sera tested at dilutions of 1:2, so a starting dilution of 1:4 is recommended.[75, 119] The main advantages of the LA test are its simplicity, availability, low cost, and the rapidity with which it may be performed (15 to 30 minutes). Its disadvantages are that it cannot be automated, one cannot use it to demonstrate VZV IgM, one must be certain of the appearance of agglutination of latex, and one must be aware of prozone reactions, which occur in 1% to 5% of sera, particularly in those with high VZV antibody titers.

SUMMARY

There have been a number of new developments in the field of VZV concerning pathogenesis, diagnosis, prevention, and treatment. These include improved understanding of how latent infection develops and is maintained, the development and, we hope, licensure of live attenuated varicella vaccine for routine use in children and in adults who have not had varicella, an increased availability of antiviral therapy for healthy and immunocompromised patients, and the development of newer diagnostic techniques, including PCR to diagnose illnesses caused by VZV and LA for rapid, sensitive, and accurate determination of immune status to VZV. Even as vaccine use becomes more and more widespread, we will continue to need effective antiviral therapy for VZV for use in immunocompromised persons and in those in whom zoster develops. Eventually it may be possible to develop either a vaccine or an antiviral drug that prevents the development of latent VZV infection. Until that time, however, VZV will remain with us, and we will continue to need an effective antiviral armamentarium, including diagnostic techniques, passive immunization, antiviral therapy, and vaccine.

REFERENCES

1. American Academy of Pediatrics: Committee on Infectious Diseases: Varicella vaccine statement. *Pediatrics* 1994, in press.
2. Preblud S, Orenstein W, Bart K: Varicella: Clinical manifestations, epidemiology, and health impact on children. *Pediatr Infect Dis* 3:505–509, 1984.
3. Hayakawa Y, Yamamoto T, Yamanishi K, et al: Analysis of varicella

zoster virus (VZV) DNAs of clinical isolates by endonuclease HpaI. *J Gen Virol* 67:1817–1829, 1986.
4. Straus SE, Reinhold W, Smith HA, et al: Endonuclease analysis of viral DNA from varicella and subsequent zoster infections in the same patient. *N Engl J Med* 311:1362–1364, 1984.
5. Williams DL, Gershon A, Gelb LD, et al: Herpes zoster following varicella vaccine in a child with acute lymphocytic leukemia. *J Pediatr* 106:259–261, 1985.
6. Arvin A, Koropchak CM, Wittek AE: Immunologic evidence of reinfection with varicella-zoster virus. *J Infect Dis* 148:200–205, 1983.
7. Gershon AA, Steinberg S, Gelb L, et al: Clinical reinfection with varicella-zoster virus. *J Infect Dis* 149:137–142, 1984.
8. Locksley RM, Flournoy N, Sullivan KM, et al: Infection with varicella-zoster virus after marrow transplantation. *J Infect Dis* 152:1172–1181, 1985.
9. Gershon AA, Steinberg S, NIAID-Collaborative-Varicella-Vaccine-Study-Group: Persistence of immunity to varicella in children with leukemia immunized with live attenuated varicella vaccine. *N Engl J Med* 320:892–897, 1989.
10. Gershon AA, LaRussa P, Steinberg S: Live attenuated varicella vaccine: Current status and future uses. *Semin Pediatr Infect Dis* 2:171–178, 1991.
11. Wilson A, Sharp M, Koropchak C, et al: Subclinical varicella-zoster virus viremia, herpes zoster, and T lymphocyte immunity to varicella-zoster viral antigens after bone marrow transplantation. *J Infect Dis* 165:119–126, 1991.
12. Feldman S, Hughes W, Daniel C: Varicella in children with cancer: 77 cases. *Pediatrics* 80:388–397, 1975.
13. Feldman S, Lott L: Varicella in children with cancer: Impact of antiviral therapy and prophylaxis. *Pediatrics* 80:465–472, 1987.
14. Shepp DH, Dandliker PS, Meyers JD: Treatment of varicella-zoster virus infection in severely immunocompromised patients: A randomized comparison of acyclovir and vidarabine. *N Engl J Med* 314:208–212, 1986.
15. Dumas AH, Geelen JLMC, Weststrate MW, et al: XbaI, PstI, and BglII restriction enzyme maps of the two orientations of the varicella-zoster virus genome. *J Virol* 40:516–526, 1981.
16. Ecker JR, Hyman RW: Varicella zoster virus DNA exists as two isomers. *Proc Natl Acad Sci U S A* 79:156–160, 1982.
17. Straus SE, Aulakh HS, Ruyechan WT, et al: Structure of varicella-zoster virus DNA. *J Virol* 40:516–526, 1981.
18. Davison AJ: Varicella-zoster virus. The Fourteenth Fleming Lecture. *J Gen Virol* 72:475–486, 1991.
19. Straus SE, Hay J, Smith H, et al: Genome differences among varicella-zoster isolates. *J Gen Virol* 64:1031–1041, 1983.
20. Gelb L: Varicella zoster virus, in Fields B: *Virology*. New York, Raven, 1990.

21. Dueland AN, Martin JR, Devlin M, et al: Acute simian varicella infection. *Lab Invest* 66:762–773, 1992.
22. Shiraki K, Okuno T, Yamanishi K, et al: Polypeptides of varicella-zoster virus (VZV) and immunological relationship of VZV and herpes simplex virus (HSV). *J Gen Virol* 61:255–269, 1982.
23. Schmidt NJ: Further evidence for common antigens in herpes simplex and varicella-zoster virus. *J Med Virol* 9:27–36, 1982.
24. Gershon A, Cosio L, Brunell PA: Observations on the growth of varicella-zoster virus in human diploid cells. *J Gen Virol* 18:21–31, 1973.
25. Gabel C, Dubey L, Steinberg S, et al: Varicella-zoster virus glycoproteins are phosphorylated during posttranslational maturation. *J Virol* 63:4264–4276, 1989.
26. Hyman RW, Ecker JR, Tenser RB: Varicella-zoster virus RNA in human trigeminal ganglia. *Lancet* 2:814–816, 1983.
27. Gilden D, Rozenman Y, Murray R, et al: Detection of varicella-zoster virus nucleic acid in neurons of normal human thoracic ganglia. *Ann Neurol* 22:337–380, 1987.
28. Croen KD, Ostrove JM, Dragovic LY, et al: Patterns of gene expression and sites of latency in human ganglia are different for varicella-zoster and herpes simplex viruses. *Proc Natl Acad Sci U S A* 85:9773–9777, 1988.
29. Mahalingham R, Wellish M, Wolf W, et al: Latent varicella-zoster viral DNA in human trigeminal and thoracic ganglia. *N Engl J Med* 323:627–631, 1990.
30. Meier JL, Holman RP, Croen KD, et al: Varicella-zoster virus transcription in human trigeminal ganglia. *Virology* 193:193–200, 1993.
31. Brunell PA: Transmission of chickenpox in a school setting prior to the observed exanthem. *Am J Dis Child* 143:1451–1452, 1989.
32. Evans P: An epidemic of chickenpox. *Lancet* 2:339–340, 1940.
33. Gordon JE, Meader FM: The period of infectivity and serum prevention of chickenpox. *JAMA* 93:2013–2015, 1929.
34. Gordon JE: Chickenpox: An epidemiologic review. *Am J Med Sci* 244:362–389, 1962.
35. Gustafson TL, Lavely GB, Brauner ER, et al: An outbreak of nosocomial varicella. *Pediatrics* 70:550–556, 1982.
36. Leclair JM, Zaia J, Levin MJ, et al: Airborne transmission of chickenpox in a hospital. *N Engl J Med* 302:450–453, 1980.
37. Moore DA, Hopkins RS: Assessment of a school exclusion policy during a chickenpox outbreak. *Am J Epidemiol* 133:1161–1167, 1991.
38. Kido S, Ozaki T, Asada H, et al: Detection of varicella-zoster virus (VZV) DNA in clinical samples from patients with VZV by the polymerase chain reaction. *J Clin Microbiol* 29:76–79, 1991.
39. Koropchak C, Graham G, Palmer J, et al: Investigation of varicella-zoster virus infection by polymerase chain reaction in the immunocompetent host with acute varicella. *J Infect Dis* 163:1016–1022, 1991.

40. Ozaki T, Miwata H, Matsui Y, et al: Varicella zoster virus DNA in throat swabs. *Arch Dis Child* 65:333–334, 1990.
41. Tsolia M, Gershon A, Steinberg S, et al: Live attenuated varicella vaccine: Evidence that the virus is attenuated and the importance of skin lesions in transmission of varicella-zoster virus. *J Pediatr* 116:184–189, 1990.
42. LaForet EG, Lynch LL: Multiple congenital defects following maternal varicella. *N Engl J Med* 236:534–537, 1947.
43. Srabstein JC, Morris N, Larke B, et al: Is there a congenital varicella syndrome? *J Pediatr* 84:239–243, 1974.
44. Gershon A: Chickenpox, measles, and mumps, in Remington J, Klein JO: *Infections of the Fetus and Newborn Infant*. Philadelphia, WB Saunders, 1994.
45. Scharf A, Scherr O, Enders G, et al: Virus detection in the fetal tissue of a premature delivery with a congenital varicella syndrome. *J Perinat Med* 18:317–322, 1990.
46. DaSilva O, Hammerberg O, Chance GW: Fetal varicella syndrome. *Pediatr Infect Dis J* 9:854–855, 1990.
47. Alexander I: Congenital varicella. *BMJ* 2:1074, 1979.
48. Paryani SG, Arvin AM: Intrauterine infection with varicella-zoster virus after maternal varicella. *N Engl J Med* 314:1542–1546, 1986.
49. Cuthbertson G, Weiner CP, Giller RH, et al: Prenatal diagnosis of second-trimester congenital varicella syndrome by virus-specific immunoglobulin M. *J Pediatr* 111:592–595, 1987.
50. Brunell PA, Kotchmar GSJ: Zoster in infancy: Failure to maintain virus latency following intrauterine infection. *J Pediatr* 98:71–73, 1981.
51. Dworsky M, Whitely R, Alford C: Herpes zoster in early infancy. *Am J Dis Child* 134:618–619, 1980.
52. Balducci J, Rodis JF, Rosengren S, et al: Pregnancy outcome following first-trimester varicella infection. *Obstet Gynecol* 79:5–6, 1992.
53. Enders G: Varicella-zoster virus infection in pregnancy. *Prog Med Virol* 29:166–196, 1984.
54. Manson MM, Logan WPD, Loy RM: *Rubella and Other Virus Infections During Pregnancy*, reports on public health and medical subjects. London, Her Majesty's Stationery Office, 1960, no. 101.
55. Siegel M: Congenital malformations following chickenpox, measles, mumps, and hepatitis. Results of a cohort study. *JAMA* 226:1521–1524, 1973.
56. Takahashi M, Gershon A: Vaccine, in Mortimer EA, Plotkin SA: *Vaccines*. 1994.
57. Takahashi M, Otsuka T, Okuno Y, et al: Live vaccine used to prevent the spread of varicella in children in hospital. *Lancet* 2:1288–1290, 1974.
58. Bogger-Goren S, Baba K, Hurley P, et al: Antibody response to

varicella-zoster virus after natural or vaccine-induced infection. *J Infect Dis* 146:260–265, 1982.

59. Hardy IB, Gershon A, Steinberg S, et al: The incidence of zoster after immunization with live attenuated varicella vaccine. A study in children with leukemia. *N Engl J Med* 325:1545–1550, 1991.
60. Martin JH, Dohner D, Wellinghoff WJ, et al: Restriction endonuclease analysis of varicella-zoster vaccine virus and wild type DNAs. *J Med Virol* 9:69–76, 1982.
61. Brunell P, Geiser C, Novelli V, et al: Varicella-like illness caused by live varicella vaccine in children with acute lymphocytic leukemia. *Pediatrics* 79:922–927, 1987.
62. Hastie IR: Varicella in immigrant nurses. *Lancet* 2:154–155, 1980.
63. LaRussa P, Lungu O, Hardy I, et al: Restriction fragment length polymorphism of polymerase chain reaction products from vaccine and wild-type varicella-zoster virus isolates. *J Virol* 66:1016–1020, 1992.
64. Kinchington PR, Ling P, Pensiero M, et al: A possible role for gpV in the pathogenesis of varicella-zoster virus. *Adv Exp Med Biol* 278:83–92, 1990.
65. Hayakawa Y, Torigoe S, Shiraki K, et al: Biologic and biophysical markers of a live varicella vaccine strain (Oka): Identification of clinical isolates from vaccine recipients. *J Infect Dis* 149:956–963, 1984.
66. Gelb LD, Dohner DE, Gershon AA, et al: Molecular epidemiology of live, attenuated varicella virus vaccine in children and in normal adults. *J Infect Dis* 155:633–640, 1987.
67. Provost PJ, Krah DL, Kuter BJ, et al: Antibody assays suitable for assessing immune responses to live varicella vaccine. *Vaccine* 9:111–116, 1991.
68. Kuter BJ, Weibel RE, Guess HA, et al: Oka/Merck varicella vaccine in healthy children: Final report of a 2-year efficacy study and 7-year follow-up studies. *Vaccine* 9:643–647, 1991.
69. White CJ, Kuter BJ, Hildebrand CS, et al: Varicella vaccine (VARIVAX) in healthy children and adolescents: Results from clinical trials, 1987 to 1989. *Pediatrics* 87:604–610, 1991.
70. Preblud SR, Orenstein WA, Koplan JP, et al: A benefit-cost analysis of a childhood vaccination program. *Postgrad Med J* 61:17–22, 1985.
71. Lieu T, Cochi S, Black S, et al: Cost-effectiveness of a routine varicella vaccination program for U.S. children. *JAMA* 271:375–381, 1994.
72. Halloran ME, Cochi SC, Lieu T et al: Epidemiologic and morbidity effects of routine immunization of preschool children with varicella vaccine in the United States. Submitted for publication.
73. Asano Y, Nagai T, Miyata T, et al: Long-term protective immunity of recipients of the Oka strain of live varicella vaccine. *Pediatrics* 75:667–671, 1985.
74. LaRussa PL, Gershon AA, Steinberg S, et al: Antibodies to varicella-

zoster virus glycoproteins I, II, and III in leukemic and healthy children. *J Infect Dis* 162:627–633, 1990.
75. Gershon A, Steinberg S, La Russa P: Measurement of antibodies to VZV by latex agglutination. *Clin Diagn Virol* 1994, in press.
76. Gershon AA, Steinberg S, NIAID-Collaborative-Varicella-Vaccine-Study-Group: Live attenuated varicella vaccine: Protection in healthy adults in comparison to leukemic children. *J Infect Dis* 161:661–666, 1990.
77. White CJ, Kuter BJ, Ngai A, et al: Modified cases of chickenpox after varicella vaccination: Correlation of protection with antibody response. *Pediatr Infect Dis J* 11:19–22, 1992.
78. Watson BM, Piercy SA, Plotkin SA, et al: Modified chickenpox in children immunized with the Oka/Merck varicella vaccine. *Pediatrics* 91:17–22, 1993.
79. White CJ: Letter to the editor. *Pediatrics* 89:354, 1992.
80. Johnson C, Rome L, Stancin T, et al: Humoral immunity and clinical reinfections following varicella vaccine in healthy children. *Pediatrics* 84:418–421, 1989.
81. Hardy IB, Gershon A, Steinberg S, et al: Incidence of zoster after live attenuated varicella vaccine. Presented at the International Conference on Antimicrobial Agents and Chemotherapy, Chicago, 1991.
82. Nader S, Bergen R, Sharp M, et al: Comparison of cell-mediated immunity (CMI) to varicella-zoster virus (VZV) in children and adults immunized with live attenuated varicella vaccine (abstract 1542). Presented at the International Conference on Antimicrobial Agents and Chemotherapy, New Orleans, 1993.
83. Arvin AM: Cell-mediated immunity to varicella-zoster virus. *J Infect Dis* 166(suppl):35–41, 1992.
84. Sharp M, Terada K, Wilson A, et al: Kinetics and viral protein specificity of the cytotoxic T lymphocyte response in healthy adults immunized with live attenuated varicella vaccine. *J Infect Dis* 165:852–858, 1992.
85. Lawrence R, Gershon A, Holzman R, et al: The risk of zoster after varicella vaccination in children with leukemia. *N Engl J Med* 318:543–548, 1988.
86. Hammerschlag MR, Gershon A, Steinberg S, et al: Herpes zoster in an adult recipient of live attenuated varicella vaccine. *J Infect Dis* 160:535–537, 1989.
87. Maretic Z, Cooray MPM: Comparisons between chickenpox in a tropical and a European country. *J Trop Med Hyg* 66:311–315, 1963.
88. Gray GC, Palinkas LA, Kelley PW: Increasing incidence of varicella hospitalizations in United States Army and Navy personnel: Are today's teenagers more susceptible? Should recruits be vaccinated? *Pediatrics* 86:867–873, 1990.
89. Nassar NT, Touma HC: Brief report: Susceptibility of Filipino nurses to the varicella-zoster virus. *Infect Control* 7:71–72, 1986.

90. Brunell PA, Novelli VM, Lipton SV, et al: Combined vaccine against measles, mumps, rubella, and varicella. *Pediatrics* 81:779–784, 1988.
91. Englund JA, Suarez CS, Kelly J, et al: Placebo-controlled trial of varicella vaccine given with or after measles-mumps-rubella vaccine. *J Pediatr* 114:37–44, 1989.
92. Arbeter AM, Baker L, Starr SE, et al: Combination measles, mumps, rubella, and varicella vaccine. *Pediatrics* 78:742–747, 1986.
93. Prober C, Kirk LE, Keeney RE: Acyclovir therapy of chickenpox in immunocompromised children—a collaborative study. *J Pediatr* 101:622–625, 1982.
94. Shepp D, Dandliker P, Meyers J: Current therapy of varicella zoster virus infection in immunocompromised patients. *Am J Med* 85(suppl 2A):96–98, 1988.
95. Arvin A: Oral therapy with acyclovir in infants and children. *Pediatr Infect Dis J* 6:56–58, 1986.
96. Dunkel L, Arvin A, Whitley R, et al: A controlled trial of oral acyclovir for chickenpox in normal children. *N Engl J Med* 325:1539–1544, 1991.
97. Wallace MR, Bowler WA, Murray NB, et al: Treatment of adult varicella with oral acyclovir. A randomized, placebo-controlled trial. *Ann Intern Med* 117:358–363, 1992.
98. Balfour HH, Rotbart H, Feldman S, et al: Acyclovir treatment of varicella in otherwise healthy adolescents. *J Pediatr* 120:627–633, 1992.
99. Landsberger EJ, Hager WD, Grossman JH: Successful management of varicella pneumonia complicating pregnancy. A report of 3 cases. *J Reprod Med* 31:311, 1986.
100. Lotshaw RR, Keegan JM, Gordon HR: Parenteral and oral acyclovir for management of varicella pneumonia in pregnancy: A case report with review of literature. *W V Med J* 87:204–206, 1991.
101. Hockberger RS, Rothstein RJ: Varicella pneumonia in adults: A spectrum of disease. *Ann Emerg Med* 115:931–934, 1986.
102. Hollingsworth HM, Pratter MR, Irwin RS: Acute respiratory failure in pregnancy. *J Intensive Care Med* 4:11–34, 1989.
103. Hankins GDV, Gilstrap LC, Patterson AR: Acyclovir treatment of varicella pneumonia in pregnancy (letter). *Crit Care Med* 15:336–337, 1987.
104. Glaser JB, Loftus J, Ferragamo V, et al: Varicella in pregnancy (letter). *N Engl J Med* 315:1416, 1986.
105. Boyd K, Walker E: Use of acyclovir to treat chickenpox in pregnancy. *BMJ* 296:393–394, 1988.
106. Smego RA, Asperilla MO: Use of acyclovir for varicella pneumonia during pregnancy. *Obstet Gynecol* 78:1112–1116, 1991.
107. White RG: Chickenpox in pregnancy (letter). *BMJ* 196:864, 1988.
108. Centers for Disease Control: ACV registry. *MMWR* 42:806, 1993.

109. Andrews EB, Tilson HH, Hurn BAL, et al: Acyclovir in pregnancy registry. *Am J Med* 85:123–128, 1988.
110. Asano Y, Yoshikawa T, Suga S, et al: Postexposure prophylaxis of varicella in family contact by oral acyclovir. *Pediatrics* 92:219–222, 1993.
111. Spring S, Laughlin C, Arvin A, et al: Varicella-zoster virus infection and post-herpetic neuralgia: New insights into pathogenesis and pain management. *J Neurol* 35:52–53, 1994.
112. Foscarnet. *Med Lett* 34:3–4, 1992.
113. Gershon A, Steinberg S, Schmidt N: Varicella-zoster virus, in Ballows A: *Manual of Clinical Microbiology*. Washington, DC, American Society for Microbiology, 1991.
114. Puchhammer-Stockl E, Popow-Kraupp T, Heinz F, et al: Detection of varicella-zoster virus DNA by polymerase chain reaction in the cerebrospinal fluid of patients suffering from neurological complications associated with chicken pox or herpes zoster. *J Clin Microbiol* 29:1513–1516, 1991.
115. Hughes P, LaRussa PS, Pearce J, et al: Transmission of varicella-zoster virus from a vaccinee with leukemia, demonstrated by polymerase chain reaction. *J Pediatr* 124:932–935, 1993.
116. Balfour HH, Edelman CK, Dirksen CL, et al: Laboratory studies of acute varicella and varicella immune status. *Diagn Microbiol Infect Dis* 10:149–158, 1988.
117. Demmler G, Steinberg S, Blum G, et al: Rapid enzyme-linked immunosorbent assay for detecting antibody to varicella-zoster virus. *J Infect Dis* 157:211–212, 1988.
118. LaRussa P, Steinberg S, Waithe E, et al: Comparison of five assays for antibody to varicella-zoster virus and the fluorescent-antibody-to-membrane-antigen test. *J Clin Microbiol* 25:2059–2062, 1987.
119. Steinberg S, Gershon A: Measurement of antibodies to varicella-zoster virus by using a latex agglutination test. *J Clin Microbiol* 29:1527–1529, 1991.
120. Williams V, Gershon A, Brunell P: Serologic response to varicella-zoster membrane antigens measured by indirect immunofluorescence. *J Infect Dis* 130:669–672, 1974.

Influenza Virus Infection in Children

Kathleen Ryan-Poirier, M.D.
Assistant Professor of Pediatrics, Division of Pediatric Infectious Diseases, University of Florida, Gainesville, Florida

Influenza is an acute respiratory illness that occurs during the winter season. Based on written historical accounts of influenza-like illness, it appears that influenza has afflicted humans for centuries and has been referred to as "the last great plague of man."[1] Although this may seem to be an overstatement in the present era of acquired immunodeficiency syndrome (AIDS), it does allow one to make several very important points about influenza. First, influenza is unique in that it has the potential to cause very serious and widespread disease, as has been witnessed in prior pandemics. Despite the fact that we have not had an influenza pandemic since 1968, both epidemiologic and genetic evidence indicates that pandemics of influenza can and will occur at some time in the future.[2] Second, the ability of influenza viruses to alter their genetic makeup to avoid host defense mechanisms and antiviral agents poses an almost insurmountable challenge to the complete control of influenza infection as has been possible with viruses such as smallpox.

INFLUENZA VIRUSES

CLASSIFICATION

Influenza viruses belong to the family *Orthomyxoviridae*, which contains three genera: influenza virus type A, influenza virus type B, and influenza virus type C (Table 1). The influenza viruses possess a segmented, single-stranded RNA genome that is termed *negative sense* because the viral genome itself is not infectious and serves as a template for the transcription of viral messenger RNA (mRNA). The RNA segments that constitute the virus genome each code for one or two viral proteins and exist as ribonucleoprotein complexes. Influenza A and B viruses contain eight genomic segments, whereas influenza C viruses contain only seven.[3]

Influenza A, B, and C viruses are distinguished from one another by differences in their nucleoprotein and matrix protein an-

Advances in Pediatric Infectious Diseases®, vol. 10

TABLE 1.
Classification of Influenza Viruses

Family	Orthomyxoviridae
Genus	Influenza
Type	A
Subtypes (human viruses)	H1N1, H2N2, H3N2
Type	B
Subtypes	None
Type	C
Subtypes	None

tigens—termed type-specific antigens. Influenza A viruses are further divided into *subtypes* based on differences in their surface glycoprotein antigens hemagglutinin (HA) and neuraminidase (NA). There are three known human influenza A virus subtypes: H1N1, H2N2, and H3N2. Influenza B and C viruses are not divided into subtypes because there is much more antigenic stability in their surface glycoprotein molecules.

The current nomenclature for influenza viruses includes the host of origin, the geographic origin, the strain number, and the year of isolation.[4] By tradition, the host of origin of human strains is not included. The description of the HA and NA of influenza A viruses is given in parentheses. For example, A/Swine/Iowa/15/30 (H1N1) would be the correct designation for a swine influenza A virus isolated in Iowa in 1930. The correct designations for a human influenza A or B virus would be A/Los Angeles/2/87 (H3N2) or B/Singapore/222/79, respectively.

VIRAL STRUCTURE AND COMPOSITION

The structures of influenza A, B, and C viruses are similar. Newly isolated viruses show variation in shape from spherical to filamentous forms, whereas viruses that have been passaged in culture tend to be predominantly spherical.[5, 6] The most striking feature of influenza virions is a layer of spikes projecting radially outward over the surface (Fig 1). The spikes of influenza A and B viruses consist individually of either HA or NA.[7] The HA spikes are the most abundant surface projection and are rod shaped when viewed by the electron microscope. Hemagglutinin derives its name from its ability to agglutinate red blood cells, and this technique is used to detect the presence of influenza in culture. The three-dimensional structure of HA, deduced by x-ray crystallographic analysis, has revealed each HA molecule to be a trimer of three identical monomers.[8] Each HA monomer contains a stalk region that is embedded in the viral envelope and a globular domain that contains the receptor-binding pocket and the major antigenic regions. Hemagglutinin is responsible for initiation of infection by attachment to host cell sialic acid–containing receptors. It also functions in the fusion of viral and endosomal membranes, which is necessary for release of the viral genome into the cell. In addition, HA is the vi-

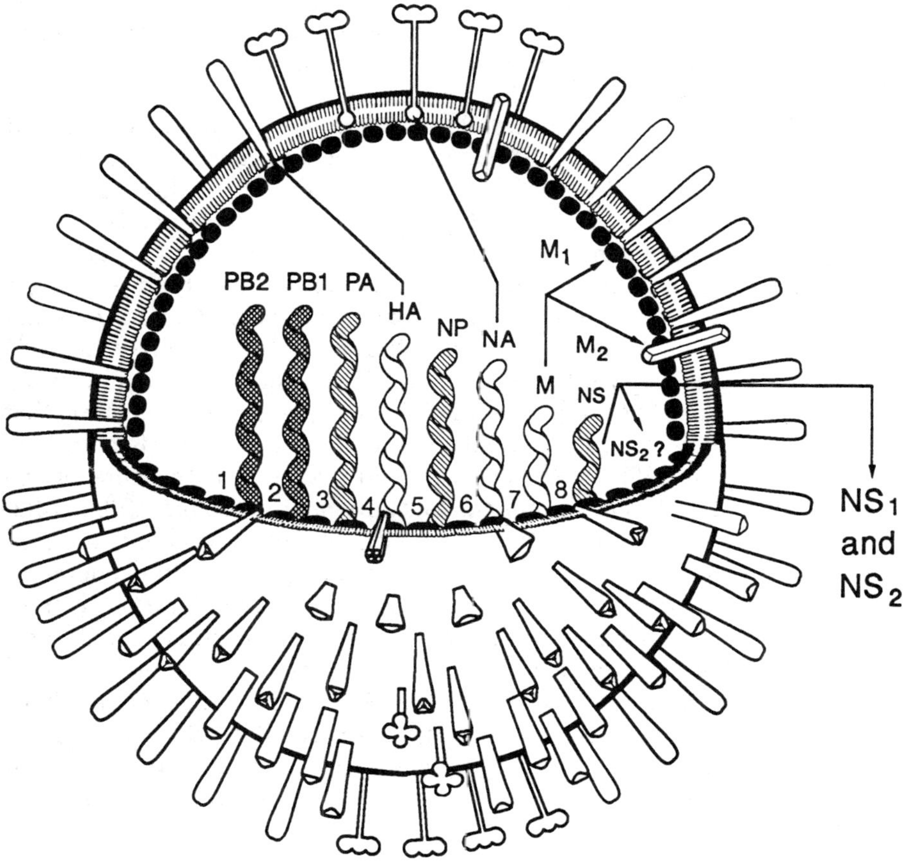

FIGURE 1.

Diagram of the influenza virion. The glycoprotein spikes consist of hemagglutinin *(HA)*, which predominates, and neuraminidase *(NA)*, which occurs in patches. Inside the lipid bilayer are eight segments of single-stranded RNA, each encoding for one or two proteins.

ral antigen that is the target for neutralizing antibodies. Neuraminidase is mushroom shaped and consists of a stalk and a box-shaped tetrameric head of four identical subunits each containing an enzyme-active center.[9] Neuraminidase, which cleaves sialic acid (neuraminic acid) residues from carbohydrates, is involved in release of progeny virus from the infected cell. Antibodies to NA are not virus neutralizing but appear to modify infection by reducing the levels of virus in the lungs and the extent of lung lesions.[10] In contrast to influenza A and B, the spikes of influenza C viruses are composed of a single glycoprotein, hemagglutinin esterase (HE), which is an integral membrane protein that displays receptor-binding activity, receptor-destroying activity (in this case an acetylesterase), and a penetration (fusion) function.[11]

The surface molecules are anchored in the virion envelope, which is derived from the plasma membrane of the host cell, and the inner surface of the envelope is lined by matrix (M1) protein, which adds rigidity to the lipid bilayer, thus providing structural integrity to the virion envelope. The M2 protein, encoded in the same RNA segment as M1, contains an extracellular region, a transmembrane region, and an intracellular tail. M2, which is thought to function as an ion channel, secondarily affects conformational changes in HA, thereby aiding in the release of progeny virus.[12, 13] M2 is present in infected cells but is not incorporated into progeny virions. The single-stranded RNA segments of the genome that are intricately associated with the nucleoprotein (NP) forming the ribonucleoprotein complexes are present within the core of the virion. The three virion-encoded polymerase proteins (PB1, PB2, and PA) are found in association with the nucleoprotein and virion RNA. The polymerase proteins are responsible for the generation of three different kinds of virus-specific RNAs. First, mRNA is transcribed from virion RNA for the production of virus-specific proteins. Then template RNA is made, from which genomic RNA, which will be incorporated into progeny virus, is generated. Two additional proteins, the nonstructural proteins NS1 and NS2 encoded by RNA segment 8 (segment 7 of influenza C), are present only in infected cells, and their function is not well defined.

HISTORY

Historical accounts of influenza-like illness in humans have provided evidence for the probable existence of influenza viruses at least as early as the period of Hippocrates. Some features of the pattern of influenza have emerged through a review of the historical data and still hold true today: (1) pandemics appear to occur at unpredictable intervals, and occasionally the disease may seem to disappear from the human population for a short length of time; (2) epidemics occur frequently (every 1 to 3 years) with varying severity; (3) there are no patterns of influenza illness that allow one to predict the occurrence of the next epidemic or pandemic; and (4) several of the epidemics seem to have begun in Asia and spread outward from that point to Russia.[14]

Isolation of the first influenza A virus in 1933 and retrospective serologic information obtained from people who survived known epidemics or pandemics have supported the historical data and provided a means to study the epidemiology of influenza virus disease. It is now evident that the influenza A pandemic of 1918, called the "Spanish flu," was caused by an influenza A virus of the H1N1 subtype. This pandemic caused at least 20 million deaths worldwide and is considered the most severe of all influenza pandemics. The H1N1 subtype of influenza A virus circulated alone in the human population until 1957. At that time it was replaced by the H2N2 subtype during the "Asian flu" pandemic. In 1968 the "Hong Kong flu" pandemic occurred and resulted in disappearance of the H2N2 subtype and appearance of the H3N2 subtype. In 1977, the H1N1 subtype reappeared in the human population with the "Russian flu" pandemic. However, unlike earlier pandemics, the H3N2 subtype did not disappear. Since 1977 the H3N2 and H1N1 subtypes of influenza A virus have cocirculated. Influenza B and C viruses cause epidemics, but to date there have been no documented pandemics caused by either of these viruses.

It is important to note that pandemics of influenza A virus will occur most commonly with the introduction of a novel subtype of HA or NA (or both) into the human population.[15] Alternatively, a pandemic can occur when a large percentage of the population consists of individuals previously unexposed to a particular subtype (and therefore highly susceptible to infection), as was the case with re-emergence of the H1N1 subtype that had been out of circulation for 20 years. It is very likely that a subtype of influenza A virus never previously encountered in the human population will suddenly appear at an undetermined time and cause widespread disease. It is also conceivable that the H2N2 subtype could reappear in the next several decades. The origin of the pandemic strains of influenza A virus has been under extensive investigation. Recent evolutionary evidence strongly suggests that new strains arise as a result of a reassortant event between a human virus and a virus from another animal species (see later).

EPIDEMIOLOGY

Influenza A, B, and C viruses are known to cause disease in humans. With the exception of several reports of influenza C viruses isolated in pigs, influenza B and C viruses are strictly human pathogens.[16] However, influenza A viruses are also readily isolated from swine, horses, and a wide variety of avian species. Pigs, horses, and the more domesticated avian species such as chickens and turkeys manifest both sporadic and epidemic respiratory disease. In contrast, wild birds (especially waterfowl) usually harbor the virus asymptomatically in the gastrointestinal tract.

There are 14 recognized influenza A virus HA subtypes and 9 recognized NA subtypes (Table 2). The 14th HA subtype was only recently discovered in ducks in Russia.[17] As mentioned earlier, only three different HA and two different NA subtypes have been isolated in humans (H1N1, H2N2, H3N2). However, all of the HA and NA subtypes have been isolated in birds. Swine and horses, like humans, become infected with a much narrower range of HA and NA subtypes. Waterfowl are therefore considered to be the reservoir of influenza A virus in nature since they harbor all subtypes of influenza A virus. Interspecies transmission of influenza virus occurs primarily from this reservoir (Fig 2).

The influenza viruses are unique among the respiratory viruses in that they undergo significant antigenic variation. Antigenic *drift* involves minor antigenic changes in the HA and NA molecules and occurs in influenza A, B, and C viruses but is most pronounced in influenza A strains.[18] This type of antigenic change occurs as a result of point mutations in the genes encoding the HA and NA molecules and leads to an accumulation of amino acid sequence changes over time. Viruses that contain mutations that allow them to escape specific antibody present in body fluid secretions and se-

TABLE 2.
Influenza A Virus Host Range

Host	Hemagglutinin Subtypes	Neuraminidase Subtypes
Humans	H1, H2, H3	N1, N2
Swine	H1, H3	N1, N2
Horses	H3, H7	N7, N8
Birds	H1–H14	N1–N9

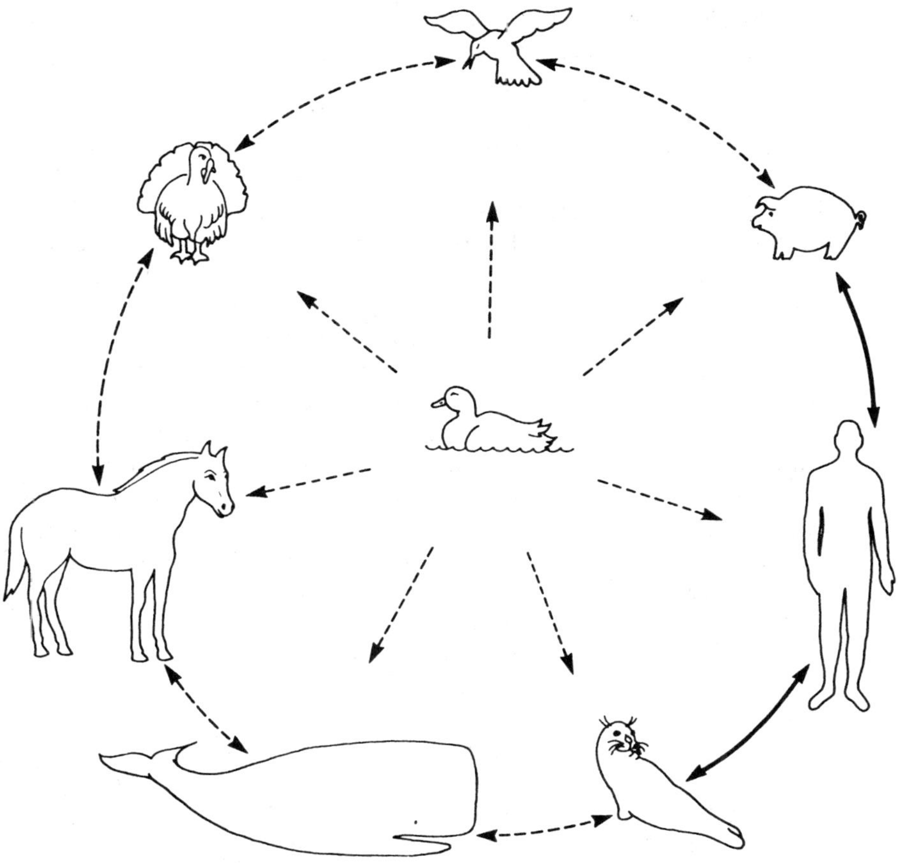

FIGURE 2.
Diagram of the "wheel of flu" depicting waterfowl as the central reservoir of influenza A virus in nature with interspecies transmission of viruses primarily from that reservoir. Viruses can also be transmitted between other species.

rum will be given a selective growth advantage. As a result, these viruses become the predominant strain within the population. As part of this pattern, widespread activity is often introduced by a "herald wave," that is, the appearance of a new strain for a few weeks at the end of one respiratory season followed by extensive epidemic spread of this strain in the next winter season.[19]

Antigenic *shift* involves major antigenic changes in the HA and NA molecules and occurs only with influenza A viruses. The changes in HA and/or NA that occur with antigenic shift can result in the appearance of pandemic viruses. Sequence information has provided ample evidence that "new" subtypes that cause pandemics in humans arise by the acquisition of a gene(s) from an animal or avian virus as the result of a genetic reassortant event. The leading hypothesis, which has gained considerable strength through intensive genetic and antigenic analysis, indicates that the reassortant event that leads to the appearance of a new subtype for humans has occurred most frequently in China.[20] This subtype then spreads rapidly to the rest of the world from its point of origin. The available data indicate that the HA and one of the internal genes (PB1) of the H3N2 subtype were derived from an avian species, whereas the remainder of the genes are those of its predecessor, the H2N2 subtype.[21] Along these lines it is perceived that the gene pool for influenza viruses is maintained to the greatest extent in avian species. Birds, because of their migratory nature, interact with a variety of animal species and transmit virus to them, or the viruses from the two species reassort. Birds could be the direct source of virus for reassortment in humans; however, it appears more likely that there is an intermediate host such as the pig, which may act as a "mixing vessel" and transmit the virus to humans.[22] Living conditions in China seem to make it particularly feasible for animal-to-human transmission of influenza virus. In the villages of rural China, pigs are sometimes raised in the same living quarters as their owners. This close contact is thought to promote interspecies transmission of the virus. Thus, owing to the extensive gene pool from which influenza viruses might draw, it is possible to imagine a wide variety of new combinations of influenza A virus that could appear in the human population.

One well-known example of interspecies transmission of influenza A virus was the outbreak of swine influenza in military recruits at Fort Dix, New Jersey, in 1976. This outbreak, which caused infection in 230 military personnel (with 1 fatal outcome), was caused by a virus indistinguishable antigenically from contemporary strains of swine influenza virus of the H1N1 subtype.[23, 24] This event was unique in that it was the first documented outbreak of an animal influenza virus in humans and occurred during the same season that the H3N2 virus A/Victoria/75 was circulating and causing disease in the human population. This outbreak caused particular concern because the 1918 H1N1 pandemic virus is considered to have been of swine origin and therefore this outbreak could have heralded the onset of a new pandemic. Because of this concern, a mass immunization program aimed at immunizing the entire U.S. population was rapidly undertaken. The swine virus never spread significantly beyond Fort Dix, and the threat of a new pandemic quickly diminished. The mechanism by which the swine virus reached humans is not known, but this episode underscores the potential significance of interspecies transmission of influenza virus.

PATHOGENESIS

Influenza virus infection is spread from person to person via the transfer of virus-containing respiratory secretions from an infected individual to a susceptible one through small-particle aerosols (<10 μm mass median diameter).[25]

The principal site of replication of influenza virus is the ciliated columnar epithelium of the middle respiratory tract, specifically the trachea and bronchi. It is not known whether the virus moves downward to this location after first attaching to epithelial cells of the nasopharynx or whether it travels upward after being deposited in the alveoli. However, virus can be recovered from both the upper and lower respiratory tracts of people naturally or experimentally infected with virus, thus indicating some replication throughout the entire respiratory tract.[26, 27] The length of the incubation period to the onset of illness or virus shedding varies, depending on the size of the viral inoculum, from 18 to 72 hours.[25] The pattern of virus shedding in children follows a typical pattern, with virus first being detected in low titer just before the onset of illness. The viral titer rises rapidly to peak at approximately $10^{4.0}$ median tissue culture infective dose ($TCID_{50}$)/mL within 48 hours. The titer remains elevated for another 24 to 48 hours and then rapidly declines to low titers.[28] Virus can often be recovered from respiratory secretions for 2 to 3 weeks.[29] Even after infectious virus can no longer be recovered, viral antigen can be detected for several days in cells and secretions of infected individuals.[30, 31] Influenza virus has only rarely been isolated from the respiratory tract without a temporally related illness compatible with influenza. Therefore an asymptomatic carrier state is not thought to be associated with influenza.

Initially there is acute diffuse inflammation of the larynx, trachea, and bronchi with mucosal injection and edema.[32] This is rapidly followed by extensive necrosis and desquamation. A loss of ciliated epithelium may be apparent as early as 24 hours after the onset of infection, and an almost complete loss of the epithelial surface with exposure of the basal cell layer may be evident, even in uncomplicated cases, within 36 to 48 hours after infection.[33]

When the lung parenchyma becomes involved, resulting in primary influenza virus pneumonia, there is also submucosal edema and hemorrhage with only a limited amount of inflammation. The alveolar epithelium may be destroyed, and there is often some component of intra-alveolar hemorrhage. A rather characteristic feature is the presence of acellular hyaline membranes lining alveolar ducts and alveoli.[32, 34] This is an uncommon finding in other viral respiratory infections. Regeneration of denuded epithelial surfaces begins rather promptly after the acute infectious process, but it may take weeks for complete recovery of cellular and ciliary function.

The detection of influenza viremia is a rare event even during the most acute stage of clinical disease.[35] This fact has made it difficult to understand the cause of the striking systemic symptoms that accompany influenza. However, there is evidence that the virus can disseminate from its initial site of invasion in the respiratory tract, which indicates that viremia may occur but may just be extremely difficult to detect. Virus has rarely been isolated from cardiac and peripheral muscle in cases of myocarditis or myositis and has been isolated from the cerebrospinal fluid or brain in patients with central nervous system involvement.[34, 36, 37] Whether the presence of the virus in blood or other tissues is responsible for the occurrence of symptoms is not clear.

CLINICAL MANIFESTATIONS

Influenza A, B, and C can produce the same constellation of clinical signs and symptoms in both children and adults. However, influenza A and B are generally considered to cause more severe disease than influenza C.[38] Disease caused by epidemic influenza A is unique in that people in all age groups are afflicted with an acute febrile upper respiratory illness. This occurs because of a more pronounced antigenic drift with influenza A that results in the absence of protective antibody levels in a significant proportion of adults as well as children. In contrast, influenza B viruses, which undergo less antigenic drift, produce more intense symptoms in children. Adults may have only a common cold with little or no constitutional symptoms if they have adequate existing antibody, unless an outbreak is caused by an antigenically distinct influenza B virus.[39] The data do suggest that nasal discharge, abdominal pain, and gastrointestinal symptoms including vomiting and diarrhea in 20% to 30% of patients are more common with influenza B virus infection.[40, 41]

The true spectrum of disease caused by influenza C has not yet been elucidated, partly because of difficulty in isolating the virus and partly because the illness produced by influenza C infection may be mild or subclinical. In one well-defined outbreak of influenza C virus in Japan, the disease in young children was characterized by temperatures of 38 to 40° C for 2 to 3 days and a prolonged period of coryza (2 weeks) accompanied by cough in 50% of the patients.[42] Adult patients during the same outbreak had a similar, although milder illness, with headache, malaise, and sore throat. In another report, young adults had symptoms of headache, myalgia, cough, conjunctivitis, and joint pain, with symptoms lasting approximately 12 days.[43] In this outbreak the influenza C virus–associated symptoms were at least as severe as those associated with influenza A infections and were more prolonged. Despite a lack of data on the clinical manifestations of influenza C virus infection, serologic evidence indicates that infection with the virus is quite common. Seropositivity rates of 64% for children up to 5 years old, 96% for 6- to 10-year-olds, 100% for 11- to 15-year-olds, and 98% for those over 16 years old have been reported.[43] Reinfection with influenza C virus appears to be common despite the demonstration of adequate antibody before reinfection.[44]

The clinical expression of infection with influenza virus may vary depending on the nature of the infecting virus and the person's age, immunologic status, and underlying medical conditions. In its classic form, influenza is "an unvarying disease caused by a varying virus" (Kilbourne) with a typical pattern of signs and symptoms. It is important to note, however, that the diagnosis of influenza is made most easily in the context of an epidemic. The simultaneous occurrence of similar cases in the community is an important diagnostic indicator. In general, following a typically short incubation period, the onset of influenza viral illness is rapid without any identifiable prodrome. Fever and a dry cough associated with intense malaise are found in greater than 90% of cases in all age groups. The degree of prostration is generally out of proportion to the respiratory symptoms. The fever and malaise last 3 to 4 days and diminish over this time period, whereas the respiratory symptoms peak during this time and then resolve slowly.

OLDER CHILDREN AND ADOLESCENTS

In older children and adolescents influenza appears in its classic form. The most frequent accompanying symptoms are a throbbing, nonlocalized headache, chills, myalgia, and sneezing. Although adolescents and adults occasionally have a productive cough, this does not necessarily predict a superimposed bacterial pneumonia. Lumbosacral backache, sore throat, conjunctival burning or discharge, and epistaxis are also encountered, whereas gastrointestinal symptoms are uncommon. The fever is usually in the range of 38 to 40° C. A biphasic fever curve can be encountered, with fever being slightly higher on approximately day 4 of illness.[45] This can occur without evidence of bacterial superinfection. Physical examination reveals nasal discharge, conjunctival infection with increased tearing, photophobia, facial flush, and a variable degree of pharyngeal erythema without exudate. In uncomplicated cases there is usually no evidence of lower respiratory tract involvement, although coarse breath sounds or faint rales may be heard in 1% to 5% of patients. Nontender cervical adenopathy may be found in 25% of patients. Hepatosplenomegaly has not been associated with influenza. Older individuals with influenza will often appear more ill than their younger counterparts. A protracted postinfluenza asthenia has been reported to occur, although complete recovery from influenza is the rule.[46]

YOUNGER CHILDREN

Acute respiratory infections in young children are a significant cause of mortality and morbidity. Influenza is thought to account for only about half of the lower respiratory tract infections that result in hospitalization of children, with respiratory syncytial virus (RSV) and the parainfluenza viruses being the most important causes.[47, 48] However, during influenza epidemics, influenza viruses supplant the other major respiratory disease viruses in the community and account for a higher proportion of hospitalizations.[49, 50] In addition, when viewed from an outpatient standpoint, influenza viruses have been found to be the most important cause of illness that necessitates young children being brought for medical care.[49]

The pattern of influenza in a younger child may include a typical influenza-like illness, a nonspecific febrile illness, or other respiratory tract syndromes such as croup, bronchitis, bronchiolitis, or pneumonitis that are indistinguishable from those caused by other respiratory pathogens. Primary infection includes high fever, with temperatures often over 39.5° C, and irritability as well as a rather toxic appearance in the majority of patients. Putto et al. reported temperatures over 39° C to be more common with influenza A infection (85%) than with influenza B infection (65%).[51] In this report the mean highest degree of fever in respiratory virus infections during hospitalization did not differ from that in defined serious bacterial infections such as meningitis, epiglottitis, sepsis, or urinary tract infection. The mean duration of fever was 5.1 to 5.2

days and did not differ significantly between influenza A and B. Of note is that 37% of patients with respiratory virus infection had fever lasting 5 days or longer.

Additional signs and symptoms include a clear nasal discharge, a hacking cough, and nonexudative pharyngitis in as many as 75% to 100% of patients.[52] Symptoms referable to the gastrointestinal tract such as anorexia, nausea, vomiting, and diarrhea can be found in as many as 40% to 50% of patients, with an inverse relation to age.[37] Vomiting tends to be a more significant finding than diarrhea.[53] Tender cervical adenitis and otitis media occur frequently (25% to 50%), as well as nonpurulent conjunctivitis. Febrile convulsions have been reported to occur as the initial symptom in children less than 3 years of age in as many as 35% to 40% of patients.[48, 53] Croup, bronchiolitis, and pneumonitis occur to a variable degree, with pneumonitis being slightly more common.[52] Pneumonitis can be particularly severe in the younger age groups and in those with underlying pulmonary or cardiac conditions.[52] A variety of central nervous system findings including apnea, opisthotonos, and seizures can also be found in approximately 20% of young children.[52] Macular, maculopapular, and petechial rashes are also encountered in a small percentage of children.

INFANTS

Influenza in infants is often unrecognized because the signs and symptoms may suggest bacterial sepsis with lethargy, poor feeding, poor peripheral perfusion, petechiae, and apneic spells.[54, 55] High fever and respiratory symptoms, primarily rhinitis, are usually present. Influenza infection does not commonly occur in the perinatal period because of the presence of maternal antibody.

LABORATORY DATA

In uncomplicated classic influenza in all age groups the leukocyte count is often normal, but leukopenia (white blood cell count, <4,500 cells/mm^3) can occur in as many as 25% of cases. The white blood cell count may indicate a relative lymphopenia or neutropenia, but a predominance of polymorphonuclear leukocytes is usually only seen with bacterial superinfection. Liver function test values may be elevated to a mild degree with influenza viral pneumonia, and the creatine phosphokinase (CPK) content may be elevated in cases with myositis. Low serum iron levels have also been noted in adults with influenza.[56] Chest radiographs may be abnormal in a small proportion of older children and adolescents without clinical evidence of pneumonia but are more frequently abnormal in young children, especially those with lower respiratory tract symptomatology.

IMMUNOCOMPROMISED CHILDREN

Influenza infection in pediatric patients with underlying pulmonary or cardiac conditions and in immunocompromised children, including those with human immunodeficiency virus (HIV) infection, is poorly defined. These patients are considered to be at risk for severe, even fatal infections with many viruses; however, systematic studies of influenza in children are lacking, with much of the available data having been accumulated in adults. Feldman et al. studied influenza infection in 20 children and young adults with cancer who were receiving immunosuppressive therapy.[57] In this study the clinical manifestations of influenza were not unusual, but the clinical course lasted twice as long (2 weeks) as in the general population. The severity of infection appeared to be unrelated to the duration of cancer therapy, to specific chemotherapeutic agents with or without irradiation, or to the status of the malignancy during infection. Complications developed in only 3 patients and were related to secondary bacterial infections with *Streptococcus pneumoniae* or *Haemophilus influenzae*, and no deaths occurred with influenza. Chemotherapy was usually withheld during the course of illness. In another study of influenza in children with cancer, the symptoms in the study patients did not differ significantly from the matched community controls, and clinical complications occurred too infrequently to analyze.[58] However, the incidence of influenza infection was higher in children with cancer (32%) than in controls (14%). In addition, the presence of an HA titer to influenza of greater than or equal to 1:32 was protective for all the control patients but did not protect 24% of the patients with cancer. Two patients with cancer required hospitalization because of fever and neutropenia, and nosocomial infection with influenza developed in 1, but none of the controls required hospitalization. In a recent report of influenza in transplant recipients (renal and bone marrow) 2 of 19 patients had severe infections whereas infections in the others were mild and self-limited.[59] One patient was a 4-year-old who contracted a fatal influenza A virus infection while in the aplastic phase after bone marrow transplantation, and the other was an adult who contracted influenza pneumonitis after renal transplantation and was treated successfully with amantadine. Another pediatric patient also contracted influenza during the aplastic phase after bone marrow transplantation and was febrile for 21 days with repeated virologic tests positive for influenza virus type A. Of note is that several of the patients in this study in whom influenza infection developed had chronic graft-vs.-host disease.

Viral respiratory pathogens, including parainfluenza viruses, RSV, and adenoviruses, have been reported to cause severe and persistent infection in children with HIV infection or severe combined immunodeficiency syndromes.[60–63] These patients often have infection with more than one viral pathogen and may have persistent infections for weeks to months. In addition, respiratory viruses have been isolated from pharyngeal ulcers and lip lesions in addition to having been recovered from nasopharyngeal secretions.[61] The patients generally have demonstrated laboratory evidence of abnormal B-cell and T-cell function as well as diminished cell-mediated immunity. The pattern of influenza in HIV-infected children is not well characterized but will likely be similar to that described for other respiratory pathogens.

COMPLICATIONS

PRIMARY VIRAL PNEUMONIA

Primary influenza pneumonia occurs in young healthy patients in nearly every epidemic but is most common in certain high-risk groups, including pregnant women and patients with cardiovascular and pulmonary disease. Patients with rheumatic heart disease are at particularly high risk.[27] Strictly speaking, influenza pneumonia is not a complication but a manifestation of the disease at the more severe end of the spectrum. Primary pneumonia usually begins within the first 48 hours of the illness and is heralded by a rapid increase in the respiratory rate with diffuse fine rales and bilateral interstitial infiltrates on chest radiography. The initial dry cough becomes productive and the sputum may be bloody. Sputum Gram stain is unrevealing, and bacterial culture of the sputum reveals normal flora whereas viral culture yields a high titer of virus. Progressive cyanosis with resultant respiratory failure is common. Patients deteriorate despite broad-spectrum antimicrobial therapy and supportive care. The mortality from this entity is quite high.

SECONDARY BACTERIAL PNEUMONIA

Secondary bacterial pneumonia associated with influenza also most commonly occurs in those patients with underlying pulmonary or cardiac disease. During the early convalescent phase of an otherwise unremarkable influenza illness, new fever and productive cough develop, with findings on physical examination and chest radiography consistent with a lobar consolidated pneumonia. *Streptococcus pneumoniae* is the organism most commonly isolated from sputum cultures, followed by *Staphylococcus aureus*, *H. influenzae*, and group A β-hemolytic streptococci. Patients generally respond to appropriate antimicrobial therapy. Staphylococcal pneumonia may be associated with the development of empyema and pneumatoceles. Combined viral-bacterial pneumonia may occur with any of the aforementioned bacteria and give a mixed clinical picture and a variable response to antibiotics. Both virus and bacteria can be isolated from the lung in combined infection. This entity, most fulminant with *S. aureus*, results in a necrotizing pneumonia with microabscesses.

MYOSITIS

A syndrome of acute myositis, also termed acute transient crural myopathy, can occur in children during the early convalescent phase of an influenza viral illness. This syndrome is most commonly seen during influenza B epidemics but can be encountered during influenza A outbreaks. The patients (usually preschool or young school-aged children) have an acute onset of muscle pain and tenderness sufficiently severe to prevent walking.[64] The gastrocnemius and soleus muscles are the primary muscles involved. Serum CPK and aspartate aminotransferase (AST) levels may be transiently elevated. Actual muscle weakness is usually not documented but can occur, and influenza virus has been isolated from a muscle biopsy specimen.[65] Complete recovery in 3 to 4 days without residual sequelae is the rule.

TOXIC SHOCK SYNDROME

Toxic shock syndrome (TSS) was first reported in association with influenza in 1986.[66] Since that time 15 additional cases have been reported (for a review see Tolan[67]). The described cases of TSS meet the case definition for TSS: isolation of *S. aureus* from various body sites shortly after an influenza-like illness. Influenza may be isolated from nasopharyngeal secretions, but serology proves to be a very useful adjunct in this setting since viral titers during the convalescent phase of illness may be below the limits of detection. Influenza B has been found in association with TSS more frequently than influenza A. The association of secondary staphylococcal infection with influenza is well recognized; therefore the occurrence of TSS in this setting is not surprising.

REYE SYNDROME

Reye syndrome has been most significantly associated with influenza and varicella infections and is slightly more common with influenza B infections. The condition, characterized by nausea, vomiting, and stupor during convalescence from the viral infection, is most common in white, male, school-aged children. The pathogenesis of Reye syndrome is obscure but is characterized by fatty degeneration of the liver and cerebral edema. This results in the findings of elevated serum transaminase and ammonia levels along with elevated central nervous system pressure but normal cerebrospinal fluid findings. There is also a strong correlation between the use of salicylates during the viral infection and the development of Reye syndrome. Therefore salicylates and salicylate-containing products should be strictly avoided in children with influenza.

Other rare complications of influenza include an acute myopathy with myoglobinuria and secondary renal failure, carditis, encephalitis, and Guillain-Barré syndrome.[68–70]

DIAGNOSIS

Isolation of influenza A or B from respiratory tract secretions inoculated into embryonated chicken eggs or tissue culture has been the standard method of diagnosing influenza. Cell lines that support the growth of influenza virus, such as primary rhesus monkey kidney (PRMK) and Madin-Darby canine kidney (MDCK), must be employed for successful isolation of the virus. Depending on the cell line used, it may be necessary to add trypsin to the tissue culture media to culture influenza. Trypsin acts to cleave the HA molecule into its active form. Nasopharyngeal swabs or washes, gargles, and tracheal aspirates or specimens obtained at bronchoalveolar lavage have been used successfully for isolation of the virus. Samples are best obtained very early in the illness when the titer of the virus in the secretions is high. The virus may be detectable as early as 72 hours after inoculation by the traditional techniques of hemadsorption or by hemagglutination using the culture supernatant. The cytopathic effect induced by influenza viruses appears more slowly or may be totally absent in certain cell lines. Blind passage of the virus will often enhance the rate of isolation. Once a hemadsorbing or hemagglutinating virus is identified in culture, the virus can be identified as influenza A or B by immunofluorescence (IF) or enzyme-linked immunosorbent assay (ELISA) using type-specific monoclonal antibody. The time from inoculation of virus into tissue culture until definitive identification of the virus usually requires at least 5 days but may take 7 to 10 days. Viral cultures are generally held for 2 weeks. Identification of the subtype of influenza A virus requires further analysis with the hemagglutination inhibition assay using subtype-specific antisera.

The shell viral technique, which involves centrifugation of the virus onto the tissue monolayer and then detection of the virus after a shorter (72-hour) period of growth by IF with type-specific monoclonal antibody, has gained wide acceptance in clinical virology laboratories in the last several years.[71] This technique provides results quickly and appears to be both sensitive and specific. Bartholoma and Forbes reported a sensitivity of 90.9% and 87.5% for fresh and frozen specimens, respectively, as compared with conventional tube cell culture.[72] In another study the sensitivity of shell vial centrifugation was found to be 82% for the detection of influenza A virus and 86% for the detection of influenza B virus (84% overall) with a specificity of 100%.[73] Even more recently a commercial kit has become available (Baxter-Bartels, Bellevue, Washington) that employs a monoclonal antibody pool for the detection of seven different respiratory viruses (influenza A and B; parainfluenza virus types 1, 2, and 3; RSV; and adenovirus) in a shell vial centrifugation assay. Specimens that are positive when the screening antibody pool is used can then be tested with individual monoclonal antibodies to the seven viruses. With this technique, Matthey et al. reported a high sensitivity (94%) and specificity (97.3%) when compared with standard cultures.[74] A similar study found the assay to be very sensitive, but there were differences in the ability of the assay to detect individual viruses.[75] For example, the shell vial assay was 94% sensitive in detecting influenza B virus but only 80% sensitive in detecting parainfluenza viruses. Of interest was the finding that the shell vial assay was more sensitive than cell culture for some specimens. Assays such as this one are unlikely to completely replace standard cell culture because optimal isolation and identification of viruses require the combination of several different techniques.

The ability to detect virus directly in clinical samples is desirable since it would allow rapid diagnosis and therefore the institution of early therapy. A new test kit for the detection of virus in clinical samples recently became available (Directigen FLU-A, Becton Dickinson, Cuckeysville, Md). This test will detect only influenza A, but it also will detect all subtypes of influenza A virus. The test employs an enzyme immunoassay membrane technique and monoclonal antibody to the nucleoprotein antigen of influenza A. It takes less than 15 minutes to perform the test, and little technical expertise is required. This test may prove to be useful in the office practice setting since it can provide a reliable diagnosis as quickly as the commonly used rapid streptococcal tests. It may also be a useful adjunctive test in clinical virology laboratories. The test has been reported to have a sensitivity of 100% and a specificity of 91.6% when compared with viral isolation in cell culture and direct IF.[76] The negative predictive value was 100% in this study, but the positive predictive value was only 62.6% when compared with cell culture and 75% when compared with IF because of false positives caused by low-intensity test kit readings. Nasopharyngeal washes and/or swabs are the best specimens for this test. The validity of the test results decreases sharply when other specimens such as gargles are used.[77] The direct detection of influenza virus in clinical samples has also been pursued with direct IF and ELISA. These procedures have not gained widespread acceptance in clinical laboratories because they are time-consuming, require a good deal of technical expertise, and have suboptimal sensitivity. The polymerase chain reaction (PCR) is another technique that is being explored for rapid identification of viruses in clinical specimens. This technique will have the advantage of being able to amplify viral nucleic acid directly from clinical samples and may therefore greatly enhance sensitivity. However, PCR has not yet been developed sufficiently for use in the clinical virology laboratory to detect influenza or other respiratory viruses.

Serologic diagnosis of an influenza virus infection can be made by using the hemagglutination inhibition, ELISA, or complement fixation assays. Paired acute and convalescent serum specimens obtained 10 to 20 days apart should be analyzed. Fourfold or greater rises in titer are considered diagnostic of infection, and a high convalescent titer (when only one specimen is available) is considered suggestive of recent infection. In office practice, serologic studies are not very useful because the results are usually not available until the patient has long since recovered from the illness. However, in the hospital setting with more critically ill patients or in those with unusual manifestations, serology still proves to be of value.

TREATMENT

Amantadine (Symmetrel) is approved in the United States for the treatment of influenza A infections in children and adults. Rimantadine (Flumadine), a close analogue of amantadine, is also effective in treating influenza A infections and has recently been approved for use in the United States. Currently there are no antiviral agents for use against influenza B or C infections. Amantadine and rimantadine disrupt the viral infectious cycle by interacting with the structural matrix protein of the virus, specifically the M2 protein component.[78] The inhibition of M2 function, which presumably acts as an ion channel, results in a secondary change in HA conformation and thereby inhibits release of progeny virus.[79]

Amantadine has been shown to be effective in reducing the symptoms and duration of acute influenza infection by as much as 50% in adults when given early in the course of the disease.[80] Rimantadine has been shown to have similar efficacy in the treatment of children.[81] Children receiving rimantadine showed significantly greater reduction in fever and improvement in daily scores for symptoms and severity of illness during the first 3 days of illness. Increased viral shedding has occurred after discontinuation of treatment with rimantadine in children when compared with placebo-treated controls.[82] The significance of this increased shedding is not clear. The primary drawback of both agents is the rapid emergence of resistant viruses that can be isolated during a single course of therapy. A rimantadine-resistant virus isolated from an index case during therapy was demonstrated to be transmitted to family members and cause clinical disease.[83] Fortunately, to date, amantadine- and rimantadine-resistant viruses have not been shown to have increased virulence. The efficacy of amantadine and rimantadine in the treatment of influenza viral pneumonia or mixed viral-bacterial pneumonia remains to be determined. Neither agent has been studied in a controlled trial for therapeutic efficacy in these situations; however, anecdotal reports indicate some efficacy.[84, 85]

The use of amantadine has been associated with central nervous system side effects, including headache, insomnia, irritability, and an inability to concentrate. These side effects have been reported to occur in 7% or more of patients, with increased incidence in the elderly.[86] In addition, there is an increased risk of seizure activity during therapy with amantadine in those patients with known seizure disorders despite therapeutic levels of anticonvulsants. These side effects are reversible with discontinuation of use of the drug. It should be noted, however, that amantadine has been used over prolonged periods of time in patients with Parkinson's disease with minimal toxicity. Rimantadine has greater antiviral activity in vitro against influenza A and is associated with fewer side effects, especially those related to the central nervous system.[87, 88] The side effect profile of rimantadine is considered to be similar to that of placebo.

Amantadine is approved for the treatment of influenza A virus infection in both adults and children, whereas rimantadine is currently approved for the treatment of influenza A virus infection in adults only. Both agents should be administered shortly after the onset of symptoms, preferably within 48 hours, for maximal efficacy. Whether antiviral therapy is effective when treatment begins beyond the first 48 hours of illness is not known. Antiviral therapy can be administered to healthy adults or children in an effort to reduce the severity and shorten the duration of influenza A illness.[89] This should generally be done in conjunction with a known or highly suspected outbreak of influenza A in the community. There are no data on the efficacy of amantadine or rimantadine therapy in high-risk individuals. Therefore, the Immunization Practices Advisory Committee (ACIP) makes no specific recommendations regarding therapeutic use of the drugs for these patients.[90] This does not preclude physicians prescribing the drugs for high-risk patients in whom influenza A infection develops. Therapy should be discontinued as soon as clinically warranted, generally 3 to 5 days, but may be continued for 7 days. A short course of treatment is recommended in the hope of diminishing the emergence of drug-resistant viral isolates. The dosage of amantadine and rimantadine should be adjusted for persons with impaired renal function, children, persons who have neuropsychiatric disorders or who take psychotropic drugs, and persons with a history of seizures.

Amantadine and rimantadine have both been approved for the chemoprophylaxis of influenza A infection in adults and children. Prophylaxis is not recommended for general use, but it is recommended in the following settings:

1. As short-term prophylaxis during an outbreak of influenza A for persons who did not receive vaccine or received vaccine after the onset of an outbreak
2. In conjunction with the vaccine in persons at high risk of complications of influenza developing and who may respond poorly to the vaccine, including those with HIV infection
3. In lieu of the vaccine when vaccine is contraindicated in a high-risk patient
4. In residents and employees of hospitals or institutions to prevent further spread of an outbreak (this should be done regardless of the vaccination status of the individuals)
5. In individuals providing care for high-risk persons in the home, hospital, or institutional setting.[89]

Chemoprophylaxis can be given for the entire influenza season (approximately 6 weeks) if necessary or can be given for shorter periods of time to cover the at-risk periods. Prophylaxis can also be given to any individual who wishes to avoid illness with influenza A. It should be stressed that chemoprophylaxis does not replace vaccination as the most effective means of preventing influenza A infection.

Ribavirin has in vitro antiviral activity against influenza A, B, and C viruses and has been shown in a limited number of trials to be effective in the treatment of uncomplicated influenza A and B when administered as small-particle aerosol therapy.[90, 91] Recently another compound (4-guanidino-2,4-dideoxy-2,3-dehydro-N-acetylneuraminic acid) that is a selective inhibitor of influenza NA has been shown to effectively inhibit a wide range of influenza A and B viruses in vitro.[92]

PREVENTION

The mainstay for the prevention of influenza has been the use of inactivated (formalin-treated) virus vaccines. The current influenza vaccines, which are produced in embryonated chicken eggs, are safe and immunogenic. The inactivated vaccines are multivalent and contain viruses representative of those currently circulating in the human population (influenza A [H3N2 and H1N1] and influenza B but not influenza C). Because the vaccine is prepared from inactivated (noninfectious) virus, it cannot cause influenza. Whole-virus, subvirion (split) virus, and purified surface antigen (subunit) preparations are available. The subvirion vaccine is made by treating the virus with ether or detergents to disrupt the viral envelope. The subunit vaccine is made from HA and NA antigens that have been cleaved from the virus and separated from other virion components in detergent-disrupted virus preparations. The composition of the vaccine is determined on a yearly basis from seroepidemiologic data gathered by the World Health Organization (WHO) from the preceding influenza season.

The overall efficacy of the vaccines is estimated to be 70% to 90% against homologous virus in healthy children and younger adults.[93] Studies have suggested that the frequency of severe illness is reduced to a greater degree than that of actual infection of the upper respiratory tract. In most children and young adults, high postvaccination hemagglutination inhibition antibody titers develop. These titers are protective against strains similar to those in the vaccine or closely related variants. Lower postvaccination antibody titers may develop in persons with certain chronic diseases, and they may therefore remain susceptible to infection of the upper respiratory tract with influenza. However, these individuals are protected from infection of the lower respiratory tract and other complications developing, thereby reducing the risk of hospitalization and death. Immunity to the vaccine components wanes significantly after several months, thus necessitating yearly vaccination in healthy as well as immunocompromised individuals. The administration of two doses at least 1 month apart is usually required for a satisfactory antibody response in previously unvaccinated children less than 9 years of age. The vaccine is administered intramuscularly in the deltoid muscle in older children and adolescents and in the anterolateral aspect of the thigh in young children. To reduce the incidence of systemic reactions only the split or subunit vaccine preparations should be used in children less than 13 years of age. The vaccine is not recommended for infants less than 6 months of age.

Widespread vaccination of the general public, especially young children in whom the attack rate is the highest, is not considered feasible or cost-effective. However, there are certain target groups in whom vaccination on a yearly basis in the autumn is strongly recommended.[93] These high risk groups include the following:

1. Adults and children who receive regular medical care for chronic cardiac or pulmonary conditions such as cystic fibrosis, bronchopulmonary dysplasia, moderately severe asthma, and chronic obstructive pulmonary disease (COPD)
2. Residents of nursing homes or other institutional care facilities
3. Healthy adults over the age of 65 years
4. Children and teenagers (6 months to 18 years of age) who are receiving long-term aspirin therapy
5. Close contacts of high-risk individuals, including household contacts and health care personnel
6. Patients with other chronic illnesses such as diabetes mellitus, metabolic or renal diseases, or hemoglobinopathies or those receiving immunosuppression.

In addition, the vaccine should be considered for pregnant women with other underlying medical conditions, patients with symptomatic HIV infection, and foreign travelers to the southern hemisphere during April to September. To minimize disruption during outbreaks, persons who provide essential community services and college students might benefit from vaccination. Finally, the vaccine should be made available to any individual who desires prophylaxis against influenza.

Although side effects have historically been considered to be significant with influenza vaccines, there are in actuality few side effects. Fewer than one third of adult vaccine recipients may have discomfort at the injection site 8 to 24 hours after vaccination that lasts for up to 2 days.[93] Respiratory disease is considered coincidental and unrelated to vaccination. Side effects in children were more prominent with the whole-virus vaccines and included a "flu-like" illness with local reactions at the site of injections. These side effects are much reduced with the use of subvirion vaccines. Therefore the use of whole-virus vaccines in children under the age of 13 is not recommended. Immediate (allergic) reactions to the vaccine rarely occur after influenza vaccination. Persons with severe egg allergy should not receive the vaccine. Guillain-Barré syndrome occurred in association with use of the 1976 swine influenza vaccine. Subsequent vaccines have not been associated with an increased frequency of Guillain-Barré syndrome.[93] Systemic vasculitis is a very rare reported complication of influenza vaccination.[94] The vasculitis can occur 2 to 20 days after vaccination, and patients have varying combinations of fever, arthralgia, myalgia, and skin lesions. The patients usually recover uneventfully, but one death has been reported in a patient with renal involvement.

Live attenuated influenza virus vaccines are being developed and appear to be promising. The advantages of a live attenuated vaccine include the possibility of administering only one dose, administration by the natural route into the respiratory tract, a wide range of antibody response, and induction of local mucosal immunity.[95] In addition, intranasal inoculation would be more cost-effective, especially in underdeveloped countries. At present there are several types of live influenza vaccines: host-range mutants, temperature-sensitive mutants, cold-adapted variants, and cold-adapted reassortants.[96] The live vaccine that has gained the widest acceptance and is currently being tested in humans is the cold-adapted reassortant type. This vaccine is prepared by obtaining the HA and NA from currently circulating strains and reassorting them with a donor virus that is cold adapted and carries the gene mutations for attenuation. There is evidence that these vaccine viruses are fully attenuated and immunogenic, do not spread even between children, and are genetically stable.[96] Trivalent vaccines of this type are being developed. In a recent study of widespread vaccination of schoolchildren in Russia with the live attenuated vaccine or inactivated vaccine it was found that the live attenuated vaccine was at least as protective if not more protective than the inactivated vaccine.[97] In addition, the live vaccine appeared to reduce the illness rates in staff and unvaccinated children, thus suggesting that viral transmission had been reduced by the vaccine.

RECENT INFLUENZA ACTIVITY

The influenza season occurs during the winter months, with a peak incidence during December, January, and February in the Northern Hemisphere. Winter circulation in the Southern Hemisphere likely maintains the viruses during the northern summer months. Influenza activity in the United States is monitored by Centers for Disease Control (CDC) surveillance systems in cooperation with state and local health departments from October through April. The CDC also receives reports of worldwide influenza activity from the WHO. There is no required reporting of influenza activity in the United States. Up-to-date information regarding influenza activity can be obtained by telephone through the CDC voice information system, through local and state health departments, and in the *Morbidity and Mortality Weekly Report.*

The predominant influenza viral isolate during the 1992–1993 season was influenza B (73%).[98] Outbreaks were reported primarily among school-aged children, and no excess occurred in influenza-associated mortality. However, widespread activity peaking during February was reported for 26 states. Although influenza type A viruses circulated at low levels initially, the number and proportion of influenza A isolates increased late in the season. More H3N2 (89%) subtype influenza A viruses were isolated during this season than H1N1 (11%) subtype viruses. Increased influenza A (H3N2) activity was concurrent with an increase in the proportion of total deaths associated with pneumonia and influenza. Worldwide influenza activity was considered to be moderate. The influenza B and influenza A (H1N1) viruses isolated during this season were antigenically similar to the virus in the 1992–1993 vaccine. Of the influenza A (H3N2) viruses isolated, 87% were not like the vaccine strain but were antigenically similar to a more recently detected variant, A/Beijing/32/92. This likely accounted for the diminished effectiveness of the 1992–1993 vaccine against the influenza A (H3N2) strains. Based on data collected from the 1992–1993 influenza season, the Food and Drug Administration Vaccines and Related Biologicals Advisory Committee recommended that the trivalent vaccine for the 1993–1994 season contain A/Texas/36/91-like (H1N1), A/Beijing/32/92-like (H3N2), and B/Panama/45/90-like viruses.[99] The only difference between this vaccine and the previous one was for the type A (H3N2) viruses.

Although sporadic cases of influenza can occur at any time, outbreaks rarely occur during the summer in the United States. Thus it was unusual for three outbreaks of influenza A (H3N2) to occur in Louisiana in August 1993.[100] The first outbreak occurred in a nursing home and affected 79 residents and 20 staff members. Twenty-five ill residents were hospitalized, and 2 had radiographic evidence of pneumonia. The second outbreak also occurred in a nursing home and affected 46% of the residents, and the third outbreak occurred among persons living and working on a dredging barge. Over half of the people on the barge were affected, and 4 were hospitalized. The virus isolated in all three of these outbreaks was antigenically similar to the influenza A (H3N2) virus that had circulated during the previous season and was included in the 1993–1994 vaccine. These early outbreaks were possible indicators of an early and more severe 1993–1994 influenza season. The CDC therefore recommended that vaccination programs begin in September rather than the routine mid-October through mid-November schedule. Influenza activity during November and early December 1993 was higher than that usually reported, with regional and widespread activity being reported in several states.[101] Widespread activity continued in January, with the deaths from pneumonia and influenza exceeding the epidemic threshold. Ninety-nine percent of the isolates were influenza type A, with the H3N2 subtype predominating. High levels of influenza activity were expected to continue throughout January 1994.

REFERENCES

1. Beveridge WIB: *Influenza: The Last Great Plague*. New York, Prodist, 1977.
2. Webster RG: On the origin of pandemic influenza viruses. *Curr Top Microbiol Immunol* 59:75–105, 1972.
3. International Committee on Taxonomy of Viruses: Fourth report. *Intervirology* 17:106–107, 1982.
4. WHO Memorandum: A revised system of nomenclature for influenza viruses. *Bull WHO* 45:119–124, 1971.
5. Chu CM, Dawson IM, Elford WJ: Filamentous forms associated with newly isolated influenza virus. *Lancet* 1:602–603, 1949.
6. Chopin PN, Murphy JS, Tamm I: Studies of two kinds of virus particles which comprise influenza A2 virus strains. III. Morphological characteristics: Independence of morphological and functional traits. *J Exp Med* 112:945–952, 1960.
7. Lamb RA: The genes and proteins of the influenza viruses, in Krug RM: *The Influenza Viruses*. New York, Plenum, 1989, pp 1–87.
8. Wilson IA, Skehel JJ, Wiley DC: Structure of the hemagglutinin mem-

brane glycoprotein of influenza at 3f resolution. *Nature* 289:366–373, 1981.
9. Varghese JN, Laver WG, Colman PM: Structure of the influenza virus glycoprotein antigen neuraminidase at 2.9f. *Nature* 303:35–40, 1983.
10. Murphy BR, Kasel JA, Chanock RM: Association of serum antineuraminidase antibody with resistance to influenza in man. *N Engl J Med* 286:1329–1332, 1972.
11. Herrler G, Rott R, Klenk H-D, et al: The receptor-destroying enzyme of influenza C virus is neuraminate-O-acetylesterase. *EMBO J* 4:1503–1506, 1985.
12. Lamb RA, Zebedee SL, Richardson CD: Influenza virus M2 protein is an integral membrane protein expressed on the infected-cell surface. *Cell* 40:627–633, 1985.
13. Wang C, Takeuchi K, Pinto LH, et al: Ion channel activity of influenza A virus M2 protein: Characterization of the amantadine block. *J Virol* 67:5585–5594, 1993.
14. Noble GR: Epidemiological and clinical aspects of influenza, in Beare AS: *Basic and Applied Influenza Research*. Boca Raton, Fla, CRC, 1982, pp 11–50.
15. Webster RG, Bean WJ, Gorman OT, et al: Evolution and ecology of influenza A viruses. *Microbiol Rev* 56:152–179, 1992.
16. Yamaoka M, Hotta H, Ito M, et al: Prevalence of antibody to influenza C virus among pigs in Hyogo Prefecture, Japan. *J Gen Virol* 72:711–714, 1991.
17. Kawaoka Y, Yamnikova S, Chambers T, et al: Molecular characterization of a new hemagglutinin, subtype H14, of influenza A virus. *Virology* 179:759–767, 1990.
18. Gorman OT, Bean WJ, Webster RG: Evolutionary processes in influenza viruses: Divergence, rapid evolution and stasis. *Curr Top Microbiol Immunol* 176:75–97, 1992.
19. Glezen WP, Couch RB, Six HR: The influenza herald wave. *Am J Epidemiol* 116:589–598, 1982.
20. Scholtissek C, Rhode W, Von Hoyningen V, et al: On the origin of the human influenza virus subtypes H2N2 and H3N2. *Virology* 87:3–20, 1978.
21. Kawaoka Y, Krauss S, Webster RG: Avian-to-human transmission of the PB1 gene of influenza A viruses in the 1957 and 1968 pandemics. *J Virol* 63:4603–4608, 1989.
22. Kida H, Shortridge KF, Webster RG: Origin of the hemagglutinin gene of H3N2 influenza viruses from pigs in China. *Virology* 162:160–166, 1988.
23. Kendal AP, Goldfield M, Noble GR: Identification and preliminary antigenic analysis of swine influenza-like viruses isolated during an influenza outbreak at Fort Dix, New Jersey. *J Infect Dis* 136:5381–5385, 1977.

24. Palese P, Shulman JL: RNA pattern of "swine" influenza virus isolated from man is similar to those of other swine influenza viruses. *Nature* 263:528–530, 1976.
25. Douglas RG Jr: Influenza in man, in Kilbourne ED: *Influenza Viruses and Influenza*. New York, Academic, 1975, p 395.
26. Couch RB, Douglas RG Jr, Fedson DS, et al: Correlated studies of a recombinant influenza virus vaccine: III. Protection against experimental influenza in man. *J Infect Dis* 124:473–480, 1971.
27. Louria DB, Blumenfeld HL, Ellis JT, et al: Studies on influenza in the pandemic of 1957–1958: II. Pulmonary complications of influenza. *J Clin Invest* 38:213–265, 1959.
28. Murphy BR, Baron S, Chelhub EG, et al: Temperature sensitive mutants of influenza virus. IV. Induction of interferon in the nasopharynx by wild-type and a temperature-sensitive recombinant virus. *J Infect Dis* 128:488, 1973.
29. Frank AL, Taber LH, Wells CR, et al: Patterns of shedding of myxoviruses and paramyxoviruses in children. *J Infect Dis* 144:433–441, 1981.
30. Berg RA, Yolken RH, Rennard SI, et al: New enzyme immunoassays for measurement of influenza A/Victoria/3/75 virus in nasal washes: A preliminary report. *Lancet* 1:851–853, 1980.
31. Ebisawa IT, Kitamoto O: Persistence of viral antigen in the nasal epithelium in complicated influenza. *Am Rev Respir Dis* 99:275–278, 1969.
32. Hers JF, Molder J: Broad aspects of the pathology and pathogenesis of human influenza. *Am Rev Respir Dis* 83(suppl):54–67, 84–97, 1961.
33. Walsh JJ, Dietlein LF, Low FN, et al: Bronchotracheal response in human influenza. *Arch Intern Med* 108:376–388, 1961.
34. Oseasohn R, Adelson JW, Kaji M: Clinicopathologic study of thirty-three fatal cases of Asian influenza. *N Engl J Med* 260:509–518, 1959.
35. Stanley ED, Jackson GG: Viremia in Asian influenza. *Trans Assoc Am Physicians* 79:376, 1966.
36. Engblom E, Ekfors TO, Meurman OH, et al: Fatal influenza A myocarditis with isolation of virus from the myocardium. *Acta Med Scand* 213:75–78, 1983.
37. Paisley JW, Bruhn FW, Lauer BA, et al: Type A2 influenza viral infections in children. *Am J Dis Child* 132:34–36, 1978.
38. Glezen WP: Morbidity associated with the major respiratory viruses. *Pediatr Ann* 19:535–542, 1990.
39. Hall WN, Goodman RA, Noble GR, et al: An outbreak of influenza B in an elderly population. *J Infect Dis* 144:297–302, 1981.
40. Lennon DR, Cherry JD, Morgenstein A, et al: Longitudinal study of influenza B symptomatology and interferon production in children and college students. *Pediatr Infect Dis J* 2:212–215, 1983.
41. DeStefano F: An outbreak of influenza B at an Indiana boarding

school: Estimate of vaccine efficacy. *Public Health Rep* 97:269–272, 1982.

42. Katagiri S, Ohizumi A, Homma M: An outbreak of type C influenza in a children's home. *J Infect Dis* 148:51–56, 1983.
43. Dykes AC, Cherry JD, Nolan CE: A clinical, epidemiologic, serologic and virologic study of influenza C virus infection. *Arch Intern Med* 140:1295–1298, 1980.
44. Homma M: Epidemiological characteristics of type C influenza. *J Cell Biochem (Suppl)* 9:278, 1985.
45. Stuart-Harris CH, Schild GC: In *Influenza. The Viruses and the Disease.* London, Edward Arnold, 1977.
46. Imboden JB, Canter A, Cluff LE: Convalescence from influenza. *Arch Intern Med* 108:393–399, 1961.
47. Kim HW, Brandt CD, Arrobio JO, et al: Influenza A and B infection in infants and young children during the years 1957–1976. *Am J Epidemiol* 109:464–479, 1979.
48. Brocklebank JT, Court SDM: Influenza A infection in children. *Lancet* 2:497–500, 1972.
49. Glezen WP, Paredes A, Taber LH: Influenza in children. *JAMA* 243:1345–1349, 1980.
50. Sugaya N, Nerome K, Ishida M, et al: Impact of influenza virus infection as a cause of pediatric hospitalization. *J Infect Dis* 165:373–375, 1992.
51. Putto A, Ruskanen O, Meurman O: Fever in respiratory virus infections. *Am J Dis Child* 140:1159–1163, 1986.
52. Cherry JD: Influenza viral infections, in Vaugh V, McKay R, Behrman R: *Nelson Textbook of Pediatrics*, ed 11. Philadelphia, WB Saunders, 1979, pp 893–897.
53. Price DA, Postlethwaite RJ, Longson M: Influenza virus A2 infection presenting with febrile convulsions and gastrointestinal symptoms in young children. *Clin Pediatr (Phila)* 15:361–367, 1976.
54. Merbalane R, Sedmak GV, Sasidharan P, et al: Outbreak of influenza in a neonatal intensive care unit. *J Pediatr* 91:974–976, 1977.
55. Dagan R, Hall CB: Influenza A virus infection imitating bacterial sepsis in early infancy. *Pediatr Infect Dis J* 3:218–221, 1984.
56. Fernandez H: Low serum iron in influenza. *N Engl J Med* 302:865, 1980.
57. Feldman S, Webster RG, Sugg M: Influenza in children and young adults with cancer. *Cancer* 39:350–353, 1977.
58. Kempe A, Hall CB, MacDonald NE, et al: Influenza in children with cancer. *Pediatrics* 115:33–39, 1989.
59. Ljungman P, Andersson J, Aschan J, et al: Influenza A in immunocompromised patients. *Clin Infect Dis* 17:244–247, 1993.
60. Frank Jr JA, Warren EW, Tucker JA, et al: Disseminated parainfluenza infection in a child with severe combined immunodeficiency. *Am J Dis Child* 137:1172–1174, 1983.

61. Josephs S, Kim HW, Brandt CD, et al: Parainfluenza 3 virus and other common respiratory pathogens in children with human immunodeficiency virus infection. *Pediatr Infect Dis J* 7:207–208, 1988.
62. Jarvis WR, Middleton PJ, Gelfand EW: Parainfluenza pneumonia in severe combined immunodeficiency disease. *J Pediatr* 94:423–429, 1979.
63. Flomberg PR, Horwitz MS: Molecular epidemiology of adenovirus type 35 infections in immunocompromised hosts. *J Infect Dis* 155:1127–1134, 1987.
64. Farrell MK, Partin JC, Bove KE, et al: Epidemic influenza myopathy in Cincinnati in 1977. *J Pediatr* 96:545–551, 1980.
65. Kessler HA, Trenholme GM, Harris AA, et al: Acute myopathy associated with influenza A/Texas/1/77 infection. Isolation of virus from a muscle biopsy specimen. *JAMA* 243:461–462, 1980.
66. Centers for Disease Control: Toxic shock syndrome associated with influenza: Minnesota. *MMWR* 35:43–144, 1986.
67. Tolan RW: Toxic shock syndrome complicating influenza A in a child: Case report and review. *Clin Infect Dis* 17:43–45, 1993.
68. Morgonsen JL: Myoglobinuria and renal failure associated with influenza. *Ann Intern Med* 80:362–363, 1974.
69. Coltman CA Jr: Influenza myocarditis. Report of a case with observations on serum glutamic oxaloacetic transaminase. *JAMA* 180:204–208, 1962.
70. Flewett TH, Hoult JG: Influenza encephalopathy and post-influenza encephalitis. *Lancet* 2:11–15, 1958.
71. Smith TF, Wold AD, Espy MJ, et al: New developments in the diagnosis of viral diseases. *Infect Dis Clin North Am* 7:183–201, 1993.
72. Bartholoma NY, Forbes BA: Successful use of shell vial centrifugation and 16 to 18 hour immunofluorescence staining for the detection of influenza A and B in clinical specimens. *Am J Clin Pathol* 92:487–490, 1989.
73. Mills RD, Cain KJ, Woods GL: Detection of influenza virus by centrifugal inoculation of MDCK cells and staining with monoclonal antibodies. *J Clin Microbiol* 27:2505–2508, 1989.
74. Matthey S, Nicholson D, Ruhs S, et al: Rapid detection of respiratory viruses by shell vial culture and direct staining by using pooled and individual monoclonal antibodies. *J Clin Microbiol* 30:540–544, 1992.
75. Rabalais GP, Stout GG, Ladd KL, et al: Rapid diagnosis of respiratory viral infections by using a shell vial assay and monoclonal antibody pool. *J Clin Microbiol* 30:1505–1508, 1992.
76. Waner JL, Todd SJ, Shalaby H, et al: Comparison of Directigen Flu-A with viral isolation and direct immunofluorescence for the rapid detection and identification of influenza A virus. *J Clin Microbiol* 29:479–482, 1991.
77. Ryan-Poirier KA, Katz JW, Webster RG, et al: Application of Directi-

gen FLU-A for detection of influenza A viruses in human and nonhuman specimens. *J Clin Microbiol* 30:1072–1075, 1992.
78. Hay AJ, Wolstenbolme AJ, Skehel JJ, et al: The molecular basis of the specific anti-influenza action of amantadine. *EMBO J* 4:3021–3024, 1985.
79. Sugrue RJ, dur Baha G, Zambon MC, et al: Specific structural alteration of the influenza hemagglutinin by amantadine. *EMBO J* 9:3469–3476, 1990.
80. Van Voris LP, Betts RF, Hayden PG, et al: Successful treatment of naturally occurring influenza A/USSR/77 H1N1. *JAMA* 245:1128–1131, 1981.
81. Thompson J, Fleet W, Lawrence E, et al: A comparison of acetaminophen and rimantadine in the treatment of influenza A infection in children. *J Med Virol* 21:249–255, 1987.
82. Breese Hall C, Dolin R, Gala CL, et al: Children with influenza A infection: Treatment with rimantadine. *Pediatrics* 80:275–282, 1987.
83. Belshe RB, Burk B, Newman F, et al: Resistance of influenza A virus to amantadine and rimantadine: Results of one decade of surveillance. *J Infect Dis* 159:430–435, 1989.
84. Little JW, Hall WJ, Douglas RG Jr, et al: Amantadine effect on peripheral airways abnormalities in influenza: A study in 15 students with natural influenza A infection. *J Intern Med* 85:177–182, 1976.
85. Hayden FG, Hall WJ, Douglas RG Jr: Therapeutic effects of aerosolized amantadine in naturally acquired infection due to influenza A virus. *J Infect Dis* 141:535–542, 1980.
86. Jackson GG, Stanley ED: Prevention and control of influenza by chemoprophylaxis and chemotherapy: Prospects from examination of recent experience. *JAMA* 235:2739–2742, 1976.
87. Tsunoda A, Maasab HF, Cochran KW, et al: Antiviral activity of alpha-methyl-1-admantane-methylamine hydrochloride. *Antimicrob Agents Chemother* 5:53–60, 1986.
88. Dolin R, Reichman RC, Madore HP, et al: A controlled trial of amantadine and rimantadine in the prophylaxis of influenza A infection. *N Engl J Med* 307:580–584, 1982.
89. Centers for Disease Control: Prevention and control of influenza. Recommendations of the Immunization Practices Advisory Committee. *MMWR* 41:1–17, 1992.
90. Gilbert BE, Wilson SZ, Knight V, et al: Ribavirin small particle aerosol treatment of infections caused by influenza strains A/Victoria/7/83 (H1N1) and B/Texas/1/84. *Antimicrob Agents Chemother* 27:309–313, 1985.
91. McClung HW, Knight V, Gilbert BE, et al: Ribavirin aerosol treatment of influenza B virus infection. *JAMA* 249:2671–2674, 1983.
92. Woods JM, Bethell RC, Coates JA, et al: 4-Guanidino-2,4-dideoxy-2,3-dehydro-N-acetylneuraminic acid is a highly effective inhibitor both of the sialidase (neuraminidase) and of growth of a wide range of

influenza A and B viruses in vitro. *Antimicrob Agents Chemother* 37:1473–1479, 1993.

93. Centers for Disease Control: Prevention and control of influenza: Part 1, vaccines. Recommendations of the Advisory Committee on Immunization Practices (ACIP). *MMWR* 42:1–14, 1993.
94. Mader R, Narendran A, Lewtas J: Systemic vasculitis following influenza vaccination; report of 3 cases and review of the literature. *J Rheumatol* 20:1429–1431, 1993.
95. Maassab HF, Heilman CA, Herlocher ML: Cold-adapted influenza viruses for use as live vaccines for man, in Mizrahi A: *Advances in Biotechnological Processes,* vol 14, *Viral Vaccines.* New York, Wiley-Liss, 1990, pp 203–242.
96. Ghendon Y: Vaccination against influenza viruses: Current status, in Mizrahi A: *Advances in Biotechnological Processes,* vol 14, *Viral Vaccines.* New York, Wiley-Liss, 1990, pp 159–201.
97. Rudenko LG, Slepushkin AN, Monto AS, et al: Efficacy of live attenuated and inactivated influenza vaccines in schoolchildren and their unvaccinated contacts in Novgorod, Russia. *J Infect Dis* 168:881–887, 1993.
98. Centers for Disease Control: Update: Influenza activity—United States, 1992–93 season. *MMWR* 42:385–387, 1993.
99. Centers for Disease Control: Update: Influenza activity—United States and worldwide, and composition of the 1993–94 influenza vaccine. *MMWR* 42:177–179, 1993.
100. Centers for Disease Control: Influenza A outbreaks—Louisiana, August 1993. *MMWR* 42:689–691, 1993.
101. Centers for Disease Control: Update: Influenza activity—United States, 1993–94 season. *MMWR* 42:1–3, 1994.

Hepatitis E

Arnold Wald, M.D.
Professor of Medicine, University of Pittsburgh, Division of Gastroenterology and Hepatology, University of Pittsburgh Medical Center, Pittsburgh, Pennsylvania

Enterically transmitted non-A, non-B (ET-NANB) hepatitis has caused large epidemics as well as smaller outbreaks and sporadic cases of viral hepatitis in many regions of the developing world. Strenuous efforts have been made to identify the causative agent and develop diagnostic tests to detect evidence of viral infection. Such efforts have culminated in characterization of hepatitis E virus (HEV), the organism responsible for most if not all cases of ET-NANB hepatitis studied to date.

EPIDEMIOLOGY

An epidemic of ET-NANB hepatitis was first documented during a large outbreak of water-borne hepatitis in New Delhi, India, in 1955. This outbreak involved an estimated 29,000 icteric cases and was associated with fecal contamination of the water supply to the city.[1] Subsequent epidemics have been described throughout Asia,[2–7] the central Asian region of the Soviet Union,[8] large parts of northern and eastern Africa,[9, 10] and Mexico[11, 12] (Fig 1). Most have been common source outbreaks of relatively short duration thought to be related to fecally contaminated water, although some outbreaks have lasted many months to several years.

Sporadic cases have also been reported in underdeveloped countries and have exhibited disease characteristics similar to those of the larger epidemics.[13] Indeed, hepatitis E is implicated in over half of sporadic cases of acute viral hepatitis in developing countries. In contrast, hepatitis E has been reported uncommonly in Europe, the United States, and other countries where sanitation systems are more developed and protection of water supplies is more secure. The few documented cases of hepatitis E reported in the United States have occurred in travelers to underdeveloped areas who have been exposed to contaminated water.[14]

Unique features of hepatitis E (ET-NANB) outbreaks have helped to distinguish it from other causes of viral hepatitis. Foremost among them is that ET-NANB hepatitis exhibits high clinical

Advances in Pediatric Infectious Diseases®, vol. 10

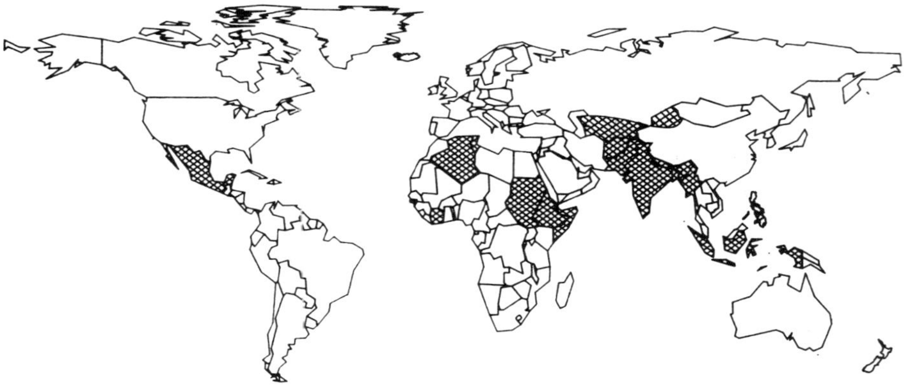

FIGURE 1.
Areas in which outbreaks of enterically transmitted non-A, non-B hepatitis (hepatitis E) have been reported. (From Hadler SC, Margolis HS: Viral hepatitis, in Evans AS: *Viral Infections of Humans: Epidemiology and Control,* ed 3. New York, Plenum, 1989, pp 351–391. Used by permission.)

attack rates among young to middle-aged adults, with the highest age-specific prevalence of clinical infection between 20 and 30 years of age. Clinical attack rates among adults have ranged from 3% to 13%, whereas among children less than 15 years of age, clinical attack rates range from 0.2% to 1.5%.[8, 12, 13] This is in contrast to hepatitis A, which occurs uncommonly in adults in these areas who, because of almost universal exposure as children to hepatitis A virus (HAV), have acquired long-lasting immunity. This suggests that hepatitis E rarely affects children, that it causes mostly subclinical infections in children, or that it commonly infects children but does not result in long-lasting immunity. In a recent prospective study of endemic acute hepatitis in a rural area of Egypt,[15] 42% of 36 children with NANB hepatitis were found to have IgG anti-HEV by enzyme-linked immunosorbent assay (ELISA). Of the 15 children who were IgG-positive, 40% had IgM anti-HEV. Similar findings were noted in acute sporadic cases of hepatitis in children living in an urban area in the Sudan.[16] This suggests that the number of overt infections of HEV in children is probably small relative to the number of subclinical infections. In the absence of readily available serologic tests and the difficulty in obtaining liver enzyme studies in large populations during these outbreaks, there are no data concerning the ratio of clinically overt to subclinical disease by age.

Another feature of hepatitis E is its relatively low secondary attack rates among exposed household contacts, perhaps suggesting that a high inoculum is required for transmission. As an example, in only 2.4% of household contacts of individuals with ET-NANB hepatitis did clinical disease develop during the 1981–1982 epidemic in Nepal, which contrasts with a secondary attack rate of 10% to 20% in HAV infections occurring in the same regions.[5] On the other hand, studies of a small Mexican outbreak of ET-NANB hepatitis found that only a minority of infected individuals used water from a stream or well thought to be fecally contaminated[12] and that contact with an individual with hepatitis from another household was an independent risk factor for the disease. This latter study suggests that person-to-person transmission is a potentially important means of infection.

Finally, ET-NANB hepatitis exhibits a disproportionately high case fatality ratio when it infects women during the third trimester of pregnancy. This is a characteristic that has not been observed with other forms of viral hepatitis. Death has been associated with fulminant hepatitis and liver failure.

HEPATITIS E VIRUS

Immune electron microscopy (IEM) has identified virus-like particles (VLPs) in stool samples of patients during the early course of several epidemics of ET-NANB hepatitis in Asia (Table 1 and Fig 2). Virus-like particles of two sizes, 27 to 30 and 32 to 34 nm, have been found,[8] but it is the larger particles that react specifically to acute-phase and convalescent sera of established cases from many different outbreaks.[17] Further evidence to support the

TABLE 1.
Properties of Hepatitis E Virus

Size	32–34 nm in diameter
Morphology	Spherical, nonenveloped
	Spikes and indentations on surface
Genome	Single-stranded, polyadenylated RNA
	Approximately 7.6 kb
	3 open reading frames
	ORF 1: nonstructural proteins
	ORF 2: structural proteins
	ORF 3: unknown function(s)

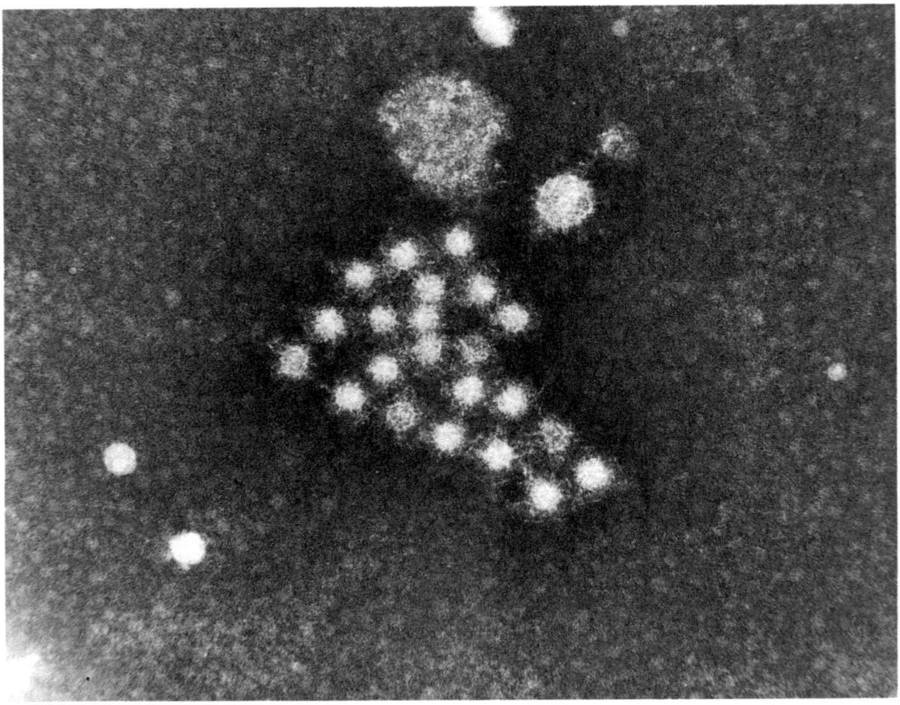

FIGURE 2.
Electron micrograph of typical 32- to 34-nm virus particles recovered from the stool of a patient with enterically transmitted non-A, non-B hepatitis in Mexico. Particles are morphologically indistinguishable from those recovered from similar cases in Borneo, India, Somalia, and Tashkent, Russia. (Courtesy of Dr. Daniel W. Bradley, Centers for Disease Control, Atlanta.)

association between the larger VLPs and ET-NANB hepatitis has been obtained from primate studies that demonstrate seroconversion following experimental infections with ET-NANB hepatitis.[8, 17] It has been hypothesized that the 27- to 30-nm VLPs may be a degradation product of the larger particles or, alternatively, represent a coexisting virus that is unrelated to ET-NANB hepatitis.[8]

Recently, the HEV genome has been cloned and sequenced.[18–20] Three open reading frames (ORFs) have been identified; ORF 1 encodes for nonstructural proteins, ORF 2 is probably responsible for synthesizing structural protein components, and ORF 3 encodes for 123–amino acid proteins of unknown function.[19] Two epitopes have been localized to the C-terminus of proteins encoded by ORF 2 and ORF 3.[21] When expressed as hybrid proteins, the two epitopes have been shown to bind antibodies present in the acute and convalescent phase of HEV-infected nonhuman primates[19] and humans.[15] These synthetic peptides are being used for the development of immunodiagnostic assays for detecting antibodies to HEV.[15] Hepatitis E virus consists of a single-stranded polyadenylated RNA virus that has not yet been officially classified. Its structure and genome organization appear to be similar to those of caliciviruses,[8] a family that has characteristics similar to those of picornaviruses.

PRIMATE STUDIES

Transmission of ET-NANB hepatitis to nonhuman primates was first reported in cynomolgus macaques in 1983[22] and subsequently in African green monkeys, tamarins, chimpanzees, and rhesus monkeys.[8] Inoculation of primates with fecal samples obtained from patients with established infection has resulted in transmission of hepatitis. Virus-like particles in the bile and stool have been documented before biochemical and clinical illness. Elevations in transaminase concentrations occur between 30 and 80 days after inoculation and are accompanied by elimination of VLPs from bile. Serum IgM and IgG antibodies appear coincident with resolution of the increase in enzyme concentration and clinical recovery.[23, 24] Histopathologic changes characteristic of acute viral hepatitis have been noted in infected animals.

These animal studies support the concept that HEV replicates in the liver and is deposited in feces via the biliary tract. The development of hepatocellular necrosis inhibits or eliminates viral replication, with disappearance of VLPs from the bile and feces when liver enzyme levels increase. The development of serum antibodies signals the end of the hepatic phase and heralds biochemical and clinical recovery. However, if seroconversion does not occur, relapsing hepatitis can ensue, although chronic hepatitis has not been demonstrated.

DIAGNOSTIC STUDIES

The diagnosis of HEV infection was initially based on detection of VLPs of 27 to 34 nm in the stools of acutely ill persons by IEM and the absence of serologic evidence of hepatitis A, B, and C, Epstein-Barr virus, and cytomegalovirus. However, this proved unsatisfactory because the required instruments are expensive and

TABLE 2.
Serologic Diagnosis of Hepatitis E Virus Infection

Fluorescent antibody blocking assay	Detects antibody that reacts with HEV* antigen in hepatocytes
Western blot assay	Recombinant antigens detect IgM and IgG antibody to HEV
ELISA*	Detects IgM and IgG antibodies by using recombinant expressed HEV antigen

*HEV = hepatitis E virus; ELISA = enzyme-linked immunosorbent assay.

many stool specimens do not contain sufficient VLPs for easy detection.

Specific antibodies that aggregate HEV particles (anti-HEV) have been detected in the sera of infected patients by IEM (Table 2). Another technique involves immunofluorescence in which a fluorescein-conjugated IgG fraction from anti-HEV serum is used to detect viral antigen in liver tissue sections of HEV-infected cynomolgus macaques.[25] More recently, encoded recombinant HEV structural proteins have been expressed in strains of *Escherichia coli* and used to detect both IgM and IgG antibodies to HEV with Western blot assays.[16, 26]

More promising diagnostic tests under development include an ELISA based on clonal recombinant HEV antigens[15, 24] to detect IgG and IgM antibodies in serum and the use of polymerase chain amplification to detect HEV in stools of acutely infected patients.[27, 28] The ELISA assay has not been approved in the United States as yet, but an assay based on the use of an IgG protein is commercially available in Asia through Genelabs Technologies, Inc., (San Antonio). The availability of the HEV ELISA in the Pacific Rim has been used to carry out epidemiologic surveys and should result in better definition of the worldwide distribution of hepatitis E.

CLINICAL FEATURES

In individual patients, hepatitis E is a self-limiting disease that resembles hepatitis A and cannot be distinguished from other forms of viral hepatitis on the basis of clinical characteristics alone. The incubation period ranges between 2 and 9 weeks, with an average of 6 weeks. As with other viral hepatidites, fever, arthralgias, nausea, and vomiting are common, and jaundice suggests the diagnosis of hepatitis, although anicteric cases are probably not uncommon. In an extremely well-characterized case of hepatitis E studied in a human volunteer who deliberately infected himself,[29] anicteric hepatitis began 30 days postinoculation. This was followed by icterus 8 days later that lasted until day 120 (Fig 3). Hepatitis E virus was detected in serum and stool during the preicteric phase by using reverse transcription/polymerase chain amplification. Serum IgG anti-HEV has persisted for 2 years after complete recovery. In this volunteer, abnormal transaminase levels lasted about 3 months, in contrast to only 2 to 3 weeks in monkeys. The presence of HEV in blood suggests that parenteral transmission of HEV can occur, as was suggested by a report of a hospital outbreak of hepatitis E.[30]

Although most patients have a mild to moderate illness, severe hepatitis with mortality rates as high as 12% has been reported.[31] However, severe disease most commonly occurs in pregnant women during their last trimester, with mortality rates averaging 20% in most epidemics and death occurring in all 9 pregnant women in one outbreak.[9] It is unclear why this is so since a predilection for severe disease in pregnant women is not characteristic of the other forms of viral hepatitis.

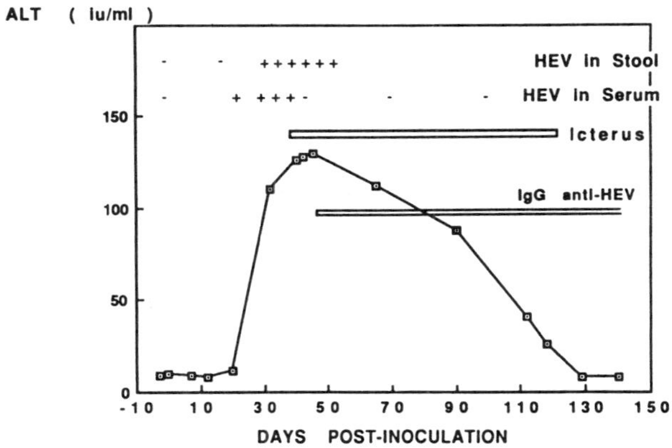

FIGURE 3.

Hepatitis E virus *(HEV)* infection in a volunteer. The aminotransferase *(ALT)* levels are plotted as international units per milliliter. Hepatitis E detection in stool and serum was by reverse transcription/polymerase chain amplification. Serum IgG anti-HEV was detected by enzyme-linked immunosorbent assay. (From Chauhan A, Jameel S, Dilawari JB, et al: *Lancet* 341:149–150, 1993. Used by permission.)

Clinically and biochemically, hepatitis E can exhibit features of hepatocellular necrosis or present a predominantly cholestatic picture. In general, clinical features correlate with liver histology, although relatively few liver biopsy studies have been reported in humans. For those who survive, recovery is complete, and there have been no reports of chronic hepatitis E infection.

PREVENTION

During epidemics of ET-NANB hepatitis, water sources should be checked for contamination and water boiled before use since there is evidence to suggest that it will reduce disease transmission. For example, boiling drinking water was associated with significantly lower attack rates of ET-NANB hepatitis in two rural villages in Mexico in 1986–1987.[12] Similar evidence for chlorination of water is not available, although it is probably useful during epidemics.[13] Immune serum globulin obtained from donors from areas of the world where hepatitis E is not endemic is unlikely to be effective for prophylaxis. Unfortunately, immunoglobulin preparations manufactured from donors living in endemic regions have not proved to be effective during epidemics of ET-NANB hepatitis in India[32] and Mexico.[13] A vaccine for hepatitis E is in the early stages of development and appears to be promising on the basis of animal studies.[33]

Travelers to endemic regions should be warned to avoid potentially contaminated water and uncooked food and cannot presume to be protected by immune serum globulin. This is particularly important for pregnant women. The diagnosis of hepatitis E should be considered in any person with acute hepatitis who has recently traveled to underdeveloped areas and who has negative serologic studies for hepatitis A, B, and C. Confirmatory assays may be done through Genelabs Technologies, Inc., San Antonio, Texas, with a non–commercially available ELISA assay and Western blot study (Dr. Patrice Yarbough, personal communication, 1994).

REFERENCES

1. Viswanathan R: Epidemiology: Infectious hepatitis in Delhi 1955–1956. *Indian J Med Res* 45(suppl 1):1–29, 1957.
2. Ramalingaswami V, Purcell RH: Waterborne non-A, non-B hepatitis. *Lancet* 1:571–573, 1988.
3. Wong DC, Purcell RH, Sreenivasan MA, et al: Epidemic and endemic hepatitis in India: Evidence for a non-A, non-B hepatitis virus aetiology. Lancet 2:876–879, 1980.
4. Khuroo MS: Study of an epidemic of non-A, non-B hepatitis: Possi-

bility of another human hepatitis virus distinct from post-transfusion non-A, non-B type. *Am J Med* 68:818–824, 1980.
5. Kane MA, Bradley DW, Shrestha SM, et al: Epidemic non-A, non-B hepatitis in Nepal. *JAMA* 252:3140–3145, 1984.
6. DeCock KM, Bradley DW, Sandford NL, et al: Epidemic non-A, non-B hepatitis in patients from Pakistan. *Ann Intern Med* 106:227–230, 1987.
7. Skidmore SJ, Yarbough PO, Gabor KA, et al: Hepatitis E virus: The cause of a waterborne hepatitis outbreak. *J Med Virol* 37:58–60, 1992.
8. Bradley DW: Enterically-transmitted non-A, non-B hepatitis. *Br Med Bull* 46:442–461, 1990.
9. Belabbes, E-H, Bougermouh A, Benatallah A, et al: Epidemic non-A, non-B viral hepatitis in Algeria: Strong evidence for its spreading by water. *J Med Virol* 16:257–263, 1985.
10. Centers for Disease Control: Enterically transmitted non-A, non-B hepatitis—East Africa. *MMWR* 36:241–244, 1987.
11. Centers for Disease Control: Enterically transmitted non-A, non-B hepatitis—Mexico. *MMWR* 36:597–602, 1987.
12. Velasquez O, Stetler HC, Avila C, et al: Epidemic transmission of enterically transmitted non-A, non-B hepatitis in Mexico, 1986–1987. *JAMA* 263:3281–3285, 1990.
13. Hadler SC, Margolis HS: Viral hepatitis, in Evans AS: *Viral Infections of Humans: Epidemiology and Control*, ed 3. New York, Plenum 1989, pp 351–391.
14. Centers for Disease Control: Hepatitis E among U.S. travelers, 1989–1992. *MMWR* 42:1–4, 1993.
15. Goldsmith R, Yarbough PO, Reyes GR, et al: Enzyme-linked immunosorbent assay for diagnosis of acute sporadic hepatitis E in Egyptian children. *Lancet* 339:328–331, 1992.
16. Hyams KC, Purdy MA, Kaur M, et al: Acute sporadic hepatitis E in Sudanese children: Analysis based on a new Western blot assay. *J Infect Dis* 165:1001–1005, 1992.
17. Bradley D, Andjaparidze A, Cook EH, et al: Aetiological agent of enterically transmitted non-A, non-B hepatitis. *J Gen Virol* 69:731–738, 1988.
18. Reyes GR, Purdy MA, Kim JP, et al: Isolation of a cDNA from the virus responsible for enterically transmitted non-A, non-B hepatitis. *Science* 247:1335–1339, 1990.
19. Tam AW, Smith MM, Guerra ME, et al: Hepatitis E virus (HEV): Molecular cloning and sequencing of the full-length viral genome. *Virology* 185:120–131, 1991.
20. Khudyakov YE, Khudyakova NS, Fields HA, et al: Epitope mapping in proteins of hepatitis E virus. *Virology* 194:89–96, 1993.
21. Yarbough PO, Tam AW, Fry KE, et al: Hepatitis E virus: Identification of type-common epitopes. *J Virol* 65:5790–5797, 1991.
22. Balayan MS, Andjaparidze AG, Savinskaya SS, et al: Evidence for a

virus in non-A, non-B hepatitis transmitted via the fecal-oral route. *Intervirology* 20:23–31, 1983.
23. Tsarev SA, Emerson SU, Tsareva TS, et al: Variation in course of hepatitis E in experimentally infected cynomolgus monkeys. *J Infect Dis* 167:1302–1306, 1993.
24. Tsarev SA, Tsareva TS, Emerson SU, et al: ELISA for antibody to hepatitis E virus (HEV) based on complete open-reading frame-2 protein expressed in insect cells: Identification of HEV infections in primates. *J Infect Dis* 168:369–378, 1993.
25. Krawczynski K, Bradley DW: Enterically transmitted non-A, non-B hepatitis: Identification of virus-associated antigen in experimentally infected cynomolgus monkeys. *J Infect Dis* 159:1042–1049, 1989.
26. Favorov MO, Fields HA, Purdy MA, et al: Serologic identification of hepatitis E virus infections in epidemic and endemic settings. *J Med Virol* 36:246–250, 1992.
27. Ray R, Aggarwal R, Salunke PN, et al: Hepatitis E virus genome in stools of hepatitis patients during large epidemic in north India. *Lancet* 338:783–784, 1991.
28. Jameel S, Durgapal H, Habibullah CM, et al: Enteric non-A, non-B hepatitis: Epidemics, animal transmission and hepatitis E virus detection by the polymerase chain reaction. *J Med Virol* 37:263–270, 1992.
29. Chauhan A, Jameel S, Dilawari JB, et al: Hepatitis E virus transmission to a volunteer. *Lancet* 341:149–150, 1993.
30. Robson SC, Adams S, Brink N, et al: Hospital outbreak of hepatitis E. *Lancet* 339:1424–1425, 1992.
31. Tandon BN, Joshi YK, Jain SK, et al: An epidemic of non-A, non-B hepatitis in North India. *Indian J Med Res* 75:739–744, 1982.
32. Joshi YK, Babu S, Sarin S, et al: Immunoprophylaxis of epidemic non-A, non-B hepatitis. *Indian J Med Res* 81:18–19, 1985.
33. Purdy MA, McCaustland KA, Krawcynski K, et al: Preliminary evidence that a trpE-HEV fusion protein protects cynomolgus macaques against challenge with wild-type hepatitis E virus (HEV). *J Med Virol* 41:90–94, 1993.

Adjuvant Therapy in Meningitis

Sheldon L. Kaplan, M.D.
Professor and Vice Chairman for Clinical Affairs, Department of Pediatrics, Baylor College of Medicine; Chief, Infectious Diseases Service, Texas Children's Hospital, Houston, Texas

A greater understanding of the molecular events underlying the pathophysiologic disturbances within the central nervous system during bacterial meningitis has led to new approaches for adjunctive treatment.[1, 2] Most of these measures relate to modulating the host response to infection, which is now thought to be a major factor in development of the neurologic sequelae following bacterial meningitis. Dexamethasone has been the predominant agent evaluated in patients to date, but other therapies have been studied in experimental models of meningitis and may ultimately be shown to be of clinical value.

PATHOPHYSIOLOGY

Cell wall components of *Streptococcus pneumoniae* and lipopolysaccharide (endotoxin) of *Haemophilus influenzae* type b, *Neisseria meningitidis*, or *Escherichia coli* are potent stimuli for the production of tumor necrosis factor (TNF) and interleukin-1β (IL-1β) by various cells within the central nervous system capable of cytokine synthesis. In fact, the levels of TNF and IL-1β in cerebrospinal fluid (CSF) from children with bacterial meningitis correlate with several of the inflammatory parameters in CSF.[3] The cytokines interact with endothelial surfaces to promote neutrophil adherence to endothelium and their transendothelial passage. Products released by neutrophils and bacteria as well as other molecules associated with the inflammatory process (prostaglandins, platelet activating factor) are injurious to the endothelium and result in alteration of the blood-brain barrier (disruption of tight intercellular junctions) leading to the development of vasogenic edema.[4] Substances released by bacteria or neutrophils (oxygen free radicals), certain cytokines, and other inflammatory mediators are toxic to neuronal cells and result in cytotoxic edema.[5] The inflammatory response also impedes normal CSF resorption by arachnoid villi, and thus an increase in CSF volume is associated with transient ventricular dilation.

The cerebral edema and greater CSF volume are the primary factors leading to increased intracranial pressure (ICP) in patients with bacterial meningitis. Cerebral blood flow (CBF) may be impaired in association with increased ICP, as well as in relation to specific vascular insults such as local vasculitis and thrombosis of intracranial vessels. In the one study of CBF in children with acute bacterial meningitis, Ashwal et al.[6] found that in 13 of 20 children total CBF was normal, although marked local variability of flow was observed. In 5 other children total CBF was significantly reduced, and in 2 brain-dead children CBF was absent. However, these children were more severely ill than the typical patient with bacterial meningitis (coma, 12; seizures, 15; paralysis, 7; cranial nerve dysfunction, 8; respiratory impairment, 10), and these results may not be generalizable to all patients. Autoregulation of CBF was preserved in these children.

The pathogenesis of hearing loss following bacterial meningitis is related to the development of bacterial labyrinthitis.[7] Bacteria may reach the cochlea via the cochlear aqueduct (which allows bacteria to move from the subarachnoid space to the cochlea)[8] or may travel with the eighth cranial nerve through the internal auditory canal. Loss of hair cells, calcification of perilymphatic channels, and/or damage to the auditory nerve results in various degrees of sensorineural hearing loss.

In children this hearing loss appears to occur early in the clinical course of meningitis since it can be detected within 24 to 48 hours of hospital admission by evoked response audiometry.[9] The factor that correlates best with the risk of deafness developing is the initial CSF glucose concentration.[10, 11] Patients with a CSF glucose level less than 20 mg/dL are more likely to suffer deafness than if the level is over 20 mg/dL for reasons that are unclear. In a rabbit model of pneumococcal meningitis following intracisternal injection of *S. pneumoniae*, hearing loss was associated with increases in protein and lactate concentrations and CSF leukocytosis, but not with CSF glucose concentrations.[12] The authors concluded that hypoglycorrhachia is not an essential factor in the development of hearing loss from meningitis. However, since the route by which the bacteria reach the CSF is not hematogenous in this model, the findings regarding glucose as a marker for deafness may not be applicable to most children with bacterial meningitis.

DEXAMETHASONE TRIALS

The efficacy and safety of corticosteroids in the adjunctive treatment of serious bacterial infections have been studied for many years. The initial trials of dexamethasone for bacterial meningitis in the late 1960s were inconclusive, but a resurgence of interest in this subject occurred following the studies of McCracken and others who helped elucidate the pathophysiologic changes that occur at a molecular level during bacterial meningitis. These concepts coupled with the knowledge that dexamethasone can modulate TNF production stimulated the Dallas group to reinitiate the study of dexamethasone in bacterial meningitis.[13, 14]

By now the details of the first two studies conducted in Dallas are well known to most physicians caring for children.[13] The studies were prospective, placebo-controlled trials in which dexamethasone plus antibiotic was compared with placebo and antibiotic in the treatment of bacterial meningitis in children. A substantial problem with the first study was that cefuroxime was chosen as the antibiotic; it is now known that cefuroxime is not an optimal agent for treating bacterial meningitis. In the second study ceftriaxone was the antibiotic employed. The timing between the first doses of dexamethasone and parenteral antibiotic was not specified. The major finding of these combined studies was that moderate to more severe bilateral hearing loss occurred in 15.5% of placebo vs. 3.3% of dexamethasone-treated children ($P < .01$). In the ceftriaxone study there were no significant differences between the two treatment groups with respect to other neurologic abnormalities at 1-year follow-up assessments (6 of 41 for placebo vs. 2 of 43 for dexamethasone-treated children).

In another trial conducted at the National Children's Hospital in Costa Rica, placebo or dexamethasone was administered 15 to 20 minutes before the first antibiotic dose.[14] This change in the timing of administration in relation to the first dose of cefotaxime was based on an impressive increase in the CSF concentrations of lipopolysaccharide and cytokines occurring within hours after a single antibiotic dose was given to rabbits with *H. influenzae* type b meningitis. A similar increase in CSF endotoxin levels occurs in children with *H. influenzae* type b meningitis 2 to 6 hours after the initial dose of ceftriaxone. By administering dexamethasone before the first dose of parenteral antibiotics it was hoped that the cytokine response would be blunted.

In the Costa Rican trial all children received cefotaxime (200 mg/kg/day) intravenously and were randomized to receive placebo or dexamethasone (0.15 mg/kg per dose every 6 hours for 16 doses). The first dose of placebo or dexamethasone was administered 15 to 20 minutes before the first parenteral dose of cefotaxime. Selected characteristics of the study patients are shown in Table 1. Complications and adverse events occurring during the hospitalization are summarized in Table 2. From a clinical standpoint the major differences were that reactive arthritis and an onset of seizures 48 hours after the start of therapy were observed less frequently and a greater number of patients had guaiac-positive stools in the dexamethasone-treated group.

The average follow-up times after discharge for the 51 dexamethasone-treated children and the 48 children who received placebo were 15.5 ± 6.3 months and 14.9 ± 6.1 months, respectively. Fifteen of 48 children (31%) in the placebo group vs. 5 of 51 (10%) in the dexamethasone-treated group had nonaudiologic

TABLE 1.
Selected Clinical Features of Children in the Costa Rican Meningitis Trial*

Characteristics	**Dexamethasone (n = 52)**	**Placebo (n = 49)**
Age (mo)	16.2 ± 17.8	19.0 ± 19.8
Duration of symptoms before therapy (hr)	24.7 ± 12.4	32.3 ± 18.0
Comatose on admission	4 (8%)	4 (8%)
Etiology		
Haemophilus influenzae type b	39 (75%)	40 (82%)
Streptococcus pneumoniae	4 (8%)	4 (8%)
Neisseria meningitidis	2 (4%)	0
Unknown or other	7 (14%)	5 (10%)

*Modified from Odio CM, Faingezicht I, Paris M, et al: *N Engl J Med* 324:1525–1531, 1991.

TABLE 2.
Complications and Adverse Events Occurring in the Costa Rican Meningitis Study*

Complication or Event	Dexamethasone (n = 52)	Placebo (n = 49)	*P* Value
Death at 48 hr	1 (2%)	1 (2%)	
Guaiac-positive stools	21 (40%)	12 (24%)	.055
Reactive arthritis	0	4 (8%)	.052
Onset of seizures 48 hr after start of therapy	2 (4%)	7 (14%)	.09

*Modified from Odio CM, Faingezicht I, Paris M, et al: *N Engl J Med* 324:1525–1531, 1991.

neurologic sequelae (P = .008). A higher incidence of moderate or more severe bilateral hearing loss occurred in the placebo group (7 of 44 [16%]), than in the dexamethasone-treated group (3 of 50 [6%]), P = .18. Eighteen of 48 (38%) in the placebo group vs. 7 of 51 (14%) in the treatment group had neurologic or audiologic sequelae 5 to 25 months or more after discharge (P = .007). It is of interest that in the first Dallas study only 15% (6 of 41) of children treated with ceftriaxone and placebo had neurologic abnormalities 1 year after discharge, a value almost identical to that found in the Costa Rican children who were treated with cefotaxime and dexamethasone.

A third trial of the efficacy of dexamethasone for bacterial meningitis in children was a multicenter study conducted in Switzerland in 14 centers.[15] All children were treated with ceftriaxone and received either dexamethasone or placebo 10 minutes before the first dose of ceftriaxone. The dose of dexamethasone was 0.4 mg/kg every 12 hours for 2 days, a regimen different from that used in the other two studies. This was based on the pharmacokinetics of dexamethasone and a desire to minimize possible side effects of steroid therapy. Selected characteristics of the patients are shown in Table 3. The children are older than those enrolled in the Dallas and Costa Rican studies, as is typically the case for children in Scandanavian studies of meningitis. Dexamethasone did not affect the parameters of inflammation in the CSF (except for higher glucose concentrations) or culture results for CSF samples obtained 24 hours after therapy was started. Eight of 55 (15%) children in the placebo group and 7 of 60 (12%) children in the dexamethasone-treated group had complications during therapy. On day 3 of treatment 11 of 39 (28%) dexamethasone-treated and 4 of 31 (13%) placebo-treated children had guaiac-positive stools ($P = .15$). Neurologic and audiologic sequelae 15 months after discharge are shown in Table 4. Although there was a trend for fewer neurologic and audiologic sequelae in the dexamethasone-treated group, there were no significant differences for any of these sequelae between the groups.

A multicenter study of dexamethasone has been conducted in six United States centers.[16] All children received ceftriaxone and either dexamethasone (0.15 mg/kg per dose every 6 hours for 16 doses) or placebo. The first dose of placebo or dexamethasone had to be given within 4 hours of the first dose of parenteral antibiotic, which may have been administered at another hospital before transfer to the study site. Auditory brain stem responses (ABRs)

TABLE 3.
Characteristics of Patients in the Swiss Multicenter Dexamethasone Study*

Characteristic	Dexamethasone (n = 60	Placebo (n = 55)
Age (yr)	3.0 ± 3.2	3.0 ± 3.2
Comatose on admission	1	1
Number with seizures	7 (12%)	7 (13%)
Etiology		
Haemophilus influenzae type b	37 (62%)	30 (55%)
Neisseria meningitidis	16 (27%)	12 (22%)
Streptococcus pneumoniae	5 (8%)	6 (11%)
No isolate	2 (3%)	7 (12%)

*From Schaad UB, Lips U, Gnehm HE, et al: *Lancet* 342:457–461, 1993. Used by permission.

TABLE 4.
Neurologic and Audiologic Sequelae at the 15-Month Follow-up in the Swiss Multicenter Dexamethasone Study*

Sequelae	Dexamethasone (n = 60)	Placebo (n = 55)	*P* Value
Neurologic			
Mild damage†	2	2	
Severe damage‡	1	3	
Total	3 (5%)	5 (9%)	.48
Audiologic			
Bilateral/ unilateral	2/1	3/5	
Mild	0	1	
Moderate	1	3	
Severe	1	1	
Deaf	1	3	
Total	3 (5%)	8 (15%)	.11
No. of Children with ≥1 sequelae	3 (5%)	9 (16%)	.07

*Modified from Schaad UB, Lips U, Gnehm HE, et al: *Lancet* 342:457–461, 1993.
†Includes ataxia, hypertonic or hypotonic extremities, and hyperactive behavior; 3 of 4 patients had mild to severe hearing loss.
‡Cerebral palsy, hemiparesis, ataxia, hydrocephalus, psychomotor retardation, and epilepsy; 4 patients with severe damage also had hearing loss of 100 dB or greater in both ears (2) or one ear (2).

were performed within 24 to 48 hours of admission when possible. Selected characteristics of the study patients are shown in Table 5. The average time between the infusion of the first dose of parenteral antibiotic and study drug was 120 (range, 0 to 240) minutes for the dexamethasone-treated children and 100 (range, 0 to 240) minutes for the placebo recipients. The hospital course of the patients was very similar, except that secondary infections developed in more patients in the dexamethasone-treated group (26/69, 38%) than in the placebo group (14/74, 19%; $P = .02$). Gastroenteritis was the predominant secondary infection in both groups.

Follow-up was available 12 months after discharge for 95 children and 6 weeks to 3 months after discharge for 29 children. At the last follow-up 4 children in the dexamethasone-treated group and 6 children in the placebo group had neurologic sequelae. In addition, there were no differences in the psychological testing results between the groups.

The final hearing results for the patients are shown in Table 6. For *H. influenzae* type b meningitis, significantly more children in the placebo group suffered bilateral deafness. There were no differences in hearing loss for the children with pneumococcal or meningococcal meningitis. Twenty-two of 121 children had bilateral moderate or more severe hearing loss when the first ABR test was performed at admission. Fourteen of these children had received placebo and 8 had received dexamethasone. There was no difference in the proportion of children in each group who remained bilaterally deaf at follow-up (3 of 8 for the treatment group and 6 of 14 for the placebo group). Thus the fact that bilateral deafness developed in more children in the placebo group with *H. influenzae* type b meningitis may reflect, by chance, that a greater number of children in the placebo group happened to be deaf earlier than in the dexamethasone-treated group. Alternately, this difference in the number of children deaf at the time of the first ABR test may mean that dexamethasone had reversed any hearing loss already present or prevented any hearing loss that was to occur in

TABLE 5.
Characteristics of Patients in the United States Multicenter Dexamethasone Study*

Characteristics	Dexamethasone (n = 69)	Placebo (n = 74)
Age (mo)	9.8	11.3
Duration of illness before admission (days)	2.0	2.0
Etiologic agent		
Haemophilus influenzae type b	44 (64%)	39 (53%)
Streptococcus pneumoniae	13	20
Neisseria meningitidis	11	13
Other	1	2

*Modified from Wald ER, Kaplan SL, Mason EO Jr, et al: *Pediatrics*, in press.

TABLE 6.
Final Audiologic Results for Children in the United States Multicenter Dexamethasone Study*

Organism	Dexamethasone	Placebo
Haemophilus influenzae type b		
Normal hearing	38	31
Unilateral deafness	5	3
Bilateral deafness	0	5†
Streptococcus pneumoniae		
Normal hearing	8	13
Unilateral deafness	2	5
Bilateral deafness	3	2
Neisseria meningitidis		
Normal hearing	11	11
Unilateral deafness	0	2
Bilateral deafness	0	0
Overall results§		
Normal hearing	58	57
Unilateral deafness	7	10
Bilateral deafness	3	7‡

*Modified from Wald ER, Kaplan SL, Mason EO Jr, et al: *Pediatrics*, in press. Used by permission.
†$P = .02$.
‡$P = .33$.
§Includes 3 children with other bacteria.

the few hours between administration of the study drug and ABR testing (median times, 17 hours for dexamethasone, 13 hours for placebo).

Preliminary results of another comparative study of dexamethasone for bacterial meningitis in children has recently been presented.[17] In a multicenter study in Canada, children were randomized to standard antibiotic therapy plus placebo or dexamethasone (0.6 mg/kg every 6 hours for 16 doses). The first dose of dexamethasone or placebo had to be administered within 24 hours of the first dose of parenteral antibiotic. The median interval between study drug and antibiotic administration was 11 hours for both groups. The clinical characteristics of the 50 children receiving dexamethasone and 51 children treated with placebo were comparable and most children had *H. influenzae* type b meningitis (58%

for the dexamethasone-treated group, 55% for those who received placebo). Neurologic and audiologic sequelae were no different at 1-year follow-up visits. One steroid-treated child with *H. influenzae* type b meningitis required surgery for gastrointestinal bleeding and bowel perforation. The authors concluded that in this study dexamethasone adjunctive therapy did not appear beneficial, but the prolonged interval between antibiotic and steroid administration may have diminished the effectiveness of dexamethasone.

Syrogiannopoulos et al.[18] compared 4 days with 2 days of dexamethasone administration in children with bacterial meningitis to test the hypothesis that a shorter course of steroids might be as efficacious but associated with fewer adverse events than the 4-day course that had been employed in the other studies. Since this 4-day duration of dexamethasone administration had been selected somewhat arbitrarily, this question is of interest. In a multicenter study conducted in Greece, dexamethasone was administered randomly to 61 children for 2 days and to 55 children for 4 days along with standard antibiotic therapy. *Neisseria meningitidis* was isolated from 35 of 61 children in the 2-day group and from 23 of 55 children in the 4-day group. *Haemophilus influenzae* type b was recovered from 20 children in the 2-day group and from 26 children in the 4-day group. No differences were found for neurologic sequelae at the 6-week follow-up between the two groups: 2 days, 3.3%, vs. 4 days, 5.9%. Similarly, hearing impairment was equivalent in the two groups: 2 days, 4.5%, vs. 4 days, 4.8%. Gross gastrointestinal bleeding occurred in 1 and 3 children receiving dexamethasone for 2 or 4 days, respectively. The authors concluded that 2 days of dexamethasone appears to be as efficacious but perhaps associated with less gastrointestinal bleeding than 4 days of dexamethasone administration.

Although no single study may have convincingly demonstrated a beneficial effect of dexamethasone for bacterial meningitis, taken in aggregate, I believe that neurologic sequelae, especially hearing impairment, are reduced by dexamethasone in *H. influenzae* type b meningitis. This is also the conclusion of two meta-analyses of the various clinical trials.[19–21] Furthermore, the American Academy of Pediatrics, the Infectious Disease Society of America, and the British Paediatric Immunology and Infectious Disease Group have established recommendations for the use of dexamethasone in bacterial meningitis due to *H. influenzae* type b, but not necessarily when caused by other organisms.[22–24] Of course, the reason for the focus on *H. influenzae* type b is that this was the predominant organism causing meningitis (60%) in almost all of the steroid studies that have been conducted.[25] However, the findings and conclusions from these studies may not be generalizable to other causes of bacterial meningitis, especially pneumococcal meningitis. This is an important point since in countries where the *H. influenzae* type b protein conjugate vaccines are employed routinely, the incidence of this form of bacterial meningitis has declined dramatically.[26]

In the prospective studies conducted to date, insufficient numbers of children with pneumococcal or meningococcal meningitis were enrolled to assess the efficacy of dexamethasone for these causes. The U.S. multicenter study had the largest number of children with pneumococcal meningitis, and no differences in outcome were noted between the dexamethasone- or placebo-treated patients. In fact, even when selected studies are combined, dexamethasone is not shown to be beneficial for pneumococcal meningitis.

The two largest studies that have addressed the efficacy of dexamethasone in pneumococcal meningitis have several deficiencies. In a prospective evaluation performed in Egypt, both children and adults were randomized to receive placebo or dexamethasone for 3 days plus intramuscular ampicillin and chloramphenicol.[27] The dose of ampicillin was somewhat low (160 mg/kg/day), and no mention was made that chloramphenicol levels were monitored. The severity of illness was very unusual since the percentage of patients comatose on admission was 79% and 69% in the dexamethasone and placebo groups, respectively. The impressive finding for pneumococcal meningitis was that the mortality rate was reduced from 40.7% (22/54) in the placebo group to 13.5% (7/52) in the dexamethasone group ($P < .02$). Thus the mortality rate was reduced threefold by dexamethasone, an amazing achievement but one that is not likely to be relevant to outcome of therapy in more modern settings of medical care. In addition, hearing loss was decreased significantly ($P < .05$) in the dexamethasone-treated group (0/45) when compared with the control group (4/32); however, hearing could not be assessed in children less than 4 years of age, and it was not clear how many of the patients with pneumococcal meningitis were children.

The other study was a retrospective review of children with pneumococcal meningitis admitted to the Children's Medical Center or Parkland Memorial Hospital in Dallas between 1984 and 1990.[28] Fifty-six children did not receive dexamethasone and 41 patients did, 27 as part of placebo-controlled trials of dexamethasone therapy. One potential important difference between the two study groups is that significantly more children not receiving dexamethasone were treated between 1984 and 1987 (44/56) as compared with dexamethasone-treated children (10/41) ($P < .001$). This may be a critical difference since the children treated in the earlier years of the study received different antibiotics (especially cefuroxime) than the children after this time, when cefotaxime and ceftriaxone were administered more frequently. Since cefuroxime appears to be associated with more neurologic sequelae of bacterial meningitis than cefotaxime or ceftriaxone, more sequelae might be expected for children treated in the earlier years of the retrospective study.[29, 30] Thus the findings of this review, namely, that fewer children in the dexamethasone-treated group (4/35) than in the control group (14/43) had adverse neurologic and/or audiologic sequelae ($P = .033$), are difficult to interpret.

Although there is no definitely convincing evidence that dexamethasone is beneficial in pneumococcal or meningococcal meningitis, are there any disadvantages for its use? Prolonged dexamethasone administration in doses higher than currently recommended for meningitis has been associated with persistently positive CSF cultures despite adequate treatment in normal children.[31] In the Dallas retrospective review, 0 of 35 non–steroid-treated and 2 of 30 steroid-treated children had a positive CSF culture 24 to 48 hours into therapy ($P = .21$). Thus steroids may have the potential to interfere with the rapid clearing of pneumococcal organisms by a β-lactam antibiotic.

More bothersome are the unknown effects of dexamethasone during treatment of meningitis caused by strains of *S. pneumoniae* resistant to penicillin and third-generation cephalosporins, a problem of growing concern.[32–34] Dexamethasone has been administered to three of eight children who had persistently positive CSF cultures for *S. pneumoniae* while receiving appropriate doses of cefotaxime or ceftriaxone.[33, 35–39] In these cases of treatment failure the minimum inhibitory concentrations (MICs) for *S. pneumoniae* CSF isolates were generally 2 μg/mL or greater. New guidelines from the National Committee for Clinical Laboratory Standards for determining the susceptibility of *S. pneumoniae* to third-generation cephalosporins have been proposed.[40] Isolates should be considered susceptible if the MIC is 0.25 μg/mL or less, intermediately susceptible if the MIC is 0.5 to 1.0 μg/mL, and resistant if the MIC is 2.0 μg/mL or greater. For meningitis isolates found to have intermediate susceptibility, the organism should be considered resistant. These new recommendations will require further clinical correlation, but in the meantime, vancomycin with or without rifampin will be administered more frequently when the possibility of encountering such isolates is considered.

Since vancomycin penetration into CSF is influenced by the inflammatory response of the host, it will not be surprising to find that the CSF concentration of vancomycin is decreased when dexamethasone is administered concomitantly to patients with bacterial meningitis.[41] The only study that remotely touches on this concern is one reported from Spain by Viladrich et al.[42] Eleven patients between 17 and 66 years of age who had pneumococcal meningitis were treated with vancomycin (7.5 mg/kg every 6 hours) and dexamethasone (0.25 mg/kg every 6 hours for 4 days). Four of the patients were thought to experience treatment failure based on a recrudescence of their illness such as a rise in temperature and recurrence of meningeal symptoms and signs after definite initial improvement. Unfortunately, repeat CSF cultures were not obtained. In view of the fact that in two of the patients dexamethasone use was discontinued before the secondary fever, the nature of the recrudescence is unclear and may have been related to inadequate vancomycin dosing and/or stopping dexamethasone therapy. Certainly more data concerning the clinical course and outcome of patients treated with vancomycin plus dexamethasone for pneumococcal meningitis are mandatory before establishing recommendations for dexamethasone administration in this circumstance.

With widespread use of the *H. influenzae* type b protein conjugate vaccine, a greater proportion of children coming to the physician with suspected bacterial meningitis will actually have viral meningitis. Frequently it is difficult to distinguish between a bacterial and viral etiology for meningitis from clinical findings or the CSF laboratory results at the time of initial evaluation. Thus many infants and children with viral meningitis will receive one or more doses of dexamethasone if steroids are administered routinely to children with suspected bacterial meningitis. The effect of dexamethasone on the course or outcome of viral meningitis is unknown. Again, no carefully controlled study has addressed this question. Waagner et al.[43] reviewed the hospital course of 32 children ultimately proved to have aseptic meningitis who received dexamethasone after being enrolled in one of the Dallas protocols. The mean age of the children was 20.5 months (range, 6 weeks to 9.5 years), and the mean number of doses of dexamethasone administered before excluding the diagnosis of bacterial meningitis was 7.4 (range, 1 to 16). The hospital course for these patients and their condition at discharge were unremarkable. Furthermore, when interviewed by phone, the parents of the children indicated that they had returned to normal activity and behavior. However, the patients were not compared with the children with aseptic meningitis who did not receive dexamethasone, and the follow-up assessment did not include testing to detect subtle neurologic effects such as behavioral or intellectual changes, which are the likely sequelae of viral meningitis.

The efficacy and safety of dexamethasone are currently being investigated in neonatal meningitis. Since cytokine release also participates in the inflammatory response associated with gram-negative enteric meningitis in neonates, the hypothesis is that modulating the neonatal response to infection may decrease neurologic sequelae.[44]

OTHER ADJUNCTIVE MEASURES

Besides some degree of restriction of intravenous fluid administration, intensive care measures to prevent alterations in blood pressure and/or ICP (30-degree elevation of the head of the bed), and aggressive treatment of seizures, no other adjunctive measures are widely advocated in the management of children with bacterial meningitis. Mannitol is recommended when symptoms and signs of severe increased ICP are present or impending herniation is suspected, but routine mannitol infusions are not included in standard management guidelines.[45] In a rabbit model of *H. influenzae* type b meningitis, a single infusion of hypertonic mannitol was associated with a transient reduction in CSF pressure and a significant reduction in CSF concentrations of lactate; the latter finding may reflect enhanced CBF and lead to reduced anaerobic metabolism.[46]

There are no clinical studies addressing the effects and outcome of mannitol infusion in the management of bacterial meningitis. Glycerol is an oral hyperosmolar agent used to combat cerebral edema and increased ICP. Investigators in Finland[47] conducted a multicenter study in which children with bacterial meningitis were all treated with ceftriaxone and randomly assigned to one of four adjunctive treatments for 3 days:

1. Dexamethasone only, 0.5 mg/kg per dose every 8 hours (n = 32)
2. Oral glycerol only, 1.5 g/kg per dose every 8 hours (n = 30)
3. Dexamethasone plus glycerol (n = 34)
4. Neither treatment (n = 26)

None of the children receiving glycerol had any neurologic abnormalities as compared with 5 (9%) of those not treated with glycerol ($P < .05$). Audiometry was assessed in 113 of 120 survivors. Severe to profound bilateral deafness occurred in four children not treated with glycerol vs. none in the glycerol-treated group ($P < .05$). Overall, glycerol was thought to be the predominant factor in reducing neurologic sequelae. This study is intriguing, but additional data regarding oral glycerol administration is mandatory before its widespread acceptance as part of routine therapy for bacterial meningitis.

NEWER ADJUNCTIVE APPROACHES

Newer approaches to anti-inflammatory treatment have been studied in experimental meningitis. Pentoxifylline is a xanthine derivative that inhibits phosphodiesterases and is widely used to improve the microcirculation of adults with chronic occlusive arterial disease. Pentoxifylline also has some anti-inflammatory properties related to modulating neutrophil adherence to endothelial cells, decreasing superoxide production by neutrophils as well as the neutrophil response to TNF, and decreasing TNF production by endotoxin stimulation of macrophages.[48] In a rabbit model of *H. influenzae* type b meningitis, concentrations of protein and lactate in CSF decreased when pentoxifylline was administered 30 minutes before ceftriaxone treatment.[49] A derivative of pentoxifylline, HWA-138, led to less cochlear inflammation in infant rats with *H. influenzae* type b meningitis treated with suboptimal antibiotic therapy.[50] There are no clinical studies of pentoxifylline in humans with bacterial meningitis; however, pentoxifylline may blunt the expected rise in TNF concentration in humans infused with endotoxin and decrease inflammation-related toxicities in patients receiving amphotericin B or bone marrow transplantation.[51–53]

Antibodies directed against the CD18 family of adhesion-promoting receptors on leukocytes have been studied in experimental meningitis. These receptors bind to ligands on endothelial cells to promote the adherence to and then transmigration of polymorphonuclear leukocytes (PMNs) between endothelial cells. Monoclonal antibodies to CD18 have been synthesized from mouse myeloma cells. When this antibody was infused intravenously into rabbits with pneumococcal meningitis, the CSF white blood cell count and protein concentrations, as well as brain weight, were reduced as compared with uninfused infected animals.[54] Similarly, anti-CD18 monoclonal antibody and dexamethasone are additive in modifying the inflammatory response of rabbits with *H. influenzae* type b meningitis treated with ceftriaxone.[55] This approach is an exciting one based on the ever-increasing knowledge of leukocyte biology and the inflammatory response. Blocking endothelial ligands such as intercellular adhesion molecule (ICAM-1) or endothelial leukocyte adhesion molecule (ELAM) are another attractive option that theoretically might be associated with a less generalized anti-inflammatory effect since the endothelial cells with increased numbers of adhesion molecules would be preferentially attracting the monoclonal agent. Anti–ICAM-1 monoclonal antibodies are currently in clinical trials for combating solid-organ transplantation rejection.[56, 57] At some point similar trials may be conducted in patients with central nervous system infections.

Undoubtedly advances in our understanding of the molecular events underlying the host response to infection will continue, and as a result newer modalities of modulating this response will be developed. It is a challenge to the clinician to evaluate the efficacy and safety of these new adjunctive measures in patients by conducting well-designed trials that can provide unambiguous answers. However, as better vaccines are developed, fewer patients with infections (especially meningitis) are available for studying the effectiveness of new interventions. Since this research is very expensive and labor-intensive, investigators must choose, more carefully than ever, those therapeutic agents that deserve further clinical evaluation.

REFERENCES

1. Sáez-Llorens X, Ramilo O, Mustafa MM, et al: Molecular pathophysiology of bacterial meningitis: Current concepts and therapeutic implications. *J Pediatr* 116:671–684, 1990.
2. Quagliarello V, Scheld WM: Bacterial meningitis: Pathogenesis, pathophysiology and progress. *N Engl J Med* 327:864–872, 1992.
3. Mustafa MM, Lebel MH, Ramilo O, et al: Correlation of interleukin-1β and cachectin concentrations in cerebrospinal fluid and outcome from bacterial meningitis. *J Pediatr* 115:208–213, 1989.
4. Patrick D, Betts J, Frey EA et al: *Haemophilus influenzae* lipopolysaccharide disrupts confluent monolayers of bovine brain endothelial cells via a serum-dependent cytotoxic pathway. *J Infect Dis* 165:865–872, 1992.
5. Täuber MG, Sachdeva M, Kennedy SL, et al: Toxicity in neuronal cells caused by cerebrospinal fluid from pneumococcal and gram-negative meningitis. *J Infect Dis* 166:1045–1050, 1992.
6. Ashwal S, Stringer W, Tomasi L, et al: Cerebral blood flow and car-

bon dioxide reactivity in children with bacterial meningitis. *J Pediatr* 117:523–530, 1990.

7. Igarashi M, Saito R, Alford BR, et al: Temporal bone findings in pneumococcal meningitis. *Arch Otolaryngol* 99:79–83, 1974.
8. Kaplan SL, Hawkins EP, Kline MW, et al: Invasion of the inner ear by *Haemophilus influenzae* type b in experimental meningitis. *J Infect Dis* 159:923–930, 1989.
9. Kaplan SL, Catlin FI, Weaver T, et al: Onset of hearing loss in children with bacterial meningitis. *Pediatrics* 73:575–578, 1984.
10. Nadol JB Jr: Hearing loss as a sequela of meningitis. *Laryngoscope* 88:739–755, 1978.
11. Dodge PR, Davis H, Feigin RD, et al: Prospective evaluation of hearing impairment as a sequela of acute bacterial meningitis. *N Engl J Med* 311:869–874, 1984.
12. Bhatt SM, Lauretano A, Cabellos C, et al: Progression of hearing loss in experimental pneumococcal meningitis: Correlation with cerebrospinal fluid cytochemistry. *J Infect Dis* 167:675–683, 1993.
13. Lebel MH, Freij BJ, Syrogiannopoulos GA, et al: Dexamethasone therapy for bacterial meningitis. Results of two double-blind, placebo-controlled trials. *N Engl J Med* 319:964–971, 1988.
14. Odio CM, Faingezicht I, Paris M, et al: The beneficial effects of early dexamethasone administration in infants and children with bacterial meningitis. *N Engl J Med* 324:1525–1531, 1991.
15. Schaad UB, Lips U, Gnehm HE, et al: Dexamethasone therapy for bacterial meningitis in children. *Lancet* 342:457–461, 1993.
16. Wald ER, Kaplan SL, Mason EO Jr, et al: Dexamethasone therapy for children with bacterial meningitis. *Pediatrics*, in press.
17. King SM, Law B, Langley J, et al: A randomized controlled trial of dexamethasone versus placebo in children with bacterial meningitis (abstract 72). Presented at the 32nd Interscience Conference on Antimicrobial Agents and Chemotherapy, Anaheim, Calif, Oct 12, 1992.
18. Syrogiannopoulos GA, Lourida AN, Theodoriodou MN, et al: Dexamethasone therapy for bacterial meningitis in children: 2- versus 4-day regimen. *J Infect Dis* 169:853–858, 1994.
19. Havens PL, Wendelberger KJ, Hoffman GM, et al: Corticosteroids as adjunctive therapy in bacterial meningitis. A meta-analysis of clinical trials. *Am J Dis Child* 143:1051–1055, 1989.
20. Geiman BJ, Smith AL: Dexamethasone and bacterial meningitis. A meta-analysis of randomized controlled trials. *West J Med* 157:27–31, 1992.
21. Havens PL: Meta-analysis Redux-steroids and meningitis revisited. *West J Med* 157:84–86, 1992.
22. American Academy of Pediatrics: Dexamethasone therapy for bacterial meningitis in infants and children, in *Report of the Committee on Infectious Diseases of the American Academy of Pediatrics*, ed 22. American Academy of Pediatrics, Elk Grove Village, Ill, 1994, pp 558–559.

23. McGowan JE Jr, Chesney PJ, Crossley KB, et al: Guidelines for the use of systemic glucocorticosteroids in the management of selected infections. *J Infect Dis* 165:1–13, 1992.
24. The Meningitis Working Party of the British Paediatric Immunology and Infectious Disease Group: Should we use dexamethasone in meningitis? *Arch Dis Child* 67:14–17, 1992.
25. Schaad UB, Kaplan SL, McCracken GH Jr: Steroid therapy for bacterial meningitis. *Clin Infect Dis,* in press.
26. Adams WG, Deaver KA, Cochi SL, et al: Decline of childhood *Haemophilus influenzae* type b (Hib) disease in the Hib vaccine era. *JAMA* 269:221–226, 1993.
27. Girgis NI, Farid Z, Mikhail IS, et al: Dexamethasone treatment for bacterial meningitis in children and adults. *Pediatr Infect Dis J* 8:848–851, 1989.
28. Kennedy WA, Hoyt MJ, McCracken GH Jr: The role of corticosteroid therapy in children with pneumococcal meningitis. *Am J Dis Child* 145:1374–1378, 1991.
29. Lebel MH, Hoyt MJ, McCracken GH Jr: Comparative efficacy of ceftriaxone and cefuroxime for treatment of bacterial meningitis. *J Pediatr* 114:1049–1054, 1989.
30. Schaad UB, Suter S, Gianella-Borradori, et al: A comparison of ceftriaxone and cefuroxime for the treatment of bacterial meningitis of infants and children. *N Engl J Med* 322:141–147, 1990.
31. Brady MT, Kaplan SL, Taber LH: Association between persistence of pneumococcal meningitis and dexamethasone administration. *J Pediatr* 99:924–926, 1981.
32. Mason EO Jr, Kaplan SL, Lamberth LB, et al: Increased rate of isolation of penicillin-resistant *Streptococcus pneumoniae* in a children's hospital and in vitro susceptibilities to antibiotics of therapeutic use. *Antimicrob Agents Chemother* 36:1703–1707, 1992.
33. Friedland IR, Shelton S, Paris M, et al: Dilemmas in the diagnosis and treatment of cephalosporin-resistant pneumococcal meningitis. *Pediatr Infect Dis J* 12:196–200, 1993.
34. Friedland IR, Paris M, Ehrett S, et al: Evaluation of antimicrobial regimens for treatment of experimental penicillin- and cephalosporin-resistant pneumococcal meningitis. *Antimicrob Agents Chemother* 37:1630–1637, 1993.
35. Sloas MM, Barrett FF, Chesney PJ, et al: Cephalosporin treatment failure in penicillin- and cephalosporin-resistant *Streptococcus pneumoniae* meningitis. *Pediatr Infect Dis J* 11:662–666, 1992.
36. Alonso J, Madrigal V, Garcia-Fuentes M: Recurrent meningitis from a multiply resistant *Streptococcus pneumoniae* treated with erythromycin. *Pediatric Infect Dis J* 10:256–257, 1991.
37. Asensi F, Pérez-Tamarit D, Otero MC, et al: Imipenem-cilastatin therapy in a child with meningitis caused by a multiply resistant pneumococcus. *Pediatr Infect Dis J* 8:895, 1989.

38. Bradley JS, Connor JD: Ceftriaxone failure in meningitis caused by *Streptococcus pneumoniae* with reduced susceptibility to beta-lactam antibiotics. *Pediatr Infect Dis J* 10:871–873, 1991.
39. Kleiman MB, Weinberg GA, Reynolds JK, et al: Meningitis with beta-lactam resistant *Streptococcus pneumoniae*: The need for early repeat lumbar puncture. *Pediatr Infect Dis J* 12:782–784, 1993.
40. NCCLS M7-A3: Minimum inhibitory concentration interpretive standard (μg/ml) for *Streptococcus pneumoniae*, vol 13, 1993.
41. McGee SM, Kaplan SL, Mason EO Jr: Ventricular fluid concentrations of vancomycin in children after intravenous and intraventricular administration. *Pediatr Infect Dis J* 9:138–139, 1990.
42. Viladrich PF, Gudiol F, Liñares J, et al: Evaluation of vancomycin for therapy of adult pneumococcal meningitis. *Antimicrob Agents Chemother* 35:2467–2472, 1991.
43. Waagner DC, Kennedy WA, Hoyt MJ, et al: Lack of adverse effects of dexamethasone therapy in aseptic meningitis. *Pediatr Infect Dis J* 9:922–923, 1990.
44. Mustafa MM, Mertsola J, Ramilo O, et al: Increased endotoxin and interleukin-1β concentrations in cerebrospinal fluid of infants with coliform meningitis and ventriculitis associated with intraventricular gentamicin therapy. *J Infect Dis* 160:891–895, 1989.
45. Kaplan SL, Fishman MA: Update on bacterial meningitis. *J Child Neurol* 3:82–93, 1988.
46. Syrogiannopoulos GA, Olsen KD, McCracken GH Jr: Mannitol treatment in experimental *Haemophilus influenzae* type b meningitis. *Pediatr Res* 22:118–122, 1987.
47. Kilpi T, Peltola H, Jauhiainen T, et al: Oral glycerol and intravenous dexamethasone in preventing hearing impairment due to childhood bacterial meningitis (abstract 1148). Presented at the 33rd Interscience Conference on Antimicrobial Agents and Chemotherapy, New Orleans, 1993.
48. Sullivan GH, Carper HT, Novick WJ, et al: Inhibition of the inflammatory action of interleukin-1 and tumor necrosis factor (alpha) on neutrophil function by pentoxifylline. *Infect Immun* 56:1722–1729, 1988.
49. Sáez-Llorens X, Ramilo O, Mustafa MM, et al: Pentoxifylline modulates meningeal inflammation in experimental bacterial meningitis. *Antimicrob Agents Chemother* 34:837–843, 1990.
50. Rodriguez AF, Kaplan SL, Hawkins EP, et al: Effect of dexamethasone or HWA-138 in combination with antibiotics in experimental *Haemophilus influenzae* type b infection. *Antimicrob Agents Chemother* 35:1980–1984, 1991.
51. Zabel P, Schönharting MM, Wolter DT, et al: Oxpentifylline in endotoxaemia. *Lancet* 2:1474–1477, 1989.
52. Bianco JA, Almgren J, Kern DL, et al: Evidence that oral pentoxifylline reverses acute renal dysfunction in bone marrow transplant re-

cipients receiving amphotericin B and cyclosporine. *Transplantation* 51:925–927, 1991.

53. Bianco JA, Applebaum FR, Nemunaitis J, et al: Phase I-II trial of pentoxifylline for the prevention of transplant-related toxicities following bone marrow transplantation. *Blood* 78:1205–1211, 1991.
54. Tuomanen EI, Saukkonen K, Sande S, et al: Reduction of inflammation, tissue damage, and mortality in bacterial meningitis in rabbits treated with monoclonal antibodies against adhesion-promoting receptors of leukocytes. *J Exp Med* 170:659–669, 1989.
55. Sáez-Llorens X, Jafari HS, Severien C, et al: Enhanced attenuation of meningeal inflammation and brain edema by concomitant administration of anti-CD18 monoclonal antibodies and dexamethasone in experimental *Haemophilus* meningitis. *J Clin Invest* 88:2003–2011, 1991.
56. Cosimi AB, Conti D, Delmonico FL, et al: In vivo effects of monoclonal antibody to ICAM-1 (CD54) in nonhuman primates with renal allografts. *J Immunol* 144:4604–4612, 1990.
57. Flavin T, Ivens K, Rothlein R, et al: Monoclonal antibodies against intercellular adhesion molecule 1 prolong cardiac allograft survival in cynomolgus monkeys. *Transplant Proc* 23:533–534, 1991.

An Update on Pediatric Immunization

Neal A. Halsey, M.D.
Professor and Division Director, Division of Disease Control, Department of International Health, The Johns Hopkins University, Baltimore, Maryland

THE PACE OF CHANGE

The pace of change in guidelines for immunizing children has increased in recent years. In the 10-year period ending in 1979, there were no significant changes in the immunization schedule for routine immunization of children. During the 1980s, *Haemophilus influenzae* type b (Hib) plain polysaccharide (PRP) vaccines were approved for use in the second year of life followed by Hib conjugate vaccines for use at 15 months of age, and a second dose of measles vaccine was added in 1989. The rate of change in immunization guidelines promises to be even faster during the 1990s. *Haemophilus influenzae* type b conjugate vaccines are now recommended for routine use in infants, and all children should receive a second dose of measles vaccine. Hepatitis B vaccine has been added to the routine schedule for infants, and new combination products have been developed for the administration of Hib conjugate with diphtheria and tetanus toxoids and pertussis vaccine (DTP). Many more combination products are under development, and several will undoubtedly be made available within the next few years. Also, in 1994 the advisory groups have made several changes in the timing of other routinely administered vaccines (Table 1).[1,2] Health care providers need to make extra efforts to keep children. Fortunately, the advisory groups are in the process of standardizing the presentation of the schedule and publishing frequent updates at standardized times.

IMPACT OF IMMUNIZATION ON DISEASE INCIDENCE

Increased attention has been paid to recent outbreaks of disease caused by measles, pertussis, and other vaccine-preventable diseases. This heightened awareness of preventable disease has helped to identify problems in our vaccine delivery system. However, we should keep these outbreaks in perspective. The wide-

TABLE 1.
Recommended Schedule for Immunization of Healthy Infants and Children*

Recommended Age†	Immunizations‡	Comments
Birth	HBV§	
1–2 mo	HBV§	
2 mo	DTP, Hib, OPV	DTP and OPV can be initiated as early as 4 wk after birth in areas of high endemicity or during outbreaks
4 mo	DTP, Hib, OPV	2-mo interval
6 mo	DTP, (Hib)¶	
6–18 mo	HBV§, OPV	
12–15 mo	Hib, MMR	MMR should be given at 12 mo of age in high-risk areas. If indicated, tuberculin testing may be done at the same visit
15–18 mo	DTaP or DTP‖	
4–6 yr	DTaP or DTP, OPV	At or before school entry. DTP or DTaP should not be given at or after the seventh birthday

Continued.

spread use of immunizations has continued to have a major impact on reducing the incidence of vaccine-preventable diseases (Fig 1).

COST-BENEFIT ANALYSIS OF IMMUNIZATIONS

Immunization remains the most cost-effective intervention available to health care providers. Formal cost-benefit analyses have revealed that most immunizations save society $2 to $14 for every dollar invested[3–8] (Table 2).

PENDING CHANGES IN THE FINANCING OF IMMUNIZATIONS

Dramatic changes in the health care system have been proposed by the current administration.[9] Increased attention will be paid to

TABLE 1 (cont.).
Recommended Schedule for Immunization of Healthy Infants and Children*

Recommended Age†	Immunizations‡	Comments
11–12 yr	MMR	At entry to middle school or junior high school unless 2 doses previously given after the first birthday
14–16 yr	Td	Repeat every 10 yr throughout life

*Adapted from *Report of the Committee on Infectious Disease.* The table is not completely consistent with all package inserts. For products used, consult the manufacturer's package insert for instructions for storage, handling, dosage, and administration. Biologicals prepared by different manufacturers may vary, and package inserts of the same manufacturer may change from time to time. Therefore the physician should be aware of the contents of the current package insert.
†These recommended ages should not be construed as absolute. For example, 2 months can be 6 to 10 weeks. However, MMR should not usually be given to children younger than 12 months. If measles vaccination is indicated, monovalent measles vaccine is recommended, and MMR should be given subsequently, at 12 to 15 months.
‡HBV = hepatitis B virus vaccine; DTP, DTaP = diphtheria and tetanus toxoids with pertussis vaccine (DTP) or with acellular pertussis vaccine (DTaP); Hib = *Haemophilus influenzae* type b conjugate vaccine; OPV = oral poliovirus vaccine containing attenuated poliovirus types 1, 2, and 3; MMR = live measles, mumps, and rubella viruses in a combined vaccine; Td = adult tetanus toxoid (full dose) and diphtheria toxoid (reduced dose) for adult use.
§An acceptable alternative to minimize the number of visits for immunization for infants of hepatitis B surface antigen–negative mothers is to administer dose 1 at age 0 to 2 months, dose 2 at age 4 months, and dose 3 at 6 to 18 months.
¶Dose 3 is not indicated if the product for doses 1 and 2 was Pedvax HIB (PRP-OMP, manufactured by Merck, West Point, Pa).
‖Should be given 6 to 12 months after the third dose of DTP, and the fourth dose is given as early as 12 months of age, provided that the interval between dose 3 and 4 is at least 6 months and DTP is given. DTaP is not currently licensed for use in children less than 15 months of age.

improving the delivery of vaccines, lowering the cost of immunizations, and modifying the methods that parents and guardians pay for vaccines. Effective October 1, 1994, all states will have the option of purchasing vaccines for children whose health insurance does not cover immunizations. The final details regarding how this program will be implemented had not been worked out at the time of this writing.

A

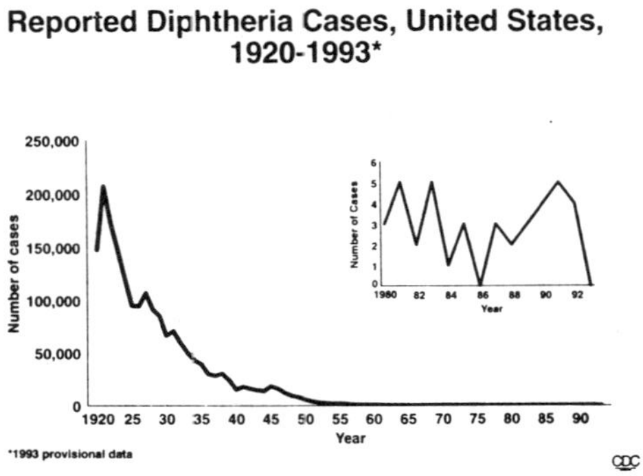

B

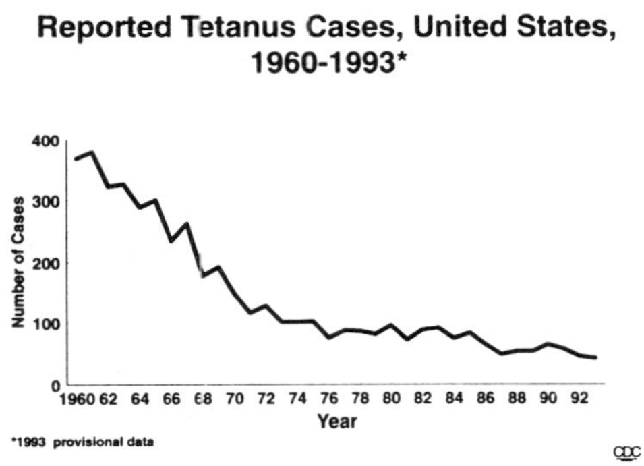

C

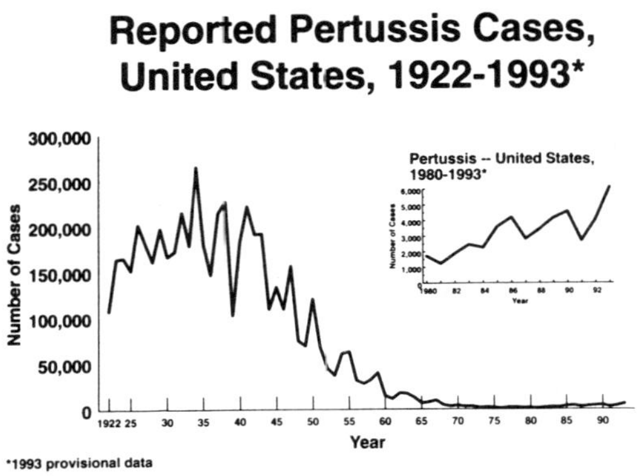

FIGURE 1.

A–I, Reported cases of Vaccine-preventable diseases in the United States. (Courtesy of Centers for Disease Control and Prevention, Atlanta.)

D Reported Poliomyelitis Cases, United States, 1920-1993*

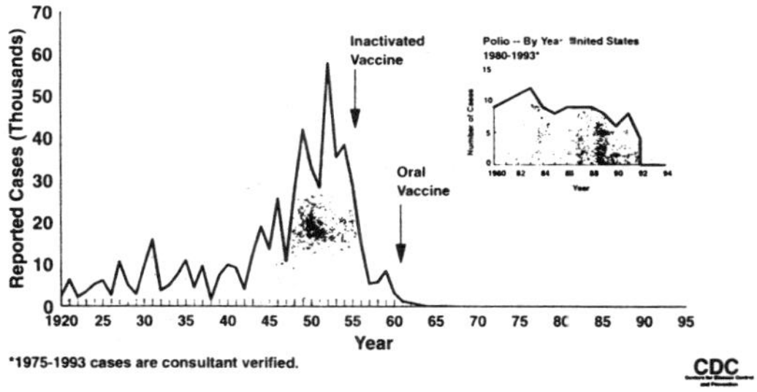

E *Haemophilus influenzae* type b Reported Cases* 1991-1993

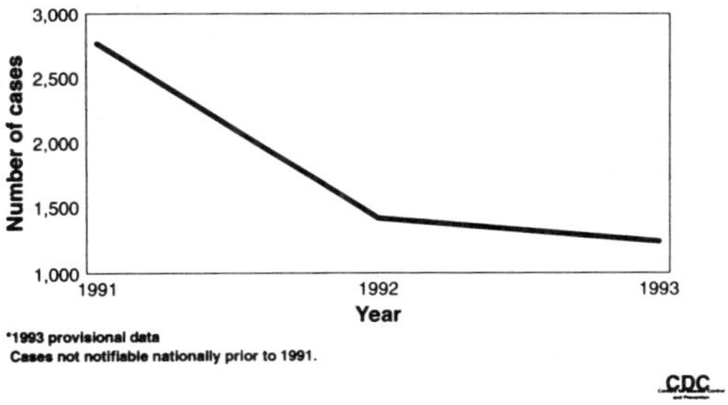

F Reported Cases of Hepatitis B, United States, 1966-1993*

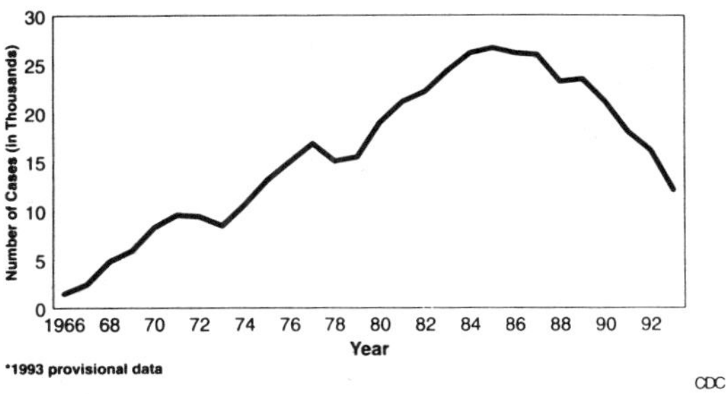

FIGURE 1 (cont.).

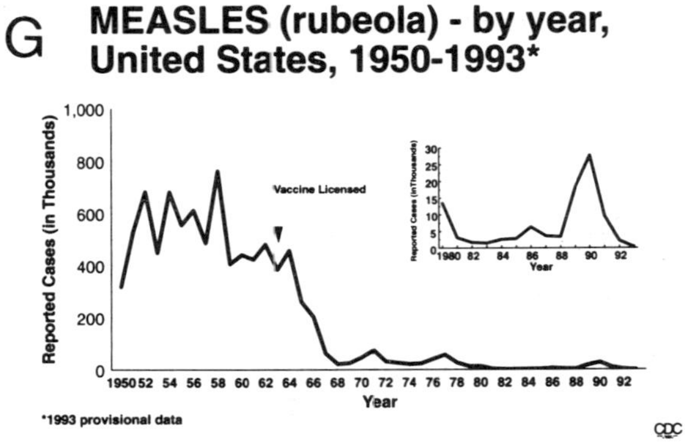

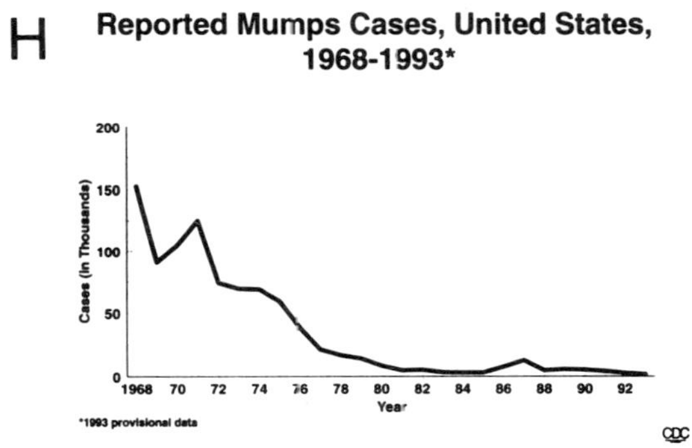

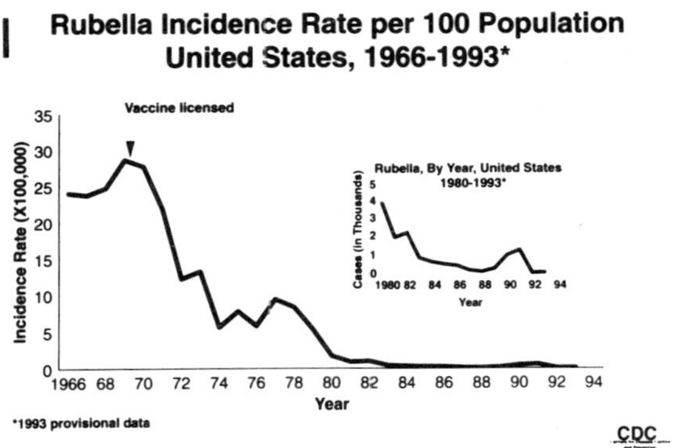

FIGURE 1 (cont.).

TABLE 2.
Cost-Benefit Ratios of a Routine Varicella Vaccination Program Compared With Other Vaccination and Preventive Programs*†

Intervention	Ratio	Source
Health care payer's perspective‡		
Varicella vaccination of children, 1 dose	0.9	Lieu et al.[3]
Pertussis, 1987 price	1.1	Office of Technology Assessment report, p. 135[4]
Haemophilus influenzae type b vaccination of children	1.3–3.4	Cochi et al.,[5] Hay and Daum[6]
Measles, mumps, rubella vaccination	3.0	White et al.[7]
Pertussis, 1984 price	11.1	Hinman and Kaplan[8]
Haemophilus influenzae vaccination of children	2.8	Hay and Daum[6]
Varicella vaccination of children, 1 dose	5.4	Lieu et al.[3]
Measles, mumps, rubella vaccination	14.4	White et al.[7]

*Adapted from Lieu TA, Cochi SL, Black SB, et al: *JAMA* 271:375–381, 1994. Used by permission.
†All estimates are adjusted to 1990 dollars. The price for one dose of varicella vaccine is $35, not including the cost of administration.
‡Health care payer's perspective includes medical costs only; ratio is the reduction in medical costs divided by the cost of the vaccination program. Societal perspective includes medical and work-loss costs; ratio is the reduction in medical and work-loss costs divided by the cost of the vaccination program.

RECENT DEVELOPMENTS IN SPECIFIC VACCINES AND VACCINE-PREVENTABLE DISEASES

PERTUSSIS

Disease

More than 6,000 cases of pertussis were reported to the Centers for Disease Control and Prevention (CDC) in 1993 (Table 3).[10, 11] This is the highest number of cases reported since 1967. The actual incidence of pertussis in 1993 was undoubtedly much higher since only about 10% of pertussis cases have been reported in many areas.[12, 13] The apparent resurgence of pertussis in the United States over the past decade (Fig 1) emphasizes the need for developing new strategies and improved vaccines for prevention of this disease. The available data indicate that the resurgence of disease was not due to any decrease in vaccine efficacy.[12] The highest incidence of pertussis has continued to be in children younger than 1 year of age, and the majority of the hospitalizations and severe disease occurred in infants less than 9 months of age.[10, 12] Forty-four percent of the cases reported in 1993 occurred in children less than 1 year of age. Three doses of pertussis vaccine are necessary to induce adequate protection against pertussis. Many of the children in whom pertussis develops contract the disease in the first few months of life before the first three doses of DTP can be given. Also, delays in delivering immunizations to infants have contributed to the high incidence in young children. Infants are often exposed to pertussis by older children and adults who have mild illnesses or are asymptomatic carriers. New strategies are needed to induce enhanced protection in older children and adults (see acellular pertussis vaccines later).

TABLE 3.
Number of Reported Cases of Diseases Preventable by Routine Childhood Vaccination—United States, December 1993 and 1992–1993*

Disease	Total Cases		No. Cases Among Children <5 yr	
	1992	1993	1992	1993
Congenital rubella syndrome	9	7	9	5
Diphtheria	3	0	1	0
Haemophilus influenzae infection	1,412	1,264	592	399
Hepatitis B	16,126	12,396	215	142
Measles	2,231	281	1,116	104
Mumps	2,485	1,640	364	275
Pertussis	3,935	6,335	2,261	3,753
Poliomyelitis, paralytic	—	—	—	—
Rubella	157	195	24	36
Tetanus	44	43	0	1

*Adapted from Centers for Disease Control and Prevention: *MMWR* 43:57–60, 1994.

Alternative Immunization Schedules in Outbreaks

During outbreaks, the American Academy of Pediatrics (AAP) and the Advisory Committee on Immunization Practices (ACIP) have endorsed the use of an accelerated schedule beginning as early as 4 to 6 weeks of age and administering the second and third doses at 30-day intervals.[1, 2] Although the final antibody titers are lower when vaccines are administered at 1-month vs. 2-month intervals, this strategy may be necessary in situations where there is continuing community-based transmission of pertussis.[14]

Vaccine Safety

Concern over possible neurologic side effects has led to decreased acceptance of whole-cell pertussis vaccine in other countries and continues to be a source of controversy in the United States. The Institute of Medicine (IOM) recently conducted a series of in-depth reviews of side effects associated with childhood vaccines.[15, 16] The initial IOM report indicated that the available evidence was insufficient to indicate a causal relationship between pertussis vaccine and chronic neurologic damage.[15] However, additional data from a 10-year follow-up of the National Childhood Encephalopathy Study (NCES) became available after the first report was published.[17, 18] The new data revealed that children who had acute neurologic disorders following DTP immunization were more likely to have long-term neurologic dysfunction 10 years after the acute episode than control children were. The IOM committee concluded that the NCES follow-up data provided evidence of only a possible relation between DTP and chronic nervous system dysfunction in children in whom a serious acute neurologic illness had developed within 7 days following DTP administration. The committee proposed three possible explanations for the association: (1) the acute and chronic neurologic changes might have been caused by DTP, (2) DTP might have triggered an acute event in children who had an underlying neurologic abnormality, or (3) DTP might have caused an acute event in children who had pre-existing conditions that would have led to chronic neurologic dysfunction even if the acute neurologic illness had not developed.

The IOM committee concluded that the balance of evidence was consistent with a causal relationship between DTP and some forms of chronic nervous system disorders in children in whom an acute neurologic disorder developed within 7 days following DTP administration. Thus physicians will need to spend extra time with parents explaining the changes in conclusions about DTP and long-term neurologic deficits. Nevertheless, the benefits from pertussis vaccine clearly outweigh the real and theoretical risks of adverse reactions.[8]

Acellular Pertussis Vaccines

The development of acellular pertussis vaccines has led to the potential for providing effective protection against pertussis with fewer side effects than occur following the administration of whole-cell DTP.[19–21] Acellular preparations (DTaP) developed by Lederle Laboratories (Pearl River, NY) and Connaught Laboratories (Swiftwater, Penn) have been licensed for use as the fourth and fifth doses for children 15 months of age or greater.[1,2] These acellular preparations have been shown to induce high levels of protection against disease caused by *Bordetella pertussis* in children vaccinated after 5 months of age or in the second year of life. The development of acellular pertussis vaccines for primary immunization of infants has been hampered by lack of knowledge of the essential antigens for inducing protective immunity. Studies in Sweden and Japan have revealed that inactivated pertussis toxin (PT) alone and PT plus filamentous hemagglutin (FHA) induce protection against disease.[21–23] Protection against milder forms of disease may have been greater with the combination of antigens than with PT alone.[23] However, some investigators believe that PT alone is all that will be needed for optimal protection.[24] At least seven different acellular products are currently being evaluated in phase III efficacy trials in Sweden, Germany, the United Kingdom, and Italy. The results from these trials are anticipated in late 1994 or early 1995. It is hoped that one or more of these products will be approved for primary immunization of infants at 2, 4, and 6 months of age.

Edwards et al.[25] have demonstrated that adults can safely receive a single injection of one of the acellular pertussis products. Significant increases in antibody concentrations to each of the vaccine components occurred in adults who received DTaP. It is not known whether booster doses of vaccines will result in decreased respiratory tract carriage or transmission of *B. pertussis*. If administering acellular pertussis vaccine to adults did result in decreased carriage of *B. pertussis* in adults, it would be reasonable to consider administering acellular pertussis vaccines at adolescence and perhaps at older ages to maintain long-term immunity to pertussis. The currently available DTaP products contain five times as much diphtheria toxoid as is normally administered in the adult tetanus-diphtheria (Td) preparations. The larger doses of diphtheria toxoid in pediatric formulations are associated with increased rates of local adverse effects in adults, so manufacturers would need to develop a special adult formulation of acellular pertussis vaccines for widespread use in adults.

DIPHTHERIA

The incidence of diphtheria in the United States has continued to decline (see Fig 1); for the first time on record there were no cases of diphtheria reported during 1993 (see Table 3).[11] However, in other countries, diphtheria continues to be a cause of significant morbidity and mortality. Several thousand cases were reported in Russia during 1993.[26] The explanation for this epidemic has not yet been determined. The potential for epidemics of diphtheria in adults exists in the United States and in other countries because serologic evidence of immunity against diphtheria wanes with increasing time since immunization.[27] Serologic surveys have shown that 20% to 40% of people more than 40 years of age in several countries do not have protective levels (0.01 IU/mL) of diphtheria antitoxin. Thus it is important for all adolescents to receive the recommended booster dose of Td at 14 to 16 years of age, and additional doses of Td should be given every 10 years. Unfortunately, tetanus toxoid alone without diphtheria toxoid is still used in some emergency rooms.

TETANUS

Disease

As with diphtheria, tetanus is also disappearing from the United States (see Fig 1). Most of the 40 to 50 cases that have occured annually in the United States have been in the few remaining adults who never received a primary series of tetanus immunization in childhood.[28] Occasional cases of neonatal tetanus have occurred in infants born to foreign-born women who delivered in the United States or came to the United States immediately after delivery. With improvements in the delivery of tetanus toxoid to women in other countries, there is a potential for elimination of neonatal tetanus as a public health problem. The World Health Organization has initiated a strategic plan to implement a global neonatal tetanus prevention program and improve the current low coverage rates for women delivering infants who have received two or more doses of tetanus toxoid.[29]

Improved Toxoids Possible

Both diphtheria and tetanus toxoids are relatively impure preparations. Only 65% to 85% of the protein in these preparations is the toxoids.[30] Improved tetanus and diphtheria toxoids could be produced through recombinant genetic technology, and highly purified preparations could be made.[30] Unfortunately, there is little financial incentive for manufacturers to invest the large amount of money required to bring these new products to market.

POLIOMYELITIS

Disease Patterns

No disease caused by wild-type poliomyelitis has occurred in the United States for more than 10 years.[31] The most important development in global poliomyelitis control has been the elimination of wild-type polio virus from Latin America. Beginning in 1985, the Pan American Health Organization launched a program to eliminate wild-type poliomyelitis by the end of 1990.[32] The last case of paralytic caused by wild-type poliomyelitis virus in Latin America was on August 23, 1991, in Peru.[33] This enormously successful campaign to eliminate poliomyelitis was accomplished through remarkable cooperation by all countries in Latin America and funding through many donor agencies. In some countries, including the United States, wild-type poliomyelitis viruses were eliminated primarily through the administration of oral poliomyelitis vaccine (OPV) in routine immunization programs. However, in several Latin American countries, national vaccine campaigns were implemented in which 95% to 100% of all children received two supplemental doses of OPV in campaigns 1 to 2 months apart each year. These efforts proved to be highly effective in interrupting the transmission of wild-type virus, and this regional program has set the stage for a global poliomyelitis eradication program.[34] The World Health Organization is currently generating resources, political will, and cooperation among nations to tackle the enormous problem of poliomyelitis in Africa and Asia.

Change in the Timing of the Third Dose of Vaccine

In the United States, three doses of OPV induce immunity to all three types of poliomyelitis in 97% to 100% of vaccinees (Table 4).[35–39] After two doses of vaccine, 5% to 10% of children are unprotected against poliomyelitis viruses type 1 or 3. There is no advantage to waiting 8 to 12 or more months between the second and third dose as has been the standard practice in the United States for more than 16 years. Therefore the ACIP and the Committee on Infectious Disease have recently recommended that the third dose can be administered at 6 to 18 months of age.[1, 2, 40] Administering the third dose earlier will provide less opportunity for transmis-

TABLE 4.
Percentage of Children With Serum Neutralizing Antibody to Poliomyelitis Types 1, 2, and 3 by the Number of Doses of Oral Poliomyelitis Vaccine Received and Schedule

		Percentage With Serum Neutralizing Antibody					
		After 2 Doses			After 3 Doses		
Study	Schedule*	p1†	p2†	p3†	p1	p2	p3
Hardy et al.[36]	2, 4, 6	93	100	91	97	100	96
Hardy et al.[36]	2, 4, 18	92	99	90	96	100	96
Faden et al.[37]	2, 4, 12	100	100	100	100	100	100
McBean et al.[38]	2, 4, 18	92	100	96	97	100	100
Modlin et al.[39]	2, 4, 15	95	100	90	96	100	98

*Age in months that oral poliomyelitis vaccine was administered.
†Poliomyelitis virus types 1, 2, and 3, respectively.

sion of wild-type viruses among young children following occasional importations from other countries.[41, 42]

Developing Countries

In developing countries the serologic response rates following OPV have been lower than the response rate in children residing in the United States.[35] Several recent studies have revealed some factors contributing to decreased response rates in developing countries.[35, 43] The OPV formulations used in developing countries have often contained lower titers of vaccine viruses, especially type 3 virus, than has been used in the United States. Improved response rates have been demonstrated after increasing the concentration of vaccine virus in the developing country formulations and/or administering supplemental doses.[35, 43, 44] The World Health Organization recommends a minimum of four doses of OPV for all children, with the first dose given at birth and subsequent doses at 6, 10, and 14 weeks of age.[45]

Vaccine-Associated Poliomyelitis

In the United States, vaccine-associated poliomyelitis has developed in a small number (three to eight) of children or adults each year.[31] The highest risk of vaccine-associated poliomyelitis occurs after the first dose of OPV when the vaccine recipients are most susceptible and most likely to transmit virus to contacts. The rates of vaccine-associated poliomyelitis have been higher in some developing countries than in the United States. Strebel et al.[46] have demonstrated a 10- to 20-fold higher rate of vaccine-associated poliomyelitis in Romanian children than has been observed in most countries. The primary factor associated with vaccine-associated poliomyelitis in this case-control study was the high number of injections of antibiotics received in the 30 days before the onset of paralysis. This study awaits validation in other countries. In the United States there has been no apparent association between injections and vaccine-associated poliomyelitis (Sutter R, personal communication, 1994).

Possible Sequential or Simultaneous Inactivated/Oral Poliomyelitis Vaccine Immunization Schedules

Sequential administration of two or more doses of inactivated poliomyelitis vaccine (IPV) followed by OPV might prevent some of the vaccine-associated cases and induce excellent intestinal immunity.[47] Several sequential schedules have induced very high levels of immunity to all three types of poliomyelitis from the simultaneous administration of IPV and OPV after one or two doses of IPV alone.[37,39,47,48] In developing countries, simultaneous IPV and OPV immunization has been shown to be highly effective in the West Bank and the Gaza Strip, and combination vaccination might be more effective than immunization with OPV alone.[43,49]

However, the use of IPV in developing countries remains controversial, in part because of the high cost.[50] Some experts are concerned that the potential use of IPV would divert too many resources from the global program and perhaps provide developing countries with an excuse for not conducting community-based mass OPV vaccination programs that have been highly effective in eliminating wild-type poliomyelitis virus. Perhaps some combination of these programs will eventually be accepted as the optimal strategy for protecting individuals from contracting poliomyelitis and eliminating transmission of wild-type virus.

Improved Oral Poliomyelitis Vaccine Possible

Studies are in progress to develop improved OPV preparations that might induce higher rates of local immunity, especially with type 3 virus.[51,52] However, introducing a new live OPV would require conducting trials in several million children to prove that the new formulation was as safe or safer than the currently available vaccine.

HAEMOPHILUS INFLUENZAE TYPE B

Disease Incidence

The licensure and widespread use of conjugate Hib vaccines have resulted in a rapid and dramatic decline in the incidence of Hib infections throughout the country (see Fig 1). Once the most common form of bacterial meningitis in children and the most common cause of acquired mental retardation in the United States, disease caused by this organism in children is now becoming rare in all areas of the country.[53] A decline in the incidence of invasive disease in infants started before the conjugate vaccine was approved for use at 2 months of age.[54] This more rapid decline than expected may be due in part to a herd immunity effect. Takela and colleagues have demonstrated in Finland[55] and in the United States[56] that vaccinated children are less likely to be carriers of Hib than unvaccinated children. Also, the Finnish investigators have demonstrated that the conjugate vaccines induce secretory IgA antibody, the presumed explanation for the inhibition of nasopharyngeal carriage.[57]

Conjugate *Haemophilus Influenzae* Type b Vaccines

There are currently four different conjugate preparations available in the United States, distributed by five different pharmaceutical companies[58, 59] (Table 5) The first conjugate vaccine to be licensed, PRP-D (ProHibit), is currently recommended only for use as a booster in children 15 months of age or older. This vaccine induces suboptimal protection against disease when administered to infants at 2, 4, and 6 months of age.[60] The other conjugate vaccines are approved for primary immunization of infants beginning at approximately 2 months of age. Following a primary series, these vaccines induce similar concentrations of serum antibodies.[61] The PRP-OMP and HbOC vaccines were shown to be highly efficacious in protecting infants against invasive Hib disease.[62, 63] PRP-T vaccines were licensed for infants primarily because they are able to induce functional antibodies in infants that were similar to the antibodies that correlated with protection in efficacy trials. The Merck, Sharp & Dohme (West Point, Penn) product (PRP-OMP) is approved for use as a two-dose primary series, and HbOC and PRP-T are approved for a three-dose primary series. The PRP-OMP vaccine induces protective levels of antibody and protection against disease following a single dose in a high proportion of children.[62] HbOC and PRP-T require two or three doses to induce protective levels of antibodies. Conjugation of the PRP to tetanus toxoid or a component of the diphtheria toxoid in HbOC converts the

TABLE 5.
Haemophilus influenzae Type b Conjugate Vaccines*

Manufacturer	Abbreviation	Trade Name	Carrier Protein
Connaught Laboratories	PRP-D†	ProHibit	Diphtheria toxoid
Lederle-Praxis	HbOC	HIBTITER	CRM197 (a nontoxic mutant diphtheria toxin)
	HbOC/DTP	Tetramune	Combination of HbOC with DTP
Merck, Sharp & Dohme	PRP-OMP	PedvaxHIB	OMP (an outer membrane protein complex of *Neisseria meningitides*)
Pasteur Merieux Vaccins (Distributed by SmithKline Beecham, and Connaught Laboratories)	PRP-T	ActHIB or OmniHib	Tetanus toxoid
Connaught Laboratories	PRP-T/DTP	OmniHib/DTP	Tetanus toxoid

*Adapted from Committee on Infectious Diseases: *Pediatrics* 92:480–488, 1993.
†PRP-D is recommended only for infants 12 months of age or older. HbOC, PRP-OMP, and PRP-T are recommended for infants beginning at approximately 2 months of age.

T-independent antibody response induced by PRP alone to a T-dependent response.[63] Granoff et al.[64] have shown that prior or simultaneous immunization with DTP may be necessary to induce an acceptable primary antibody response to Hib conjugate vaccines that use either diphtheria or tetanus toxoids as the carrier protein. Therefore, for the unusual infants who do not receive the first dose of DTP at the same time that the first dose of Hib vaccine is administered, PRP-OMP vaccine should be given.

Interchangeability of *Haemophilus Influenzae* Type b Conjugate Vaccines

Because of the varying characteristics of these vaccines and the different methods of production, concern was raised about the ability to "mix and match" the different vaccines in a primary vaccine series. However, several studies have demonstrated that the PRP-OMP or the HbOC vaccines primed for subsequent secondary antibody responses to second and third doses of the alternate vaccine or PRP-T.[65–67] The interchangeability of these vaccines for primary immunization has been endorsed by both the ACIP and the Committee on Infectious Diseases of the AAP.[1, 2, 59]

Manufacturers are investigating the potential for using similar conjugation technologies to develop conjugate pneumococcal vaccines that might be effective for use in children as young as 2 months of age.[68]

HEPATITIS B

Disease Incidence and Mortality From Hepatitis B Infections

The incidence of hepatitis B infections in the United States has declined slowly in the 12 years since the first hepatitis B vaccines were licensed (see Fig 1). Between 5,000 and 6,000 deaths occur

TABLE 6.
Deaths Caused by Vaccine-Preventable Disease Before Routine Immunization of Children in the United States*

Disease	Years	Death/Year
Measles	1960–1962	400–500
Haemophilus influenzae type b	1986–1988	800–1,000
Hepatitis B	1987–1990	5,000–6,000

*From Centers for Disease Control and Prevention: National Vaccine Program, Atlanta, Ga.

TABLE 7.
Recommended Doses of Hepatitis B Vaccines*

Population	Recombivax (MSD)†		Engerix-B (SK)	
	μg	mL	μg	mL
Infants of HBsAg-negative mothers and children <11 yr	2.5	0.5 (was 2.5)	10	0.5
Infants of HBsAg-positive mothers (HBIG [0.5 mL] should also be given)	5	0.5	10	0.5
Children and adolescents 11–19 yr	5	0.5	20	1.0
Adults ≥20 yr	10	1.0	20	1.0
Dialysis patients and other immunosuppressed persons	40	1.0	40	2.0

*Adapted from American Academy of Pediatrics, Committee on Infectious Diseases: Universal hepatitis B immunization. *Pediatrics* 89:795–799, 1992.
†MSD = Merck, Sharp & Dohme; SK = SmithKline Biologicals; HBsAg = hepatitis B surface antigen; HBIG = hepatitis B immune globulin.

every year in the United States from chronic liver disease and/or hepatocellular carcinoma induced by hepatitis B virus (HBV) infections.[69] Thus the deaths from hepatitis B infections in the United States are five to ten times more than those from Hib in the 1970s or measles in the 1950s before the vaccines to prevent those diseases were licensed (Table 6).

Vaccines

In the United States the original plasma-derived hepatitis B vaccine has been replaced by vaccines produced by using recombinant genetic techniques. The two products available in the United States (Table 7) are recommended for use in different doses and volumes for infants born to hepatitis B surface antigen (HBsAg)-positive or HBsAg-negative mothers.[1, 69, 70] Merck, Sharp & Dohme has recently released a vaccine formulation containing 2.5 μg of antigen in 0.5 mL. The original pediatric formulation had 2.5 μg in 0.25 mL. Since the different concentrations of vaccine available could lead to confusion, physicians should order the vaccines by the dose in micrograms, and note the specific manufacturer. These vaccines are considered equivalent by the Food and Drug Administration (FDA) and the advisory committees when the products are used in accordance with the manufacturers' recommendations.

Strategy to Prevent Disease: Universal Infant Immunization

The continuing high rates of hepatitis B infections in the United States despite the availability of effective vaccines for more than 10 years led to a change in the strategy to control hepatitis B infections in the United States.[69–71] The advisory committees now recommend the routine administration of three doses of hepatitis B vaccine to infants and young children as part of the routine immunization schedule.

Some physicians who care for children have had a difficult time recognizing the importance of vaccinating children to prevent hepatitis B infections because most of the complications of chronic hepatitis B infections are seen in adults. The strategy of vaccinating infants and children to prevent serious disease and premature death in adults is not unique to hepatitis B vaccine. Our routine childhood rubella immunization program has proved to be highly effective in preventing rubella and congenital rubella syndrome in young adults. Similarly, the administration of a primary series of tetanus toxoid in infancy helps provide long-term immunity against tetanus.

Universal infant immunization is only one part of a comprehensive strategy to eliminate hepatitis B as a public health problem in the United States.[69] Universal adolescent immunization was considered as an alternative approach that might have a more rapid impact on the epidemiology of hepatitis B infections than infant immunization.[70, 71] One province of Canada has initiated a universal preadolescent strategy, and the results to date indicate a high success rate for immunizing 10- to 11-year-old children in school settings (Scheifele D, personal communication, 1994). In the United States we have not had an effective program for delivering preventive services to adolescents, especially those in high-risk groups. However, adolescents should be immunized whenever resources permit since they are at increased risk.

The high rate of becoming a chronic carrier when hepatitis B infection is acquired in childhood was an additional factor considered by the committees when they recommended universal hepatitis B immunization. In the United States, approximate 26% of all of the chronic carriers have acquired their infections in early childhood even though only 8% of all infections occurred during childhood. The universal infant strategy should prevent most cases of chronic carriage, especially if the first dose of vaccine is given at birth.[69]

Duration of Immunity

Hepatitis B vaccination has been shown to protect for 9 or more years against the development of an HBsAg chronic carrier state.[72, 73] Ongoing longitudinal studies will determine the need for booster doses of vaccines for children immunized in infancy. The currently available data indicate that 20% or more individuals may have serum antibody concentrations to HBsAg (anti-HBs) decrease to below the presumed postvaccination protective level (10 mIU/mL) 6 to 10 years after primary immunization. However, immune-competent individuals are still protected against clinical disease and the development of the HBsAg carrier state when they have been exposed to hepatitis B virus infections.[72–74] Although there are inadequate data to recommend booster doses at this time, immunized populations will be monitored to determine whether a single supplemental dose of hepatitis B vaccine at either 4 to 6 years and/or at adolescence might be necessary to help ensure persistence of immunity throughout adult life.

Infants Born to Hepatitis B Surface Antigen–Positive Mothers

The recommendations for the management of infants born to HBsAg-positive mothers remain unchanged. These infants should receive a single 0.5-mL dose of hepatitis B immune globulin (HBIG) and the first dose of hepatitis B vaccine as soon as possible after birth.[1, 2, 69, 70] Note that the recommended dose of vaccine for these infants is larger than the dose recommended for infants born to HBsAg-negative mothers (see Table 7). These infants should complete the primary series of vaccination at 1 and 6 months of age. Hepatitis B immune globulin preparations in countries outside the United States often have the dose given in international units rather than in volume as is the custom in the United States. The U.S. standard immune globulin preparation was developed before the international unit standard was developed by the World Health Organization. Unpublished studies by the FDA indicate that the standard 0.5-mL dose of HBIG should provide at least 100 IU of anti-HBs, an amount approximately equivalent to the minimum recommendation for products made outside of the United States (Finlayson J, personal communication, 1994).

Infants Born to Unscreened Mothers

Infants born to mothers whose surface antigen status is unknown should receive the first dose of hepatitis B vaccine at birth in the dose recommended for infants born to surface antigen—positive mothers.[69, 70] The mother should be screened for HBsAg, and if found positive, the infant should receive HBIG as soon as possible. If the mother is negative for HBsAg, then the infant should complete the primary series as per the standard recommendations.

Immunization Schedules for Term Infants Born to Hepatitis B Surface Antigen–Negative Mothers

Hepatitis B vaccine has been shown to be highly effective in a variety of immunization schedules.[71] The AAP and the ACIP have recommended two alternative immunization schedules, with the AAP encouraging the routine immunization of the first dose at birth (Table 8).[69–71]

Several alternative effective schedules have allowed physicians to fit hepatitis B immunization into routine clinic visits without the need for administering more than three injections at any one visit or extra clinic visits (see Table 8). The administration of hepatitis B vaccine at birth has occasionally led to longer than recommended intervals before the child received the second or third doses of vaccine. Intervals of up to 10 months between the second and third doses of hepatitis B vaccine are associated with an excellent antibody response, and the longer the interval between the second and third dose, the higher the final geometric mean antibody concentration.[75] Although intervals of longer than 2 months

TABLE 8.
Hepatitis B Immunization Schedules for Infants Born to Hepatitis B Surface Antigen–Negative Women*

Schedule	Age (mo)
Recommended	
a†	0, 1–2, 6–18
b	2, 4, 6–18
Alternative, effective schedules adopted by some pediatricians	
d	0.5, 2, 6
e	1, 6, 18
f	6, 9, 15
g	9, 12, 18

*Adapted from Halsey NA: *Pediatr Infect Dis J* 12:449, 1993.
†Preferred by the American Academy of Pediatrics.

between the first and second doses have not been studied carefully, the advisory committees suggest that it is not necessary to restart the immunization schedule for children who have had longer than the recommended 1- to 2-month interval between doses. Ongoing studies of longer than 2 months between the first and second doses should provide information regarding additional alternative immunization schedules.

The development of new combination products will undoubtedly enhance the ability to introduce hepatitis B vaccine and other new vaccines under development into the routine schedule. Hepatitis B vaccine has been successfully combined with at least one Hib conjugate vaccine, and studies are under way to evaluate combination products, including DTP, IPV, and hepatitis B in the same syringe.

Low-Birth-weight or Premature Infants

Premature or low-birth-weight infants immunized at birth appear to have a somewhat lower antibody response than term infants in some but not all studies.[76–78] Since infants born to HBsAg-negative mothers are not at immediate risk of contracting hepatitis B infections, it is prudent to wait until either hospital discharge (if the infants weigh greater than 2,000 g) or approximately 2 months of age before initiating hepatitis B vaccination for infants with birth weight less than 2,000 g.[78] Premature infants born to HBsAg-positive mothers should be immunized at birth as described earlier.

MEASLES

Disease Incidence

The resurgence of measles in 1989–1991 resulted in more than 55,000 cases of measles, 11,000 hospitalizations, and 150 deaths (see Fig 1).[11, 79, 80] This epidemic was an obvious setback in the efforts to completely eliminate measles transmission in the United States. However, the widespread use of measles vaccine has resulted in more than a 99% reduction in the incidence of measles in most years as compared with disease transmission in the prevaccine era.

The increased efforts at measles control has resulted in a significantly lower incidence of measles in the last 2 years. An all-time low of 281 cases of measles was reported to the CDC in 1993 (see Table 3). During the first 7 months of 1994, 772 cases of measles were reported, indicating continuing measles transmission and the need to intensify control efforts.

Moving?

I'd like to receive my ***Advances in Pediatric Infectious Diseases*** without interruption.
Please not the following change of address, effective:

Name: ______________________________

New Address: ______________________________

____

City: ____________________ State: ________ Zip: ________

Old Address: ______________________________

____

City: ____________________ State: ________ Zip: ________

Reservation Card

Yes, I would like my own copy of ***Advances in Pediatric Infectious Diseases***. Please begin my subscription with the current edition according to the terms described below.* I understand that I will have 30 days to examine each annual edition. If satisfied, I will pay just $64.95 plus sales tax, postage and handling (price subject to change without notice).

Name: ______________________________

Address: ______________________________

City: ____________________ State: ________ Zip: ________

Method of Payment

❍ Visa ❍ Mastercard ❍ AmEx ❍ Bill me ❍ Check (in US dollars, payable to Mosby, Inc.)

Card number: ____________________ Exp date: ____________

Signature: ______________________________

LS-0908

*Your *Advances* Service Guarantee:

When you subscribe to *Advances*, we'll send you an advance notice of future volumes about two months before they publish. This automatic notice system is designed to take up as little of your time as possible. If you do not want *Advances*, the advance notice makes it quick and easy for you to let us know your decision, and you will always have at least 20 days to decide. If we don't hear from you, we'll send you the new volume as soon as it's available. And, of course, *Advances* is yours to examine free of charge for 30 days (postage, handling and applicable sales tax are added to each shipment.).

NO POSTAGE
NECESSARY
IF MAILED
IN THE
UNITED STATES

BUSINESS REPLY MAIL

FIRST CLASS MAIL PERMIT No. 762 CHICAGO, IL

POSTAGE WILL BE PAID BY ADDRESSEE

Chris Hughes
Mosby-Year Book, Inc.
200 N. LaSalle Street
Suite 2600
Chicago, IL 60601-9981

NO POSTAGE
NECESSARY
IF MAILED
IN THE
UNITED STATES

BUSINESS REPLY MAIL

FIRST CLASS MAIL PERMIT No. 762 CHICAGO, IL

POSTAGE WILL BE PAID BY ADDRESSEE

Chris Hughes
Mosby-Year Book, Inc.
200 N. LaSalle Street
Suite 2600
Chicago, IL 60601-9981

Factors Contributing to 1989–1991 Epidemic

LOW VACCINATION COVERAGE.—The highest incidence rates of measles occurred in pre–school-aged children, especially in children less than 15 months of age.[79] Since this was the recommended age for routine measles vaccination, almost all of these children were unvaccinated. However, the majority of children older than 15 months of age in whom measles developed were also unvaccinated. In 1992 a survey indicated that 83% of 2-year-old children in the United States had received their first dose of measles-mumps-rubella (MMR) vaccine.[11] However, studies in several inner-city populations revealed that only 50% to 70% of children had received measles vaccine by the time they were 2 years old.[81] Factors contributing to the low rates of completing measles immunization at the recommended age have included the inadequate quality and quantity of vaccine delivery services.[11] Efforts are under way to improve the accessibility to vaccines in public clinics.

VACCINATION OF CHILDREN WITH MINOR ILLNESSES.—Health care providers have often withheld vaccines from children with minor illnesses.[82, 83] Most studies have demonstrated that children with mild respiratory tract infections or diarrhea have responded to measles vaccine as well as children without minor illnesses.[84, 85] In a study involving more than 2,000 children, more than 98% of all children with minor illnesses responded to measles vaccine.[85] Children with fever had a slightly lower response rate than children who did not have fever in one study, but these differences were very small, and more than 97% of the children responded to the vaccine. Therefore children with minor illnesses can be effectively vaccinated against measles.[1, 2, 86]

INCREASED SUSCEPTIBILITY TO MEASLES DURING INFANCY.—A second factor contributing to the recent epidemic in very young children has been the lower level of passively derived maternal antibodies in children born to vaccinated mothers as compared with children born to mothers who had natural measles.[87–89] Standard-titer attenuated measles vaccines induce serum antibody concentrations that are fourfold to sixfold lower than the concentrations following natural measles.[90] Since infants born to vaccinated mothers receive lower antibody concentrations, the infants become susceptible to measles and measles vaccine at a younger age than children whose mothers had natural measles. More than 25% of all the children with measles during 1989 and 1990 were younger than 15 months of age.[79] Several recent unpublished studies have revealed that we can effectively vaccinate children born to mothers with vaccine-derived immunity at 12 months of age (Atkinson W, personal communication, 1994). Because of these data, the AAP and the ACIP now recommend that measles vaccine may be given at 12 months of age as an option to the usual recommendation of 15 months.[1, 2] In areas where measles has been a problem in pre–school-aged children and especially in urban inner-city areas where vaccine coverage has been low, the ACIP strongly encourages the administration of measles vaccine at 12 months of age.[2]

Age for Administering the Second Dose of Measles-Mumps-Rubella Vaccine.—In spite of the widespread transmission of measles in pre–school-aged children, the incidence of measles in school-aged children and college students was lower in 1989–1991 than would have been expected based on disease transmission patterns in the early 1980s.[79] Undoubtedly, the recommendations for administering a second dose of measles vaccine have contributed to the improved control of measles in older age groups. The AAP continues to recommend that the second dose be administered at 11 to 12 years of age unless two doses have been administered to children when they were 12 months of age or older.[1] The choice of 11 to 12 years was based in part on the observations that a small percentage of vaccinated children will have waning immunity following one dose of vaccine.[91, 92] The ACIP has continued to recommend that the second dose of measles vaccination be administered at school entry (4 to 6 years of age).[2, 86] Both committees recommend that young adults entering college should have received two doses of measles vaccine, and during measles outbreaks, children and young adults born in 1957 or later should receive a second dose of measles vaccine. Both committees recommend that the second dose of measles vaccine be MMR whenever possible.

High-Titer Measles Vaccines.—During the 1980s, efforts were made to develop more effective vaccines for immunizing children at 6 months of age, an age when passively acquired maternal antibodies usually interfere with vaccination. Studies in several developing countries revealed that increasing the dose of measles vaccine from approximately 3,000 infectious units per dose to 50,000 to 300,000 infectious units per dose resulted in significantly improved serologic response rates at 6 months of age.[93–95] This improvement in serologic response rates in young infants was not associated with any increased incidence of the usual side effects, including fever and rash, within the 2 to 3 weeks following vaccination. However, careful follow-up studies conducted in Guinea-Bissau, Senegal, and Haiti revealed that female children who had received the high-titer vaccines had significantly higher subsequent mortality than female infants who had received lower-titer vaccines.[96–99] There were no differences in mortality by vaccine dose among the male vaccinees. The biological mechanism to explain this phenomenon has not been explained, but the high-titer vaccines could have induced some alterations in the host's ability to respond to other infections.[100, 101] Natural measles is associated with increased delayed mortality in some countries.[102]

These studies resulted in withdrawal of the World Health Organization recommendation for use of the vaccine at 6 months of age.[97] Standard-titer measles vaccines have induced excellent protection against measles and significant reductions in mortality in all countries, including the same developing countries where the high-titer vaccines had been used.[103–105] Increased efforts will need to be made, especially in developing countries, to identify the optimal means to use standard-titer measles vaccines.

Measles Eradication Program in Latin America.—The Pan American Health Organization has coordinated efforts in the English-speaking Caribbean to interrupt measles transmission by administering a supplemental dose of measles vaccine for all children 1 to 15 years of age.[106, 107] These efforts were initiated in 1991 and have been highly successful in reaching more than 90% of the target children. Recently, Brazil and other South American countries have participated in this effort, and this approach shows significant promise for future global measles control in developing countries.

MUMPS

Disease Incidence

The incidence of mumps has continued to be very low in recent years (see Fig 1).

Mumps Vaccine and Meningoencephalitis

Investigations in Japan, Canada, and the United Kingdom have revealed that the Urabe strain of mumps vaccine has caused aseptic meningitis and the rate has been significantly higher than the rate following the Jeryl Lynn strain that is used in the MMR vaccine distributed in the United States.[108] Public health officials in the United Kingdom and Canada have recently withdrawn their support for use of the Urabe strain of mumps vaccine. If other countries follow this lead, there is a potential for having only a single manufacturer of mumps vaccine and MMR. Optimally, other mumps vaccine strains will be developed or manufacturers will acquire the right to produce the Jeryl Lynn strain of mumps vaccine so that multiple manufacturers will be able to provide MMR vaccines.

Duration of Immunity

Some concern has been raised over the duration of immunity from mumps vaccine because occasional outbreaks have occurred in highly immunized populations. In a recent study, mumps vaccine was found to be 83% (95% confidence interval [CI] = 57%, 94%) effective.[109] The routine administration of a second dose of mumps vaccine as part of MMR at either 4 to 6 years or 11 to 13 years of age should help ensure optimal protection against mumps.

RUBELLA

Disease Incidence

The recent resurgence of measles in the United States was accompanied by an increased incidence of rubella in 1990–1991 (see Fig 1) and congenital rubella syndrome. The intensified efforts to control measles through the use of MMR vaccine have also resulted in further declines in the incidence in rubella; fewer than 200 cases of rubella were reported during 1992 and 1993 in the United States (see Table 3).

Rubella Vaccine and Arthritis

The RA 27/3 strain of rubella vaccine has proved to be highly safe and effective. However, rubella vaccines have been associated with acute arthritis in a small percentage of vaccinees for many years.[110] The rate, however, is much lower than the rate following infection by the wild-type rubella virus. Recently, Tingle et al.[111] have argued that rubella vaccine may cause recurring or chronic arthritis for several months or years following vaccination. After a detailed review of the available data, the IOM committee recently concluded that the "Evidence is consistent with a causal relation" for the RA 27/3 strain of rubella vaccine and chronic arthritis.[15] Therefore physicians are probably obligated to inform vaccine recipients that there is a remote possibility of arthritis following the administration of rubella vaccine, but as with most other adverse events, the risk is much lower than that following the natural disease.

VARICELLA

Disease Incidence

In the absence of a vaccine, more than 90% of people acquire varicella by the time they are 18 to 24 years of age.[112–114]

Varicella Vaccine

Clinical studies with varicella vaccines have been under way for more than 20 years. The virus used in the preparation of vaccines was isolated by Professor Takahashi in Japan and named the Oka strain.[115] This vaccine has been licensed in Europe for use in children in remission from leukemia and has been available in the United States under a compassionate release for the same purpose for several years. Recurring rumors of the pending licensure of varicella vaccine and premature statements of the almost immediate availability of the vaccine have haunted public health officials and infectious disease experts for the past decade. At the time of this writing, the FDA is once again considering licensure, and the long-awaited varicella vaccine could soon be approved for routine use in children and adults in the United States.

Antibody Response to Vaccine

Approximately 97% of young children who receive a single dose of vaccine show evidence of serologic immunity as compared with 82% to 90% of adolescents and young adults.[116–119] Following the second dose of vaccine, 97% to 99% of adolescents and adults have an antibody response. The concentration of serum antibodies following vaccinations that correlates with long-term protection against varicella has not been determined precisely, but several antibody assays have been used to determine susceptibility to varicella, including indirect fluorescent antibody (IFA), fluorescent antibody to membrane antigen (FAMA), neutralization, latex agglutination (LA), indirect hemagglutination, immune adherence hemagglutination, radioimmunoassay, and enzyme-linked immunosorbent assay (ELISA). The ELISA and LA are the most practical for routine screening. The complement fixation assay is not sufficiently sensitive to be used for screening for susceptibility.

Side Effects Associated With Varicella Vaccine

Live attenuated varicella vaccine induces a mild rash illness in approximately 4% of seronegative children.[116–119] In addition, a local injection site rash consisting of a small number or papules or vesicles has been observed in 3% to 4% of children, presumably from virus spillage along the needle track. The majority of children in whom a body rash developed in the few weeks following varicella vaccine have had 10 or fewer skin lesions as compared with a mean of 300 or more lesions in children who had natural varicella. The lesions tend to be small and papular as compared with the vesicular rash seen in children with clinical varicella. Parents have described the rash as resembling mosquito bites. As with most other live viral vaccines and placebo control groups as well, varicella vaccine has been associated with temperatures of 100° F and higher in 10% to 20% of children in the 3 to 4 weeks following vaccination. The illnesses following vaccine administration have been mild and usually considered insignificant by the parents.

In one child a transient arthritis developed 13 days after vaccination (White J, personal communication, 1994). Since natural varicella is occasionally associated with arthritis, this arthritis was probably caused by the vaccine. No serious events have been reported following more than 9,000 doses of vaccine given to children.

Varicella vaccine will not be recommended for routine administration to immunocompromised individuals. Patients who are receiving aerosol or intermittent steroids will be eligible to receive varicella vaccine. Many experts have recommended withholding the use of steroids for 1 to 2 weeks before vaccination and 2 to 3 weeks after vaccination to minimize any potential for adverse events. Physicians should refer to the specific advisory committee guidelines for details.

Varicella vaccine has been used extensively in children with acute lymphocytic leukemia and continues to be available under a compassionate release approved by the FDA for children who have been in continuous remission for 1 or more years and who have an absolute lymphocyte count of 700 cell/mm^3 or higher and a platelet count of 100,000 cells/mm^3 or greater. When children with leukemia have been immunized, transmission to their household contacts has been observed in as many as 17% of the susceptible children (White J, personal communication, 1994). Fortunately, the vaccine virus appears to have retained its attenuation characteristics after replication in the leukemic children since the household contacts who acquired varicella infections had subclinical disease or illnesses with very mild rash. When healthy children have been immunized, no clinical signs of varicella-like illnesses have developed in their household contacts, but a small number of asymptomatic seroconversions have occurred.

Vaccine Efficacy

The efficacy of varicella vaccine for preventing clinical illness has been 96% to 100% in the first 2 years following vaccination.[120] Its efficacy against any clinical disease following household exposure was lower. Breakthrough cases of varicella in vaccines following exposure to persons with varicella have occurred at a rate of approximately 2% to 3% per year. These breakthrough cases have been much milder than natural varicella; the median number of skin lesions in breakthrough cases was only 53 vs. approximately 300 for children with natural varicella, and temperatures over 100° F were recorded in only 12% of the breakthrough cases as compared with 57% of the children with natural varicella.[121]

The rate of zoster developing among vaccinated leukemic children has been significantly lower than the rate in leukemic children who have had natural varicella.[122] In at least one instance, vaccine-like virus has been identified in a zoster lesion from a child with leukemia (White J, personal communication, 1994). Thus there is evidence that the varicella-zoster vaccine virus may persist in dorsal root ganglia as has been demonstrated for the wild-type varicella-zoster virus. Preliminary data suggest that the virus identified in the zoster lesions has retained its attenuated characteristics, and there has been no evidence of transmission from people with postvaccination zoster to their contacts. The available data regarding the incidence of zoster in healthy children and adults following vaccination are insufficient to determine whether vaccinees will be less likely for zoster to develop than people who have been infected with the wild-type virus.[123]

Vaccine Recommendations

Both the ACIP and the Committee on Infectious Diseases (COID) have voted to recommend the administration of a single dose of this vaccine for children 12 to 18 months of age as part of the routine immunization schedule if and when a license is granted by the FDA. The advisory committees have also recommended that children 18 months to 13 years of age who do not have a history of having had clinical varicella receive a single dose of varicella vaccine. Persons 13 years of age and older should receive two doses of vaccine separated by 4 to 8 weeks to ensure optimal immunity. Varicella vaccine is available as a lyophilized preparation and must be stored at freezer temperatures (−10° F or colder); the freezer compartment of a frost-free refrigerator/freezer is acceptable.

Combined Measles-Mumps-Rubella-Varicella Vaccine

Within several years, the manufacturer anticipates combining varicella vaccine with measles, mumps, and rubella to make a combination product (MMR-V). Preliminary studies have shown that the four live viruses can be combined in a single preparation, but if all of the conditions are not carefully controlled, there can be interference. Therefore physicians should not mix the monovalent varicella vaccine with MMR. However, the vaccines can be administered simultaneously at separate sites without any evidence of interference. Also, limited available data indicate that varicella vaccine can probably be administered simultaneously with either IPV or live OPV without evidence of interference. Definitive studies are in progress.

Vaccine Cost and Cost-Benefit Data

The cost of the vaccine was not available at the time of preparation of this manuscript. However, this vaccine will probably be more expensive than other vaccines routinely recommended for vaccination of all children. A detailed cost-benefit analysis has been done based on an assumed cost of $35 per dose.[3] When both direct health care costs and the indirect benefits to society from prevention of work lost by parents who have to stay home and care for sick children were considered, the overall benefit-to-cost ratio of varicella vaccination was approximately 5:1. This compares favorably with other childhood vaccines (see Table 2). The high public demand for a vaccine to prevent varicella is anticipated to be a major factor in the rapid acceptance of this vaccine for routine use. Also, vaccination of susceptible health care workers will undoubtedly result in significant cost savings for hospitals and other health care facilities where the prevention and management of nosocomial varicella has been a significant problem for many years.

THE IMMUNIZATION SCHEDULE

The addition of more vaccines to the recommended routine schedule for children has resulted in an increasingly complex set of recommendations for health care providers. Efforts are under way to simplify the schedule, but this process will take some time.[124] The COID and the ACIP are actively working together to improve the presentation of the schedule to try to unify the presentation of recommendations to avoid the perception of conflicting advice from advisory bodies. Manufacturers are actively developing several new combination products that are intended to lead to a decreased need for the number of injections at each of the routine visits. Products under active development include additional DTP/Hib products (two are now available), DTP/IPV, DTP/HBV, Hib/HBV, and similar products using DTaP in place of the whole-cell DTP. Flexibility will be needed on the part of the FDA to allow for interchangeability of these products in various schedules, and physicians will need to be aware of the need for monitoring changes in the immunization schedule.[125]

The AAP has recently agreed to publish an updated immunization schedule at least once every 12 months in the January issue of *Pediatrics.* This should help physicians keep up with anticipated additional changes in the recommendations for immunizing children.

REFERENCES

1. American Academy of Pediatrics (AAP): In Peter G, Halsey N, Pickering L, et al: *Report of the Committee on Infectious Disease,* ed 23. Elk Grove Village, Ill, American Academy of Pediatrics, 1994.
2. Centers for Disease Control and Prevention: General recommendations on immunization. Recommendations of the Advisory Committee on Immunization Practices (ACIP). *MMWR* 43(RR-1), 1994.
3. Lieu TA, Cochi SL, Black SB, et al: Cost-effectiveness of a routine varicella vaccination program for US children. *JAMA* 271:375–381, 1994.
4. *Healthy Children: Investing in the Future,* Washington, DC, US Congress, Office of Technology Assessment, Publication OTA-H-345, 1988.
5. Cochi SL, Broome CV, Hightower AW: Immunization of US children with *Haemophilus influenzae* type b polysaccharide vaccine. *JAMA* 253:521–529, 1985.
6. Hay JW, Daum RS: Cost-benefit analysis of *Haemophilus influenzae* type b prevention: conjugate vaccination at eighteen months of age. *Pediatr Infect Dis J* 9:246–252, 1990.
7. White CC, Koplan JP, Orenstein WA: Benefits, risks and costs of immunization for measles, mumps and rubella. *Am J Public Health* 75:739–744, 1985.
8. Hinman AR, Kaplan JP: Pertussis and pertussis vaccine. *JAMA* 251:3109–3113, 1984.
9. Omnibus Budget Reconciliation Act of 1993. PL 103-66.
10. Centers for Disease Control and Prevention: Resurgence of pertussis—United States, 1993. *MMWR* 42:952–960, 1993.
11. Centers for Disease Control and Prevention: Reported vaccine-preventable diseases—US 1993, and the Childhood Immunization Initiative. *MMWR* 43:57–60, 1994.
12. Farizo KM, Cochi SL, Zell ER, et al: Epidemiological features of pertussis in the United States, 1980–1989. *Clin Infect Dis* 14:708–719, 1992.
13. Sutter RW, Cochi SL: Pertussis hospitalizations and mortality in the United States, 1985–1988: Evaluation of the completeness of national reporting. *JAMA* 267:386–391, 1992.
14. Orenstein WA, Weisfeld J, Halsey NA: Diphtheria and tetanus toxoids and pertussis vaccine combined, in Halsey NA, deQuadros C: *Recent Advances in Immunization: A Literature Review,* Scientific Publication No 451. Washington, DC, Pan American Health Organization, 1983, pp 30–51.

15. Howson CP, Howe CJ, Fineberg HV (eds): *Adverse Effects of Pertussis and Rubella Vaccines: A report of the Committee to Review the Adverse Consequences of Pertussis and Rubella Vaccines.* Washington, DC, National Academy Press, 1991.
16. Institute of Medicine, Division of Health Promotion and Disease Prevention: In Stratton KR, Howe CJ, Johnston RB Jr: *Adverse Events Associated With Childhood Vaccines: Evidence bearing on causality.* Washington, DC, National Academy Press, 1994.
17. Miller D, Madge N, Diamond J, et al: Pertussis immunization and serious acute neurological illnesses in children. *BMJ* 307:1171–1176, 1993.
18. Institute of Medicine Committee to Study New Research on Vaccines: *DPT Vaccine and Chronic Nervous System Dysfunction. A New Analysis.* Washington, DC, National Academy Press, 1994.
19. Englund JA, Glezen WP, Barreto L: Controlled study of a new five-component acellular pertussis vaccine in adults and young children. *J Infect Dis* 166:1436–1441, 1992.
20. Englund JA, Decker MD, Edwards KM, et al: Acellular and whole-cell pertussis vaccines as booster doses: A multicenter study. *Pediatrics* 93:37–43, 1994.
21. Cherry JB: Acellular pertussis vaccines: A solution to the pertussis problem. *J Infect Dis* 168:21–24, 1993.
22. Storsaeter J, Olin P: Relative efficacy of two acellular pertussis vaccines during years of passive surveillance. *Vaccine* 8:142–144, 1992.
23. Blackwelder WC, Storsaeter J, Olin P, et al: Acellular pertussis vaccine: Efficacy and evaluation of clinical case definitions. *Am J Dis Child* 145:1285–1289, 1991.
24. Robbins JB, Pittman M, Trollfors B, et al: *Primum non nocere:* A pharmacologically inert pertussis toxoid alone should be the next pertussis vaccine. *Pediatr Infect Dis J* 12:795–807, 1993.
25. Edwards KM, Decker MD, Graham BS, et al: Adult immunization with acellular pertussis vaccine. *JAMA* 269:53–56, 1993.
26. Lumio J, Jahkola M, Vuento R, et al: Diphtheria after visit to Russia. *Lancet* 342:53–54, 1993.
27. Galazka AM: *Immunological Basis for Immunization for Diphtheria.* Geneva, Switzerland, World Health Organization, 1993.
28. Centers for Disease Control and Prevention: Summary of notifiable diseases, United States, 1992. *MMWR* 41:577, 1992.
29. Expanded Programme on Immunization: Global Advisory Group. *Wkly Epidemiol Rec* 63:9–13, 1988.
30. Levin MM, Hone DM, Stocker BAD, et al: *New and improved vaccines against typhoid fever,* in Woodrow GC, Levin MM: *New Generation Vaccines.* New York, Marcel Dekker, 1990, p 251.
31. Strebel PM, Sutter RW, Cochi SL, et al: Epidemiology of poliomyelitis in the United States one decade after the last reported case of indigenous wild virus–associated disease. *Clin Infect Dis* 14:568–579, 1992.
32. deQuadros CA, Andrus JK, Olivé J-M, et al: Eradication of poliomy-

elitis: Progress in the Americas. *Pediatr Infect Dis J* 10:222–229, 1991.
33. Expanded programme on immunization: Progress towards global eradication of poliomyelitis, 1988–1993. *MMWR* 43, 499–503, 1994.
34. Wright PF, Kim-Farley RJ, deQuadros CA, et al: Strategies for the global eradication of poliomyelitis by the year 2000. *N Engl J Med* 325:1774–1779, 1991.
35. Patriarca PA, Wright PF, John TJ: Factors affecting the immunogenicity of oral poliovirus vaccine in developing countries: Review. *Rev Infect Dis* 13:926–939, 1991.
36. Hardy GE, Hopkins CC, Linnemann CC, et al: Trivalent oral poliovirus vaccine: A comparison of two infant immunization schedules. *Pediatrics* 45:444–448, 1970.
37. Faden H, Modlin JF, Thoms ML, et al: Comparative evaluation of immunization with live attenuated and enhanced-potency inactivated trivalent poliovirus vaccines in childhood: Systemic and local immune response. *J Infect Dis* 162:1291–1297, 1990.
38. McBean AM, Thoms ML, Albrecht P, et al: Serologic response to oral polio vaccine and enhanced-potency inactivated polio vaccines. *Am J Epidemiol* 128:615–628, 1988.
39. Modlin JF, Halsey NA, Thoms ML, et al: Serum neutralizing antibody response to three experimental sequential IPV-OPV immunization schedules (abstract 1239). Presented at the 33rd Interscience Conference on Antimicrobial Agents and Chemotherapy, New Orleans, October 1993, p 346.
40. Committee on Infectious Diseases: Administration of the third dose of OPV at 6–18 months of age. *Pediatrics* 1994, in press.
41. Centers for Disease Control and Prevention: Isolation of wild poliovirus type 3 among members of a religious community objecting to vaccination—Alberta, Canada, 1993. *MMWR* 42:337–339, 1993.
42. Centers for Disease Control and Prevention: CDC update: Poliomyelitis outbreak, 1992. *MMWR* 41:917–919, 1992.
43. Mornier BJ, van Loon FP, Rhodes PH, et al: Immunogenicity of a supplemental dose of oral versus inactivated poliovirus vaccine. *Lancet* 341:1545–1550, 1993.
44. Richardson G, Linkins R, Eames M, et al: Immunogenicity of oral poliovirus vaccine (OPV) given in mass campaigns versus routine immunization programs (abstract 1237). Presented at the 33rd Interscience Conference on Antimicrobial Agents and Chemotherapy, New Orleans, 1993, p 346.
45. Kim-Farley R, Expanded Program on Immunization Team: Global immunization. *Annu Rev Public Health* 13:223–237, 1992.
46. Strebel P, Combiescu A, Nedelcu N, et al: Excess risk of vaccine-associated paralytic poliomyelitis (VAPP), Romania 1984–92 (abstract 1650). Presented at the 33rd Interscience Conference on Antimicrobial Agents and Chemotherapy, New Orleans, 1993, p 420.
47. McBean AM, Modlin JF: Rationale for the sequential use of inactivated poliovirus vaccine and live attenuated poliovirus vaccine for

routine poliomyelitis immunization in the United States. *Pediatr Infect Dis J* 6:881–887, 1987.
48. Modlin JF, Onorato IM, McBean AM, et al: The humoral immune response to type 1 oral poliovirus vaccine in children previously immunized with enhanced potency inactivated poliovirus vaccine or live oral poliovirus vaccine. *Am J Dis Child* 144:480–484, 1990.
49. Lasch EE, Abed Y, Marcus O, et al: Combined live and inactivated poliovirus vaccine to control poliomyelitis in a developing country—five years after. IABS Congress on Use and Standardization of Combined Vaccines, Amsterdam, The Netherlands, 1985. *Dev Biol Stand* 65:137–143, 1986.
50. Patriarca PA, Foege WH, Swartz TA: Progress in polio eradication. *Lancet* 342:1461–1464, 1993.
51. Murray MG, Kuhn RJ, Arita M, et al: Poliovirus type 1 type 3 antigenic hybrid virus constructed in vitro elicits type 1 and type 3 neutralizing antibodies in rabbits and monkeys. *Proc Natl Acad Sci U S A* 85:3203, 1988.
52. Minor PD, Almond JW: New and improved vaccines against poliomyelitis, in Woodrow GC, Levine MM: *New Generation Vaccines*. New York, Marcel Dekker, 1990.
53. Adams WG, Deaver KA, Cochi SL, et al: Decline of childhood *Haemophilus influenzae* type b (Hib) disease in the Hib vaccine era. *JAMA* 269:221–226, 1993.
54. Murphy TV, White KE, Pastor P, et al: Declining Incidence of *Haemophilus influenzae* type b disease since introduction of vaccination. *JAMA* 269:246–248, 1993.
55. Takela AK, Eskola J, Leinonen M, et al: Reduction of oropharyngeal carriage of *Haemophilus influenzae* type b (Hib) in children immunized with Hib conjugate vaccine. *J Infect Dis* 164:982–986, 1991.
56. Takela AK, Santosham M, Almedio-Hill J, et al: Vaccination with *Haemophilus influenzae* type b meningococcal protein conjugate vaccine reduces oropharyngeal carriage of *Haemophilus influenzae* type b among American Indian children. *Pediatr Infect Dis J* 12:593–599, 1993.
57. Kauppi M, Rönnberg PR, Saarinen L, et al: Mucosal antibody concentrations after immunization with *Haemophilus influenzae* type b (Hib) conjugate vaccine. Presented at the seventh International Congress of Mucosal Immunity, Prague, Czechoslovakia, Aug 16–20, 1992.
58. Committee on Infectious Diseases: *Haemophilus influenzae* type b conjugate vaccines: Recommendations for immunization with recently and previously licensed vaccines. *Pediatrics* 92:480–488, 1993.
59. Centers for Disease Control and Prevention: Recommendations for use of *Haemophilus* b conjugate vaccines and a combined diphtheria, tetanus, pertussis, and *Haemophilus* b vaccine. Recommenda-

tions of the Advisory Committee on Immunization Practices (ACIP). *MMWR* 42:1–15, 1994.

60. Committee on Early Childhood, Adoption, and Dependent Care: The pediatricians's role in promoting the health of patients in early childhood education and/or child care programs. *Pediatrics* 92:489–492, 1993.
61. Granoff DM, Anderson EL, Osterholm MT, et al: Differences in the immunogenicity of three *Haemophilus influenzae* type b conjugate vaccines in infants. *J Pediatr* 121:187–194, 1992.
62. Santosham M, Wolff M, Reid R, et al: The efficacy in Navajo infants of conjugate vaccine consisting of *Haemophilus influenzae* type b polysaccharide and *Neisseria meningitides* outer-membrane protein complex. *N Engl J Med* 324:1767–1772, 1991.
63. Black SB, Shinefield HR, Fireman B, et al: Efficacy in infancy of oligosaccharide conjugate *Haemophilus influenzae* type b (HbOC) vaccine in a United States population of 61,080 children. *Pediatr Infect Dis J* 10:97–104, 1991.
64. Granoff DM, Rathore MH, Holmes SJ, et al: Effect of immunity to the carrier protein on antibody responses to *Haemophilus influenzae* type b conjugate vaccines. *Vaccine* 11(suppl):46–51, 1993.
65. Greenberg DP, Leiberman JM, Marcy SM, et al: Safety and immunogenicity of mixed sequences of *Haemophilus influenzae* type b (Hib) conjugate vaccines in infants (abstract 997). *Pediatr Res* 33:169, 1993.
66. Daum RS, Milewski WM, Ballanco GA: Interchangeability of H. influenzae type b vaccines for the primary series ("mix and match")—a preliminary analysis (abstract 976). *Pediatr Res* 33:166, 1993.
67. Anderson EL, Decker MD, Edwards KM, et al: Interchangeability of conjugated *Haemophilus influenzae* type b (HiB) vaccines in infants (abstract 493). *Pediatr Res* 33:85, 1993.
68. Steinhoff ME, Edwards K, Deyserling H, et al: A randomized comparison of three bivalent S. *pneumoniae* glycoprotein conjugate vaccines in young children: Effect of polysaccharide size and linkage characteristics. *Pediatr Infect Dis J* 13:368–374, 1994.
69. Centers for Disease Control and Prevention: Hepatitis B virus: A comprehensive strategy for eliminating transmission in the United States through universal childhood vaccination. Recommendations of the Immunization Practices Advisory Committee (ACIP). *MMWR* 40:1–25, 1991.
70. Hall C, Halsey NA, Committee on Infectious Diseases: Universal hepatitis B immunization. *Pediatrics* 89:795–800, 1992.
71. Halsey NA: Discussion of Immunization Practices Advisory Committee/American Academy of Pediatrics' recommendations for universal hepatitis B vaccination. *Pediatr Infect Dis J* 12:446–449, 1993.
72. Hadler SC, Francis DP, Maynard JE, et al: Long-term immunogenicity and efficacy of hepatitis B vaccine in homosexual men. *N Engl J Med* 315:209–214, 1986.

73. Wainwright RB, McMahon BJ, Bulkow LR, et al: Duration of immunogenicity and efficacy of hepatitis B vaccine in a Yupik Eskimo population. *JAMA* 261:2362–2366, 1989.
74. Margolis HS, Alter MJ, Hadler SC: Hepatitis B: Evolving epidemiology and implications for control. *Semin Liver Dis* 11:84–92, 1991.
75. Hadler SC, Monson MA, Lugo DR, et al: Effect of timing of hepatitis B vaccine dose on response to vaccine in Yucpa Indians. *Vaccine* 7:106–110, 1989.
76. Lau Y-L, Tam AYC, Ng KW, et al: Clinical and laboratory observations: Responses of preterm infants to hepatitis B vaccine. *J Pediatr* 121:962–965, 1992.
77. Chirico G, Belloni C, Gasparoni A, et al: Hepatitis B immunization in infants from HBsAg negative mothers. *Pediatrics* 92:717–719, 1993.
78. Committee on Infectious Diseases: Update on timing of hepatitis B vaccination for premature infants and for children with lapsed immunization. *Pediatrics* in press.
79. Gindler JS, Atkinson WL, Markowitz LE et a: Epidemiology of measles in the United States in 1989 and 1990. *Pediatr Infect dis J* 11:841–846, 1992.
80. Robertson SE, Markowitz LE, Berry DA, et al: A million dollar measles outbreak: Epidemiology, risk factors, and a selective revaccination strategy. *Public Health Rep* 107:24–31, 1992.
81. Centers for Disease Control and Prevention: Retrospective assessment of vaccination coverage among school-aged children—selected US cities, 1991. *MMWR* 41:103–108, 1992.
82. Szilagyi PG, Rodewald LE, Humiston SG, et al: Missed opportunities for childhood vaccinations in office practices and the effect of vaccine status. *Pediatrics* 91:1–7, 1993.
83. Hughart N, Guyer B, Stanton B, et al: Do child health care provider practices conform to the new CDC standards for pediatric immunization practices? *Arch Pediatr Adolesc Med* 1994, in press.
84. Halsey NA, Boulos R, Andre J, et al: Factors influencing the response to measles vaccine in 6–12 month old Haitian infants. *N Engl J Med* 313:544–549, 1985.
85. Atkinson W, Markowitz L, Baughman A, et al: Serologic response to measles vaccination among ill children (abstract 422). Presented at the 32nd Interscience Conference on Antimicrobial Agents and Chemotherapy, Anaheim, Calif, Oct 12, 1992, p 181.
86. Measles prevention: Recommendations of the Immunization Practices Advisory Committee (ACIP). *MMWR* 38(suppl 9):1–13, 1989.
87. Pabst HF, Spady DW, Marusyk RG, et al: Reduced measles immunity in infants in a well-vaccinated population. *Pediatr Infect Dis J* 11:525–529, 1992.
88. Lennon JL, Black FL: Maternally derived measles immunity in the era of vaccine protected mothers. *J Pediatr* 108:671–676, 1986.

89. Jenks PJ, Caul EO, Roome PCH: Maternally derived measles immunity in children of naturally infected and vaccinated mothers. *Epidemiol Infect* 101:473–476, 1988.
90. Krugman S: Further attenuated measles vaccine: Characteristics and use. *Rev Infect Dis* 5:477–481, 1983.
91. Reyes MA, Franky de Borrero M, Roa J, et al: Measles vaccine failure after documented seroconversion. *Pediatr Infect Dis J* 6:848–851, 1987.
92. Mathias R, Meekison J, Arcan T, et al: The role of secondary vaccine failures in measles outbreaks. *Am J Public Health* 79:475–478, 1989.
93. Markowitz LE, Sepulveda J, Diaz-Ortega JL, et al: Immunization of six month-old infants with different doses of Edmonston-Zagreb and Schwarz measles vaccines. *N Engl J Med* 322:580–587, 1990.
94. Job JS, Halsey NA, Boulos R, et al: Successful immunization of infants at 6 months of age with high dose Edmonston-Zagreb measles vaccine. *Pediatr Infect Dis J* 10:303–311, 1991.
95. Berry S, Hernandez H, Kanashiro R, et al: Comparison of high titer Edmonston-Zagreb, Biken-CAM and Schwarz measles vaccines in Peruvian infants. *Pediatr Infect Dis J* 11:822–827, 1992.
96. Garenne M, Leroy O, Beau JP, et al: Child mortality after high titer measles vaccines: Prospective study in Senegal. *Lancet* 338:903–907, 1991.
97. Expanded Programme on Immunization: Safety of high-titer measles vaccines. *Wkly Epidemiol Rec* 67:357–361, 1992.
98. Aaby P, Knudsen K, Whittle H, et al: Long-term survival after Edmonston-Zagreb measles vaccination: Increased female mortality rate. *J Pediatr* 122:904–908, 1993.
99. Holt EA, Moulton LH, Siberry GK, et al: Differential mortality by measles vaccine titer and sex. *J Infect Dis* 168:1087–1097, 1993.
100. Ward BJ, León ME, Halsey NA, et al: *Possible Mechanisms of Immunologic Changes After High Titer Measles Vaccination*, in *Vaccines 93: Modern Approaches to New Vaccines Including AIDS*. Cold Spring Harbor, NY, Cold Spring Harbor Laboratory Press, 1993, pp 329–335.
101. León ME, Ward B, Kanashiro R, et al: Immunological parameters two years after high titer measles immunization in Peruvian children. *J Infect Dis* 168:1097–1105, 1993.
102. Hull HF, Williams PJ, Oldfield F: Measles mortality and vaccine efficacy in rural West Africa. *Lancet* 1:972–975, 1983.
103. Aaby P, Pedersen IR, Knudsen K, et al: Child mortality related to seroconversion or lack of seroconversion after measles vaccination. *Pediatr Infect Dis J* 8:197–200, 1989.
104. Koenig MA, Khan MA, Wojtyniak B, et al: Impact of measles vaccination on childhood mortality in rural Bangladesh. *Bull WHO* 68:441–447, 1990.
105. Holt E, Boulos R, Halsey N, et al: Childhood survival in Haiti: The

protective effect of measles vaccination. *Pediatrics* 85:188–194, 1990.

106. Plan to eliminate indigenous transmission of measles in the English-speaking Caribbean countries. *Bull Pan Am Health Organ* 24:240–246, 1990.
107. Pan American Health Organization: Measles elimination in the Americas. *Bull Pan Am Health Org* 26:271–275, 1992.
108. Institute of Medicine, Division of Health Promotion and Disease Prevention: Adverse events associated with childhood vaccines: Evidence bearing on causality, measles and mumps vaccines, in Howson CP, Howe CJ, Fineberg HV: *Adverse Effects of Pertussis and Rubella Vaccines: A report of the Committee to Review the Adverse Consequences of Pertussis and Rubella Vaccines.* National Academy Press, Washington, DC, 1991, pp 131–135.
109. Hersh BS, Fine PE, Kent K, et al: Mumps outbreak in a highly vaccinated population. *J Pediatr* 119:187–193, 1991.
110. Polk BF, Modlin JF, White JA, et al: A controlled comparison of joint reactions among women receiving one or two rubella vaccines. *Am J Epidemiol* 115:19–25, 1982.
111. Tingle AJ, Allen M, Petty RE, et al: Rubella-associated arthritis. I. Comparative study of joint manifestations associated with natural rubella infection and RA 27/3 rubella immunisation. *Ann Rheum Dis* 45:110–114, 1986.
112. Wharton M, Fehrs L, Cochi SL, et al: Health impact of varicella in the 1980s (Abstract 1138). Presented at the 30th Interscience Conference on Antimicrobial Agents and Chemotherapy, Atlanta, October 21–24, 1990.
113. Kelly PW, Petruccelli BP, Stehr-Green P, et al: The susceptibility of young adult Americans to vaccine-preventable infections. A national serosurvey of US Army recruits. *JAMA* 266:2724–2729, 1991.
114. Gershon AA, Raker R, Steinberg S, et al: Antibody of varicella-zoster virus in parturient women and their offspring during the first year of life. *Pediatrics* 58:692–696, 1976.
115. Takahashi M, Otsuka T, Okuno Y, et al: Live vaccine used to prevent the spread of varicella in children in hospital. *Lancet* 2:1288–1290, 1974.
116. Arbeter AM, Starr SE, Plotkin SA: Varicella vaccine studies in healthy children and adults. *Pediatrics* 78(suppl):748–756, 1986.
117. Johnson CE, Shurin PA, Fattlar D, et al: Live attenuated varicella vaccine in healthy 12- to 14-month-old children. *Pediatrics* 81:512–518, 1988.
118. White CJ, Kuter BJ, Hildebrand CS, et al: Varicella vaccine (VARIVAX) in healthy children and adolescents: results from clinical trials, 1987–1989. *Pediatrics* 87:604–610, 1991.
119. Gershon AA, Steinberg SP, LaRussa P, et al: Immunization of healthy adults with live attentuated varicella vaccine. *J Infect Dis* 158:132–137, 1988.

120. Weibel RE, Neff BS, Kuter BJ, et al: Live attenuated varicella vaccine, efficacy trial in healthy children. *N Engl J Med* 310:1409–1415, 1984.
121. Watson BM, Piercy SA, Plotkin SA, et al: Modified chickenpox in children immunized with the Oka/Merck varicella vaccine. *Pediatrics* 91:17–22, 1993.
122. Hardy I, Gershon AA, Steinberg SP, et al: The incidence of zoster after immunization with live attenuated varicella vaccine. *N Engl J Med* 325:1545–1550, 1991.
123. White CJ: Letters to the editor. *Pediatrics* 318:354, 1992.
124. Halsey NA: A possible approach to simplification of the US immunization schedule. Presented at the 26th National Immunization Conference St. Louis, Mo, 1992, pp 191–193.
125. Halsey NA: Proceedings of the "Combined Vaccines and Simultaneous Administration: Current Issues and Perspectives." Practical considerations regarding the impact on immunization; schedules of the introduction of new combined vaccines. New York Academy Press, 1994 (in press).

Use of Prophylactic Antibiotics in Children

Camille N. Bitar, M.D.
Division of Infectious Diseases, Department of Pediatrics, Louisiana State University School of Medicine, and Tulane University School of Medicine, New Orleans, Louisiana

Russell W. Steele, M.D.
Division of Infectious Diseases, Department of Pediatrics, Louisiana State University School of Medicine, and Tulane University School of Medicine, New Orleans, Louisiana

Shortly after the discovery of antimicrobials in the 20th century, the concept of chemoprophylaxis was introduced with the assumption that an antibiotic that eradicates an infection should also be able to prevent disease. Although most data have confirmed the efficacy of prophylaxis for many well-defined indications, some applications have actually led to an increase in infection, e.g., penicillin prophylaxis for meningococcal disease was associated with a higher incidence of secondary disease.[1] Therefore, any recommendation must be supported by well-designed clinical studies.

In general, prophylaxis works best when directed at a single specific pathogen to either prevent the progression of infection or eradicate colonization before disease becomes clinically established. Benefit is also most likely when the antibiotics used for prophylaxis have the following additional attributes: safety, low low propensity for generating antibiotic resistance, and achievement of adequate serum concentrations at a tolerable and cost-effective dosage. Patient compliance is also a critical issue.

Situations in which the efficacy of chemoprophylaxis has been established will be reviewed in this chapter, with particular emphasis on those clinical circumstances or diseases encountered most frequently in ambulatory practice (Table 1).

RECURRENT ACUTE OTITIS MEDIA

It is estimated that 30% of a pediatrician's time is spent in managing various aspects of otitis media. Even more important than treat-

TABLE 1.
Infections or Disease for Which Antimicrobial Chemoprophylaxis Has Been Established

Otitis media
Recurrent urinary tract infection
Rheumatic fever
Bacterial endocarditis
Neonatal group B streptococcal infection
Infections in pediatric acquired immunodeficiency syndrome
Bacterial meningitis
Meningococcal disease
Haemophilus influenzae type b disease
Asplenia
Tuberculosis
Traveler's diarrhea
Malaria
Influenza A
Pertussis
Surgical procedures
Pneumocystis carinii

ment of acute episodes is recognition of those children with persistent middle ear effusions since this may result in delay of psychomotor and language development or permanent conductive hearing loss.[2, 3] It should also be appreciated that recurrent acute otitis media (RAOM) is a common source of discomfort in children, parental anxiety, and cost for acute medical care.

With the high incidence of RAOM and frequent sequelae, a variety of strategies have been examined for prevention that employ various combinations of prophylactic antibiotics,[4–6] ventilation-tubes,[7] steroids, and nonsteroidal anti-inflammatory agents.[8–10] Vaccines and immunoglobulin have also been investigated.[11–13] Of all approaches, a regimen of prophylactic antibiotics alone followed by ventilation tubes only for the more recalcitrant cases appears most rational.[4–7, 9–12, 14] A 7-day course of steroids (0.5 to 1.0 mg/kg/day divided every 12 hours) with antibiotics after antibiotics alone have failed has also been shown to be of benefit before beginning a longer course of prophylactic treatment.[15]

Recurrent acute otitis media is defined as three episodes of infection within a 6-month period or four within 12 months. Data now exist that support the efficacy of ampicillin[4] and sulfisoxazole[5, 6] in reducing acute attacks of otitis media and in clearing middle ear effusions. Additional studies have suggested that ventilation tubes in combination with prophylactic antibiotics may be necessary for some patients.[4, 7] However, most investigators agree that a trial of chemoprophylaxis is warranted before any decision for ventilation tube placement.[7, 14]

Trimethoprim-sulfamethoxazole (TMP/SMX) is equally effective as other regimens and is associated with a very low incidence of adverse reactions.[6, 14] However, the pharmaceutical companies that manufacture TMP/SMX have not requested approval from the Food and Drug Administration for this prophylactic indication, and a disclaimer emphasizing this restriction appears in the current *Physicians' Desk Reference.*

The only theoretical adverse consequence of long-term prophylaxis is selection of antibiotic-resistant pathogens in the respiratory tract. This has been observed in some studies[14] but not in others.

Other strategies for the prevention of RAOM do not appear to be effective. These include immunoglobulin,[11] antihistamines, and decongestants.[16]

TABLE 2.
Antibiotic Prophylaxis for Recurrent Otitis Media (OM)

Candidates for therapy
3 episodes of OM within 6 mo
4 episodes of OM within 12 mo
Chemoprophylaxis
Sulfisoxazole, 35 mg/kg/dose once or twice daily
or
Amoxicillin, 20 mg/kg/day divided or once daily
Duration of therapy
90 days following the last episode of OM
or
During the winter months
or
For the duration of each new upper respiratory infection
Consider ventilating tubes
Failure of chemoprophylaxis alone
Poor compliance

Table 2 summarizes a practical approach for the management of children with RAOM based on the current literature.

RECURRENT URINARY TRACT INFECTION

Recurrent infections are observed in 30% to 50% of children with urinary tract infections (UTIs), with approximately 90% of these occurring within 3 months after the initial episode. Eighty percent of recurrences are new infections by different fecal-colonic bacterial species that have become resistant to recently administered antibiotics. The recurrence rate is not altered by extending the duration of treatment. Failure to eradicate an organism from the urine suggests an anatomic or physiologic defect. These patients require suppressive antibiotics until the underlying abnormality resolves or is surgically corrected (Fig 1). Recurrent UTI, if unrecognized, may lead to serious renal injury, hypertension, or end-stage renal disease.[17–19]

The anatomic status of the upper urinary tract and the presence or absence of vesicoureteral reflux (VUR) can have an important bearing on the long-term treatment chosen. Vesicoureteral reflux has been reported in up to 50% of children with UTI, and chemoprophylaxis is an integral part of the management of these patients[20, 21] (see Fig 1). Posterior urethral valves also predispose to infection and renal damage, but the value of antimicrobial prophylaxis is not as clear for this anatomic defect.[22]

Children who have three or more UTIs in a 12-month period

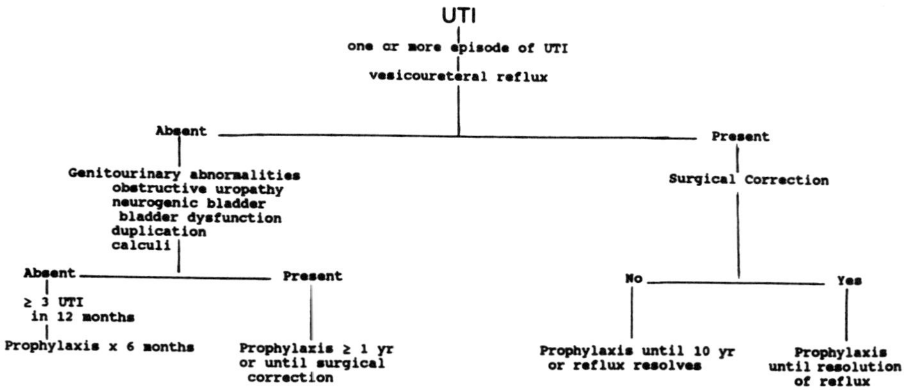

FIGURE 1.
Algorithm for the prevention of urinary tract infection (UTI).

TABLE 3.
Antibiotic Prophylaxis for Recurrent Urinary Tract Infection

Antibiotic	Daily Dosage
Trimethoprim/sulfomethoxazole (TMP/SMX)	2 mg of TMP/10 mg of SMX/kg as a single bedtime dose *or* 5 mg TMP/25 mg SMX twice per week
Nitrofurantoin	1–2 mg/kg divided q24h
Sulfisoxazole	10–20 mg/kg divided q12h
Nalidixic acid	30 mg/kg divided q12h
Methenamine mandelate	75 mg/kg divided q12h

may need chronic suppressive antibiotic therapy for 3 to 6 months to allow repair of intrinsic bladder defense mechanisms. Girls with frequent UTIs tend to have asymptomatic recurrences. Children with recurrent UTI and anatomic defects or reflux may need suppressive antibiotics for as long as the defect exists (see Fig 1). Resistance to antibiotics commonly develops, however, because of R′ factors in fecal-colonic bacteria in patients receiving long-term suppressive therapy.

Other methods for decreasing reinfections of the lower urinary tract include avoiding bubble bath and detergents in the bath water, wiping the perineal area from front to back after voiding or defecation, increasing water intake, emptying the bladder every 3 to 4 hours during the day, and wearing cotton panties that have no permanent or aniline dyes. Agents that have been shown to be efficacious for chronic suppressive therapy include the sulfonamides, TMP/SMX, nitrofurantoin, fluoroquinolones, nalidixic acid, and oxolinic acid (Table 3). Previously, sulfonamides were the preferred agents, but with the recognition of increased resistance among coliform bacteria, the combination of TMP/SMX appears superior. A unique advantage of the trimethoprim component is its ability at relatively low dosages to reduce colonization of Enterobacteriaceae in the urethral orifice, thus diminishing the incidence of ascending reinfection.[23, 24]

Nitrofurantoin has been effectively used as prophylaxis for recurrent UTI in infants and children. Although it is active against most strains of *Escherichia coli*, it is inactive against many isolates of *Proteus, Pseudomonas, Klebsiella*, and *Enterobacter*. Resistance rarely develops with this agent.[24–26] Pulmonary, neurologic, and hepatic adverse effects have been reported, but these are rare.[27]

The fluoroquinolones (ciprofloxacin and norfloxacin) are effective chronic therapy for recurrent UTI but should not be used in pregnant women or prepubertal children because of potential cartilage damage.

Nalidixic acid and oxolinic acid are both bactericidal for most of the common gram-negative uropathogens. Oxolinic acid has been associated with central nervous system (CNS) toxicity. Moreover, rapid and frequent development of bacterial resistance has been reported in many series.[28, 29]

RHEUMATIC FEVER

Although the incidence of rheumatic fever has markedly declined in the United States during the last two decades, periodic outbreaks have recently been reported in widespread regions, thus suggesting a change in epidemiologic patterns.[30, 31] During the same time period, rheumatic fever and rheumatic heart disease have remained relatively more common in developing countries.[32]

The strategy for prevention of rheumatic fever, which has remained consistent since the 1950s, is directed at reducing both the initial attacks of streptococcal infection (primary prevention) and recurrent attacks of acute rheumatic fever (secondary prevention).

Primary prevention is best achieved with immediate and appropriate antimicrobial therapy against group A, β-hemolytic streptococcal (GABHS) upper respiratory tract infections. Recommended therapy consists of intramuscular benzathine penicillin G, 600,000 units for children who weigh less than 60 lb and 1.2 million units for those over 60 lb. Phenoxymethyl penicillin (penicillin V), 250 mg three times daily for 10 days orally, is considered equivalent. For patients allergic to penicillin, erythromycin, 20 to 40 mg/kg/day orally divided twice daily is recommended. Oral cephalosporins are acceptable alternatives for penicillin-allergic patients, except those who have had true anaphylactic reactions to penicillin. Sulfonamides and TMP/SMX are not effective for primary prevention; they do, however, have a role in secondary prevention.

Failure of primary prevention has been observed in asymptomatic patients and in mild cases of streptococcal tonsillopharyngitis, as well as in patients with poor compliance or those less likely to seek medical attention for minor illnesses.[33]

After the initial attack of acute rheumatic fever, patients are highly susceptible to recurrent episodes following GABHS infection. Continuous antimicrobial prophylaxis has been shown to prevent or at least significantly reduce the recurrence of rheumatic fever and rheumatic heart disease.[34, 35]

The risk of recurrence is increased in economically disadvantaged populations and decreases as the time interval since the most recent attack lengthens. Risk is also higher with a history of multiple previous episodes, carditis, or increased exposure to GABHS infection as seen among school teachers, health workers, military recruits, and parents of young children.[33]

The best regimen for secondary antimicrobial prophylaxis is intramuscular benzathine penicillin G, 1.2 million units (>60 lb) or 600,000 units (<60 lb) at 3- to 4-week intervals. For high-risk patients, this antibiotic should be given every 3 weeks.[36–38] Oral penicillin V, 250 mg twice daily, and oral sulfadiazine, 500 mg (<60 lb) or 1.0 g (>60 lb) daily, are also recommended, but the risk of recurrence is somewhat higher with these oral regimens as compared with injectable penicillin, even with optimal compliance.[39] For patients allergic to penicillin and sulfa, oral erythromycin, 250 mg twice daily, is an effective alternative.

At present there is no consensus as to when antimicrobial prophylaxis can be safely discontinued. In general, secondary prevention should be continued for at least 5 years after the last episode of rheumatic fever and until the patient has reached early adulthood. At this time, some authorities recommend changing from parenteral to oral prophylaxis.[33, 40] Recent data have also supported discontinuation of prophylaxis in low-risk young adults as long as they are maintained under adequate medical follow-up.[41]

The continuous, long-term use of penicillin theoretically increases the risk of penicillin allergy. However, data reported from the International Rheumatic Fever Study Group indicated similar rates of serious penicillin allergy in rheumatic patients receiving long-term prophylaxis as compared with children without rheumatic fever who received short-term parenteral penicillin.[42]

Patients with rheumatic heart disease also require subacute bacterial endocarditis prophylaxis before dental and surgical procedures as outlined in the following sections.

BACTERIAL ENDOCARDITIS

Infective endocarditis is a potentially life-threatening disease that has decreased in incidence as a consequence of chemoprophylactic intervention. Early diagnosis and therapeutic intervention have also contributed to a decline in mortality by 80% over the past 50 years.

Patients with congenital or acquired heart disease are at an increased risk for endocarditis developing following well-defined medical, dental, and surgical procedures. Antimicrobial prophylaxis is recommended by both the American Heart Association and the Committee on Infectious Diseases of the American Academy of Pediatrics for use perioperatively at times when the risk of bacteremia from defined procedures is high.[43–45] Table 4 lists those congenital or acquired cardiac conditions for which endocarditis prophylaxis is or is not recommended.[43, 46, 47]

Mitral valve prolapse is a common disorder but is a relatively low risk factor for endocarditis. Definitive data to provide guidance and management are particularly limited. Patients with this condition associated with mitral regurgitation or thickened and/or redundant mitral valve leaflets are at a higher risk for bacterial endocarditis.[48–50] The current consensus is that these patients should receive antimicrobial prophylaxis.

DENTAL PROCEDURES AND UPPER RESPIRATORY TRACT SURGICAL PROCEDURES

Table 5 summarizes the procedures (dental and surgical) for which endocarditis prophylaxis generally is or is not indicated.[51, 52] Decisions should be individualized according to the risk introduced

TABLE 4.
Endocarditis Prophylaxis Related to Cardiac Conditions

Prophylaxis recommended
Prosthetic cardiac valves (including biosynthetic valves)
Most congenital cardiac malformations
Surgically constructed systemic pulmonary shunts
Rheumatic and other acquired valvular dysfunction
Idiopathic hypertrophic subaortic stenosis
Previous history of bacterial endocarditis
Mitral valve prolapse with insufficiency or with thickened valve leaflets
Prophylaxis not recommended
Isolated secundum atrial septal defect
Patients in whom a ventricular septal defect has closed spontaneously
Postoperative atrial septal defect, patent ductus arteriosus, patients with a ventricular septal defect in whom there is no residual shunt

TABLE 5.
Endocarditis Prophylaxis For Specific Procedures

Prophylaxis is indicated
All dental procedures likely to induce gingival or mucosal bleeding, including routine professional cleaning
Tonsillectomy and/or adenoidectomy
Surgical procedures or biopsy involving respiratory mucosa
Rigid bronchoscopy
Incision and drainage of infected tissue
Genitourinary and gastrointestinal procedures involving surgery or instrumentation
Prophylaxis is not indicated
Dental procedures not likely to induce gingival or mucosal bleeding, including simple adjustment or orthodontic appliances, spontaneous shedding of deciduous teeth, or fillings above the gum line
Endotracheal intubation
Tympanostomy tube insertion
Flexible bronchoscopy
Cardiac catheterization
Cesarean section
Therapeutic abortion

by the procedure and the predisposition to infection for the specific cardiac defect. Because α-hemolytic (viridans) streptococci are most commonly implicated in endocarditis following dental procedures, prophylaxis should be specifically directed against these organisms.[53] Certain upper respiratory tract procedures may also cause bacteremia with organisms having similar antibiotic susceptibilities to those producing bacteremia following dental procedures.[43, 54, 55] Therefore the same regimens are recommended.

Table 6 contains suggested regimens of prophylaxis for dental procedures and instrumentation of the upper respiratory tract.[43, 44, 46, 47] In those patients at particularly high risk for endocarditis (e.g., those with prosthetic heart valves or surgically constructed systemic pulmonary shunts), parenteral prophylactic antibiotics are favored (Table 7).

GENITOURINARY AND GASTROINTESTINAL TRACT SURGERY AND INSTRUMENTATION

Data are inadequate to support specific recommendations to cover the entire range of invasive diagnostic and therapeutic procedures.

TABLE 6.
Recommended Prophylactic Antibiotic Regimens for Dental-Respiratory Tract Procedures in Low-Risk Patients

Category	Antibiotic Regimen
Oral regimens	Amoxicillin, 50 mg/kg (max, 3 g) po 1 hr before the procedure, then 25 mg/kg (max, 1.5 g) 6 hr after the initial dose
	or
	Penicillin, 1 g (<60 lb) or 2 g (>60 lb) po 1 hr before the procedure, then 0.5 g (<60 lb) or 1 g (>60 lb) 6 hr after the initial dose
Parenteral regimens	Ampicillin, 50 mg/kg (max, 2 g) IM or IV ½ hr before the procedure, then ampicillin, 25 mg/kg (max, 1 g) IV or IM, or amoxicillin, 25 mg/kg (max, 1.5 g) po 6 hr after the initial dose
	or
	Penicillin G, 50,000 units/kg (max, 2 million units) IM or IV ½ hr before the procedure, then 25,000 units/kg (max, 1 million units) IM or IV 6 hr after the initial dose
Penicillin allergic: oral regimens	Erythromycin ethylsuccinate, 20 mg/kg (max, 800 mg) po 2 hr before the procedure, then 10 mg/kg (max, 400 mg) 6 hr after the initial dose
or	*or*
Rheumatic fever on penicillin prophylaxis: oral regimens	Erythromycin stearate, 20 mg/kg (max, 1 g) po 2 hr before the procedure, then 10 mg/kg (max, 500 mg) 6 hr after the initial dose
	or
	Clindamycin, 10 mg/kg (max, 300 mg) po 1 hr before the procedure, then 5 mg/kg (max, 150 mg) 6 hr after the initial dose
Penicillin allergic: parenteral regimen	Clindamycin phosphate, 10 mg/kg (max, 300 mg) IV 1 hr before the procedure, then 5 mg/kg (max, 150 mg) 6 hr after the initial dose

Based on the limited data available, the American Heart Association recommends prophylaxis for the following: cystoscopy, prostatic surgery, urethral catheterization, urinary tract surgery, vaginal hysterectomy, gallbladder surgery, colonic surgery, esophageal dilatation, sclerotherapy for esophageal varices, colonoscopy, upper gastrointestinal endoscopy with biopsy, or proctosigmoidoscopic biopsy.[43] Thus patients at risk for bacterial endocarditis who are undergoing such procedures should receive prophylactic antibiotics as outlined later.

Bacteremia less often accompanies other genitourinary and gastrointestinal tract procedures, and endocarditis has rarely if ever developed subsequent to these procedures.[43, 54, 55] These include percutaneous liver biopsy, upper gastrointestinal endoscopy or proctosigmoidoscopy without biopsy, barium enema, uncomplicated vaginal delivery, and brief (in and out) bladder catheterization with sterile urine.

Enterococci (e.g., *Streptococcus faecalis*) are most frequently responsible for endocarditis following genitourinary and gastrointestinal tract surgery or instrumentation.[53] Although gram-negative bacillary bacteremia may follow such procedures, these organisms are only rarely responsible for endocarditis. Table 8 contains suggested regimens of prophylaxis for genitourinary and gastrointestinal procedures for both standard- and special-risk patients as adapted from the current American Heart Association recommendations.[43, 44, 46, 47]

TABLE 7.
Recommended Prophylactic Antibiotic Regimen and Dosages for Dental-Respiratory Tract Procedures for Special-Risk Patients

Category	Antibiotic Regimens
Non–penicillin allergic	Ampicillin, 50 mg/kg (max, 2 g) IM or IV *plus* Gentamicin, 2.0 mg/kg (max, 80 mg) IM or IV ½ hr before the procedure, then amoxicillin, 25 mg/kg (max, 1.5 g) po 6 hr after the initial dose or ½ the parenteral regimen dose 8 hr after the initial dose
Penicillin allergic	Vancomycin, 20 mg/kg (max, 1 g) IV starting 1 hr before the procedure. Repeat dose not necessary.

TABLE 8.
Recommended Prophylactic Antibiotic Regimens and Dosages for Genitourinary/Gastrointestinal Procedures in Standard- and Special-Risk Patients

Category	Antibiotic Regimen
Non–penicillin allergic	Ampicillin, 50 mg/kg (max, 2 g) IM or IV *plus* Gentamicin, 2.0 mg/kg (max, 80 mg) IM or IV ½ hr before the procedure, then amoxicillin, 25 mg/kg (max, 1.5 g) po 6 hr after the initial dose or ½ the parenteral regimen dose 8 hr after the initial dose
Penicillin allergic	Vancomycin, 20 mg/kg (max, 1 g) IV starting 1 hr before the procedure *plus* Gentamicin, 2.0 mg/kg (max, 80 mg) IM or IV 1 hr before the procedure, then ½ the parenteral regimen dose 8 hr after the initial dose

CARDIAC SURGERY

Patients undergoing open heart surgery, especially with placement of prosthetic heart valves or prosthetic intravascular or intracardiac materials, are at risk for bacterial endocarditis.[54, 56] Endocarditis associated with open heart surgery is most often due to *Staphylococcus aureus*, coagulase-negative staphylococci, or diphtheroids.[53, 57] Streptococci, gram-negative bacteria, and fungi are less common. Penicillinase-resistant penicillins or "first-generation" cephalosporins are most often selected, although the choice of antibiotic should be influenced by each hospital's antibiotic susceptibility data. Prophylaxis should be started immediately before the operative procedure and continued for no more than 2 days postoperatively to minimize the emergence of resistant microorganisms. The effects of cardiopulmonary bypass and compromised postoperative renal function on serum antibiotic levels should be considered and doses timed appropriately before and during the procedure.

NEONATAL GROUP B STREPTOCOCCAL INFECTION

Intrapartum administration of intravenous penicillin or ampicillin to group B streptococcus (GBS)-colonized mothers has been shown to decrease vertical transmission of the bacterium and prevent neonatal disease.[58–64] This occurs whether the mother is lightly or heavily colonized and has been documented in both low-risk and high-risk neonates. Risk factors only vary the incidence of disease in untreated pregnancies and therefore the relative benefits of chemoprophylaxis.

Early studies reported efficacy of ampicillin given every 6 hours in reducing colonization of neonates from 46% to 58% in untreated women to 0% to 7% of treated mothers.[60, 65] More importantly, absolute elimination of early-onset disease was seen as compared with 7% (9 of 136) of those with invasive disease among infants whose mothers were not treated.[65] Perhaps the best-designed and most-quoted study was published in 1986.[59] This randomized, controlled trial examined selective intrapartum ampicillin (2-g loading dose followed by 1 g every 4 hours until delivery) in colonized high-risk women. Neonatal colonization was reduced from 51% to 9% and bacteremia from 6% to 0%. After cultures were obtained from neonates, those whose mothers received chemoprophylaxis were given four doses of intramuscular ampicillin, 50 mg/kg per dose at 12-hour intervals. Additional studies later confirmed protective efficacy.[58, 63, 64] Collectively these data strongly support maternal intrapartum chemoprophylaxis, and this strategy for preventing GBS infection has been endorsed by the American Academy of Pediatrics[66] and by the American College of Obstetricians and Gynecologists.[67] There is, however, some disagreement between these two organizations as to the cost-effectiveness of its routine implementation.[68]

Until an efficacious GBS vaccine is developed, selective intrapartum chemoprophylaxis for colonized high-risk pregnant women should be encouraged. This will require that physicians offering obstetric services arrange some mechanism for culturing GBS.

All pregnant women should be screened at 26 to 28 weeks' gestation for GBS by using a single swab specimen from the lower portion of the vagina and anorectum and employing appropriate selective broth medium for transport and solid media for final recovery. Results of this culture should be recorded and readily available at the time that the mother begins labor.

There are two exceptions to the prerequisite that colonization is required for treatment: maternal GBS bacteriuria and neonate with previous invasive GBS disease. The former circumstance is appropriate since bacteriuria is strongly predictive of heavy genital colonization and early-onset disease, and the latter history is known to be an independent variable highly associated with neonatal GBS sepsis.

Risk factors include the following:

1. Onset of labor less than 37 weeks' gestation
2. Rupture of membranes less than 37 weeks' gestation
3. Maternal fever or other signs suggestive of bacterial infection
4. Multiple births
5. Maternal diabetes
6. Rupture of membranes beyond 18 hours

For the latter category, a decision should be made by the obstetrician 12 hours after the membranes have ruptured as to whether labor is likely to continue more than 6 additional hours.

HUMAN IMMUNODEFICIENCY VIRUS INFECTION

There are four potential secondary infections in pediatric acquired immunodeficiency syndrome (AIDS) that warrant prophylaxis: bacteremia/sepsis, *Pneumocystis carinii* infection, tuberculosis, and *Mycobacterium avium-intracellulare* infection.[69, 70] Table 9 summarizes criteria for these indications and currently recommended treatment.

Intravenous immunoglobulin has been used in infants and children infected with human immunodeficiency virus (HIV), with encouraging reports of its efficacy in preventing bacterial sepsis and decreasing the number of hospitalizations.[71, 72]

Pneumocystis carinii pneumonia (PCP), the most common infection in pediatric AIDS and often the first manifestation of disease, warrants an early primary prevention strategy. Trimethoprim-sulfamethoxazole is currently the drug of choice for prophylaxis, with dapsone or aerosolized pentamidine reserved as alternatives for patients intolerant of TMP/SMX.[73–79]

Although the incidence of *Mycobacterium tuberculosis* infection in pediatric patients with AIDS is considerably lower than in adults, a prevention strategy should be considered for children living in an environment of high tuberculosis (TB) prevalence. The World Health Organization (WHO) currently recommends the administration of bacille Calmette-Guérin (BCG) vaccine for HIV-infected patients in high TB prevalence areas. However, disseminated BCG infection has been reported in children with symptomatic HIV infection who have received this vaccine.[80, 81] *Mycobacterium avium-intracellulare* complex (MAC) infection has been recognized with increased frequency and is associated with high morbidity and short survival. Prophylaxis is recommended for adult patients with AIDS, and many experts also recommend treatment for children seen in centers where MAC is commonly encoun-

TABLE 9.
Routine Prophylaxis for Children Infected with Human Immunodeficiency Virus

Clinical Syndrome	Indications		Prophylaxis and Dosage
Bacterial sepsis	Hypogammaglobulinemia Abnormal antibody formation Serious bacterial infection *or* Presumed bacterial pneumonia × 2		IVIG,* 400 mg/kg/mo
Pneumocystis carinii pneumonia	Age (yr)	$CD4+$ cells/mm^3	TMP/SMX $150\ mg/m^2/day$ TMP po divided bid on 3 consecutive days (M, T, W) each week *or* Dapsone, 1 mg/kg/day po (max, 100 mg) *or* Aerosolized pentamidine
	<1	<1,500 (20%)	
	1–2	<750 (20%)	
	2–6	<500 (20%)	
	>6	<200 (20%)	
Tuberculosis	At birth (when immune function is near normal) for neonates born to HIV-positive mothers if high risk for TB		BCG vaccine
MAI/MAC	Same as in PCP		Rifabutin 5 mg/kg/day po (max, 300 mg, once daily)

*IVIG = intravenous immune globulin; TMP/SMX = trimethoprim/sulfamethexazole; BCG = bacille Calmette-Guérin; TB = tuberculosis; PCP = *Pneumocystis carinii* pneumonia; MAI/MAC = *Mycobacterium avium-intracellulare* complex.

TABLE 10.
Suggested Antimicrobial Therapy for Suppressive or Secondary Prevention of Opportunistic Infections in Patients Infected with Human Immunodeficiency Virus

Clinical Syndrome for Which Initial Therapy Has Been Completed	Prophylaxis
Oral and esophageal candidiasis	Clotrimazole, fluconazole, or ketoconazole
Toxoplasma cerebritis	TMP/SMX* or pyrimethamine plus sulfadiazine
Cytomegalovirus	High-dose acyclovir, ganciclovir, or foscarnet
Herpes simplex	Acyclovir or vidarabine
Cryptococcosis	Fluconazole or ketoconazole

*TMP/SMX = trimethoprim/sulfamethoxazole.

tered. Rifabutin has been approved for prophylaxis. Additional options currently under investigation include azithromycin, clarithromycin, and biological-response modifiers.[82–84]

Other clinical syndromes and opportunistic infections in patients with HIV may require suppressive or secondary prevention since recurrence of these diseases is common (Table 10).[85–89]

Primary prophylaxis against HIV following exposure to contaminated needles is still controversial.[90–92] The risk for HIV-1 transmission associated with a single parenteral exposure to a contaminated needle is 0.37%. The only available therapy is zidovudine (AZT), but its efficacy for prophylactic use has not been established.

BACTERIAL MENINGITIS

The most common causes of bacterial meningitis in the United States at all ages beyond the neonatal period are *Neisseria meningitidis*, *Streptococcus pneumoniae*, and *Haemophilus influenzae*. Previously the latter etiology constituted the majority of cases in early childhood. However, introduction of the *H. influenzae* type b (Hib) polysaccharide vaccine in 1985 and the conjugated vaccine in 1988 has led to a marked decline in the incidence of invasive Hib disease.[93, 94]

In identified index cases of meningococcal and Hib invasive disease there is an increase in the rate of nasopharyngeal carriage of the organisms among household and other intimate contacts and a significantly increased incidence of disease.[95–97] Antimicrobial prophylaxis is therefore recommended for these contacts. Approximately 50% of all secondary cases of invasive disease occur in the first week after contact, and 25% occur during the second week, so chemoprophylaxis should be administered as soon as possible. There is no evidence that *S. pneumoniae* produces secondary household spread.

MENINGOCOCCAL DISEASE

The secondary attack rate for household contacts of meningococcal meningitis or meningococcemia is 1 per 250 (0.4%). Rifampin prophylaxis at a dose of 20 mg/kg/day (maximum, 1,200 mg) divided every 12 hours for 2 days effectively eliminates this risk. Half this dose (10 mg/kg/day) may be used in neonates. Soft contact lenses should be removed because rifampin causes permanent staining. Prophylaxis is also recommended for other groups that have had intimate contact with these patients. Pregnancy is a contraindication to rifampin, but ceftriaxone, 250 mg intramuscularly as a single dose, may be substituted.

Tables 11 and 12 list the high-risk contacts and the available alternatives for chemoprophylaxis of meningococcal disease.[44, 96–99] The fluoroquinolones are effective as prophylaxis for contacts with meningococcal disease; however, they are not licensed for prepubertal children and pregnant women.[100] Penicillin G and chloramphenicol, despite their efficacy for treatment of meningococcal meningitis, are not effective in eradicating oropharyngeal carriage of *N. meningitidis*.

HAEMOPHILUS INFLUENZAE TYPE B DISEASE

The risk to household contacts of a child with invasive *H. influenzae* disease is 600 times higher than that in the general population

TABLE 11.
High-Risk Contacts of Meningococcal Disease

All household contacts
Nursery or day care center contacts
Hospital personnel and individuals who had intimate exposure to oral secretions from the index case

TABLE 12.
Antibiotics for Meningococcal Prophylaxis

Antibiotic Prophylaxis	Dosage	Comments
Rifampin	<1 mo: 5 mg/kg twice daily po for 2 days >1 mo: 10 mg/kg twice daily po for 2 days (max, 600 mg/dose)	Contraindicated for pregnant women Orange-red urine Stains contact lenses
Sulfisoxazole	2 mo–1 yr: 500 mg daily po for 2 days 1 yr–12 yr: 500 mg twice daily po for 2 days >12 yr: 1 g twice daily po for 2 days	Contraindicated for pregnant women during the third trimester and infants younger than 2 mo
Ceftriaxone	<12 yr: 125 mg IM as single dose >12 yr: 250 mg IM as a single dose	Safe for pregnant women Better compliance
Fluoroquinolones	Single adult po dose	Contraindicated for pregnant women and children younger than 18 yr
Minocycline	100 mg twice daily po for 5 days	Contraindicated for pregnant women and children younger than 8 yr

and is age dependent;[96] the secondary attack rate for young infants less than 1 year is 6%; 1 to 4 years of age, 2.1%; and 4 to 6 years, 0.5%. The risk to unimmunized contacts in day care centers has not been fully determined but appears to be great enough to warrant prophylaxis for children attending these centers and for adult personnel once there have been two cases of *H. influenzae* systemic disease within 60 days.[44, 101, 102] Rifampin prophylaxis for culture-positive individuals has been shown to reduce the oropharyngeal carriage of *H. influenzae* by 97%. Rifampin at a dose of 20 mg/kg (maximum, 600 mg) once daily for 4 days eradicates the oronasopharyngeal carriage of Hib in the majority of contacts.[99, 103] For infants younger than 1 month of age, the dose should be reduced to 10 mg/kg once daily for 4 days. The index case should also receive chemoprophylaxis before discharge.

ASPLENIA

Asplenia may be congenital, postsurgical, or functional, the latter primarily resulting from sickle cell disease or other hemoglobinopathies. Regardless of the cause, patients are susceptible to invasive infection caused by encapsulated bacteria, particularly *S. pneumoniae* but occasionally Hib and *N. meningitidis*.[104–106] Continuous antibody prophylaxis in addition to vaccination for pneumococci and *H. influenzae* has been an effective strategy for reducing the incidence of fatal postsplenectomy infections. However, protection is not absolute, and there are several reports of fatal postsplenectomy pneumococcal sepsis in patients who had received pneumococcal vaccine and were currently receiving appropriate antimicrobial prophylaxis regimens.[107–110] Adequate levels of penicillin for pneumococci can be achieved with oral penicillin V at doses at 125 mg three times daily for children younger than 5 years and 250 mg three times daily for children 5 years of age and older. Although somewhat more expensive, amoxicillin has certain advantages over the penicillin regimen when given at a dose of 20 mg/kg/day. Because of more consistent absorption from the gastrointestinal tract, higher serum concentrations are achieved, and in addition, amoxicillin has excellent activity against most strains of *H. influenzae*. The more pleasant taste of amoxicillin suspension also increases compliance. Some authorities suggest that various antibiotics should be rotated for long-term prophylaxis to prevent the emergence of resistant organisms.[111] Consideration may also be given to the use of TMP/SMX in a dose of 4 mg TMP/kg/day for children younger than 5 years of age since this antibiotic offers enhanced coverage for *H. influenzae*. The required duration of antimicrobial prophylaxis in asplenic patients has not yet been defined. Some recommend continuation during the patient's entire lifetime,[112] whereas others have suggested long-term prophylaxis during the adult years only if there are additional high-risk factors.[44] Asplenic patients and patients with sickle cell disease who are 2 years of age or older should receive pneumococcal vaccine (23-valent polysaccharide vaccine), and a second dose should be given 3 to 5 years later to children who would be younger than 10 years old at revaccination.[44, 113, 114] The polysaccharide conjugate *Haemophilus* and meningococcal vaccines should also be given routinely.

For elective splenectomy, pneumococcal vaccination should preferably be given 2 weeks before surgery because this will result in a more vigorous immune response likely resulting from the contribution of immunologically reactive splenic lymphocytes.[115]

TUBERCULOSIS

Tuberculosis remains the most common serious infectious disease worldwide and accounts for 10 to 12 million new infections and 3 million deaths per year. As a consequence of the AIDS epidemic, TB has undergone a change in epidemiology that necessitates a more defined and effective strategy for chemoprophylaxis and vaccination. Multiple randomized placebo-controlled trials of isoniazid chemoprophylaxis have been completed and published during the past four decades, and all have shown a protective effect.[116–118] Skin testing and a history of exposure were the most critical determinants for initiation of prophylaxis. More recently, recommendations have included tuberculin skin test–negative individuals at high-risk of infection (Table 13). Table 14 summarizes recent changes in interpretation of the Mantoux skin test that are based on the risk of disease in relation to different clinical and historical circumstances.[119–122]

Patients who receive BCG vaccine may react to Mantoux test antigen, but an induration of 15 mm or greater should usually be

TABLE 13.
Children Who Should Receive Isoniazid Prophylaxis

Children	Duration of Treatment
Asymptomatic skin test reactor with normal chest x-ray findings	9 mo
Skin test–negative household contact of an active case	3 mo (then repeat the skin test)
Previously skin test–positive children who are immune suppressed (malignancy, corticosteroid, or immunosuppressive therapy)	For the duration of immune suppression

TABLE 14.
Definition of a Positive Mantoux Skin Test (5 Tuberculin Units of Purified Protein Derivative) in Children

- Reaction size of $\geq$5 mm
  - Children in close contact with known or suspected infectious cases of tuberculosis
    - Households with active cases
    - Households with previously active cases if
      - Treatment cannot be verified as adequate before the exposure
      - Treatment was initiated after a period of contact with the child
      - Reactivation is suspected
  - Children suspected to have tuberculous disease
    - Chest roentgenogram consistent with active or previously active tuberculosis
    - Clinical evidence of tuberculosis
  - Children with underlying conditions that put them at high risk of acquiring severe tuberculosis
    - Immunocompromised conditions
    - HIV infection
- Reaction size of $\geq$10 mm
  - Children at increased risk of dissemination
    - Young age <4 yr old
    - Other medical risk factors: Hodgkin's diseases, lymphoma, diabetes mellitus, chronic renal failure, malnutrition
  - Increased environmental exposure
    - Those from or whose parent have emigrated from high-prevalence regions of the world
    - Children frequently exposed to the following adults
      - HIV infected
      - Homeless persons
      - Users of intravenous and other street drugs
      - Poor and medically indigent city dwellers
      - Residents of nursing homes
      - Migrant farm workers
- Reaction size of $\geq$15 mm
  - Children $\geq$4 yr old without any risk factors

considered to have resulted from TB exposure for these individuals.

Isoniazid remains the drug of choice for TB chemoprophylaxis following skin test conversion[116, 117, 119, 123, 124] and is given at a dose of 10 mg/kg (maximum, 300 mg) once daily. When compliance cannot be ensured, a regimen consisting of 20 mg/kg (maximum, 900 mg) twice weekly under direct health care worker observation is recommended. For infants and children, therapy should be continued for 9 months. For HIV-infected patients a minimum of 12 months of therapy is recommended.[119, 125] Compliance remains a significant problem in TB-preventive therapy, and for noncompliant individuals who have received less than 80% of the recommended medication, a new full course of chemoprophylaxis should be implemented.

The recommended chemoprophylactic therapy for contacts of patients with isoniazid-resistant *M. tuberculosis* infection is rifampin at an oral dose of 10 mg/kg (maximum, 600 mg) once daily. For isoniazid- and rifampin-resistant *M. tuberculosis*, pyrazinamide with ethambutol or pyrazinamide with ciprofloxacin (for postpubertal contacts only) is suggested.[125]

TRAVELER'S DIARRHEA

Traveler's diarrhea usually occurs during the first week of travel and is generally a mild self-limited disease. The incidence is highest among persons visiting Latin America, Africa, Asia, and the Middle East. Numerous organisms are responsible, with the vast majority being due to enterotoxigenic *E. coli* in Americans who travel to Mexico or South America. *Giardia* is a more likely pathogen for travelers to the Soviet Union.

If meticulous attention is paid to avoiding potentially contaminated food and water, the incidence of infection is extremely low. Prophylactic antibiotics are no longer routinely recommended because their use leads to the rapid development of bacterial resistance.[126, 127] Antimicrobial therapy should be reserved for symptomatic cases or for individuals entering an extremely high-risk area (poor sanitation) and who will be remaining there for more than 5 days. Recommended antibiotics are TMP/SMX, trimethoprim alone, and the quinolones ciprofloxacin or norfloxacin (for patients older than 18 years).[128–130] It is most practical to allow travelers to bring appropriate medication with them if they are staying for more than 5 days, but with instructions to begin therapy only if symptoms occur. Loperamide, an antimotility medication, is safe and can be combined with antibiotics for more effective symptomatic care. Bismuth subsalicylate has also been shown to be a useful adjunct to antimicrobial therapy in adults.

For infants and children less than 2 years of age, prophylaxis is not recommended. Once asymptomatic, these young patients should be given fluids with a higher electrolyte content such as that contained in oral rehydration solutions.[130, 131]

MALARIA

Primary prevention of malaria relies on a combination of personal protective measures and antimicrobial prophylaxis. International

TABLE 15.
Recommended Antibiotic Regimens and Dosage for Malaria Prevention

Category	Antibiotic Regimen
Non–chloroquine-resistant malaria strains (*Plasmodium vivax, P. ovale, P. malariae,* and chloroquine-sensitive *P. falciparum*)	Chloroquine phosphate, 5 mg/kg (max, 300 mg) base (equivalent to 8.3 mg/kg; max, 500 mg salt) once/wk starting 2 wk before travel to a malarious area and continuing during travel until 4 wk after leaving the area *or* Hydroxychloroquine sulfate, 5 mg/kg (max, 310 mg) base (equivalent to 6.5 mg/kg; max, 400 mg salt) once/wk starting 2 wk before travel to a malarious area and continuing during travel until 4 wk after leaving the area
P. vivax and *p. ovale* endemic areas (relapse prevention)	Chloroquine phosphate or hydroxychloroquine sulfate, same dose and regimen as above *plus* Primaquine, 0.3 mg/kg/day (max, 15 mg/day) for 14 days after leaving the malarious area
Chloroquine-resistant malaria strain (chloroquine-resistant *P. falciparum*)	Mefloquine hydrochloride (tablet, 250 mg) <15 kg: not recommended 15–19 kg: ¼ tab/wk 20–30 kg: ½ tab/wk 31–45 kg: ¾ tab/wk >45 kg: 1 tab/wk Starting 1 wk before travel and continuing during travel until 4 wk after leaving the malarious area *or*

(continued)

TABLE 15 (continued).

	Chloroquine phosphate, same dose and regimen as above *plus* Pyrimethamine/sulfadoxine (tablet, 25 mg/500 mg) <1 yr: ¼ tab 1–3 yr: ½ tab 4–8 yr: 1 tab 9–14 yr: 2 tab >14 yr: 3 tab Given as a single dose for self-treatment for febrile disease when medical facility unavailable *or* Doxycycline (alone) ≤8 yr: contraindicated >8 yr: 2 mg/kg (max, 100 mg/day) once/day starting 1–2 days before travel and continuing during travel until 4 wk after leaving the malarious area

travelers visiting malaria endemic areas should be encouraged to avoid exposure to mosquitoes, use insect repellents and pesticides, and wear long pants and long-sleeved shirts. For most malarious areas, oral chloroquine is the drug of choice for primary prophylaxis.[131, 132] For travel to regions reporting chloroquine-resistant *Plasmodium falciparum*, mefloquine alone or chloroquine plus pyrimethamine/sulfadoxine or doxycycline should be used (Table 15).[132–135]

INFLUENZA A INFECTION

Prophylaxis is recommended for all with medical problems that would result in more extensive infection once influenza developed and for all individuals with increased exposure to potential outbreaks. Influenza vaccine remains the primary means for prevention of influenza infection in such high-risk individuals. However, during influenza outbreaks, rimantidine or amantadine is indicated for those who have not been immunized but have been exposed to active disease.[44, 136–138] Once vaccine is given, antiviral therapy need only be continued for 14 days. In extremely high-risk individuals, the combination of vaccine plus rimantadine offers maximum protection, 90% vs. 70% for either alone. The dosage for both antiviral agents is 5 to 8 mg/kg/day (maximum, 200 mg/day) given orally once daily or divided into two doses.

PERTUSSIS

Prophylactic erythromycin is effective in preventing symptomatic disease as well as eradicating colonization in contacts of pertussis cases. Although immunization affords protection in 70% to 80% of recipients, prophylaxis should be offered to immunized as well as unimmunized family, day care center, or hospital contacts during outbreaks of pertussis.[44, 139–143] Erythromycin is given orally at 50 mg/kg/day (maximum, 1.5 g) divided three times daily for 14 days.

SURGICAL AND WOUND INFECTION

The most common use of antibiotics in hospitals is for surgical prophylaxis. Abundant randomized clinical trials have well demonstrated their benefit.[144, 145] This includes clean, clean-contaminated, contaminated, or infected surgical procedures. Major shortcomings are risks of drug toxicity, emergence of resistant organism, and superinfections. Chemoprophylaxis should be initiated before the surgical procedure for maximum efficacy[146] so that peak serum levels are achieved during the operation and for a short time after. The duration of antibiotic administration should not exceed 48 hours.[146–150] Most surgical procedures require specific regimens directed at pathogens previously shown to cause postoperative infection (Table 16).[147–154]

PNEUMOCYSTIS CARINII INFECTION

In addition to HIV infection, malignancies of the reticuloendothelial system such as leukemia and lymphoma under treatment, organ transplantation, congenital immunodeficiency, and immunosuppression predispose children to *Pneumocystis carinii* infection.[155] Trimethoprim-sulfamethoxazole remains the drug of choice for primary and secondary prevention of such infection.[156–158] The dosage regimen is the same as outlined earlier for HIV infection (see Table 9).

TABLE 16.
Recommended Antimicrobial Prophylaxis for Certain Surgical Procedures

Surgical Procedure	Prophylactic Antibiotic
Tonsillectomy and adenoidectomy	No available data
Tympanostomy	Gentamicin eardrops
Cleft palate repair	po TMP/SMX,* sulfisoxazole, or ampicillin
Major head and neck surgery	IV cefazolin, ampicillin, or gentamicin plus clindamycin
Eye surgery	Gentamicin or tobramycin ophthalmic drops or Cefazolin subconjunctival injection
Cardiothoracic and vascular surgery	IV cefazolin, oxacillin, or vancomycin
Inguinal hernia repair	No available data
Appendectomy	IV cefoxitin, cefazolin, or metronidazole
Colon surgery	po erythromycin plus neomycin, IV cefoxitin, cefazolin, or metronidazole
Gastroduodenal surgery	IV cefazolin
Biliary tract surgery	IV cefazolin or gentamicin
Elective splenectomy	Pneumococcal vaccine before the procedure
Penetrating abdominal trauma	IV cefoxitin
Urinary tract obstructive	po TMP/SMX, ampicillin, or nitrofurantoin
Ruptured viscus	Cefoxitin ± gentamicin or clindamycin plus gentamicin
Abortion	
First trimester	IV/IM penicillin G or po doxycycline
Second trimester	IV cefazolin, IV/IM penicillin G, or po metronidazole
Orthopedic surgery	IV cefazolin or vancomycin
Cerebrospinal fluid shunting procedures	IV cefazolin, oxacillin, or TMP/SMX
Gastrostomy	IV cefazolin, vancomycin, or clindamycin
Burns	IV or po penicillin plus 0.5% silver nitrate or 10% mafenide acetate cream

*TMP/SMX = trimethroprim/sulfamethoxazole.

REFERENCES

1. Artenstein MS, Lamson TH, Evans JR: Attempted prophylaxis against meningococcal infection using intramuscular penicillin. *Mil Med* 132:1009–1011, 1967.
2. Teele DW, Klein JO, Rosner B, et al: Otitis media with effusion during the first three years of life and the development of speech and language. *Pediatrics* 74:282–287, 1984.
3. Paradise JL: Antimicrobial prophylaxis for recurrent acute otitis media. *Ann Otol Rhinol Laryngol* 101:33–36, 1992.
4. Casselbrant ML, Kaleida PH, Rockette HE, et al: Efficacy of antimicrobial prophylaxis and of tympanostomy tube insertion for prevention of recurrent acute otitis media: Results of a randomized clinical trial. *Pediatr Infect Dis J* 11:278–286, 1992.
5. Liston TE, Foshee WS, Pierson WD: Sulfisoxazole chemoprophylaxis for frequent otitis media. *Pediatrics* 71:524–530, 1983.
6. Gutman LT: Prophylactic use of trimethoprim-sulfamethoxazole in children with recurrent otitis media. *Pediatr Infect Dis J* 11:685, 1992.
7. Liston TE: Prevention of recurrent otitis media. *Pediatr Infect Dis J* 11:897–898, 1992.
8. Varsano IB, Volovitz BM, Gussman JE: Effect of naproxen, a prostaglandin inhibitor, on acute otitis media and persistence of middle ear effusion in children. *Ann Otol Rhinol Laryngol* 98:389–392, 1989.
9. Berman S, Nuss R, Roark R, et al: Effectiveness of continuous vs. intermittent amoxicillin to prevent episodes of otitis media. *Pediatr Infect Dis J* 11:63–67, 1992.
10. Bergus GR: Staving off acute otitis media. When is prophylaxis with antibiotics desirable? *Postgrad Med* 90:99–106, 1991.
11. Jorgensen F, Andersson B, Larsson S, et al: Nasopharyngeal bacterial flora in otitis prone children treated with immunoglobulin. *Acta Otolaryngol (Stockh)* 112:530–538, 1992.
12. Heikkinen T, Ruuskamem O, Waris M, et al: Influenza vaccination in the prevention of acute otitis media in children. *Am J Dis Child* 145:445–448, 1991.
13. Sloyer JL, Ploussard JH, Howie VM: Efficacy of pneumococcal polysaccharide vaccine in preventing acute otitis media in infants in Huntsville, Alabama. *Rev Infect Dis* 3(suppl):119, 1981.
14. Sih T, Moura R, Caldas S, et al: Prophylaxis for recurrent acute otitis media: A Brazilian study. *Int J Pediatr Otorhinolaryngol* 25:19–24, 1993.
15. Berman S, Grose K, Nuss R, et al: Management of chronic middle ear effusion with prednisone combined with trimethoprim-sulfamethoxazole. *Pediatr Infect Dis J* 9:533–538, 1990.
16. Woolbert LF: Do antihistamines and decongestants prevent otitis media? *Pediatr Nurs* 16:265–267, 1990.

17. Kass EJ: Acute and recurrent urinary tract infections in children. *Prim Care* 12:607–620, 1985.
18. Jodal U: The natural history of bacteriuria in childhood. *Infect Dis Clin North Am* 1:713–729, 1987.
19. Holland NH, Jackson EC, Kazee M, et al: Relation of urinary tract infection and vesicoureteral reflux to scars: Follow-up of thirty-eight patients. *J Pediatr* 116(suppl):65–71, 1990.
20. Shapiro ED: Infections of the urinary tract. *Pediatr Infect Dis J* 11:165–168, 1992.
21. Jodal U, Koskimies O, Hanson E, et al: Infection pattern in children with vesicoureteral reflux randomly allocated to operation or long term antimicrobial prophylaxis. The international reflux study in children. *J Urol* 148:1650–1652, 1992.
22. Mochon M, Kaiser BA, Dunn S, et al: Urinary tract infections in children with posterior urethral valves after kidney transplantation. *J Urol* 148:1874–1876, 1992.
23. Hanson E, Hansson S, Jodol U: Trimethoprim-sulfadiazine prophylaxis in children with vesicoureteral reflux. *Scand J Infect Dis* 21:201–204, 1989.
24. Stamay TA, Condy M, Mibara G: Prophylactic efficacy of nitrofurantoin macrocrystals and trimethoprim-sulfamethoxazole in urinary infections. Biologic effect on the vaginal and rectal flora. *N Engl J Med* 296:780–783, 1977.
25. Lohr JA, Nunley DH, Howards SS, et al: Prevention of recurrent urinary tract infections in girls. *Pediatrics* 59:562–565, 1977.
26. Brendstrup L, Hjelt K, Petersen KE, et al: Nitrofurantoin versus trimethoprim prophylaxis in recurrent urinary tract infection in children. A randomized, double blind study. *Acta Paediatri Scand* 79:1225–1234, 1990.
27. McCracken GH Jr: Options in antimicrobial management of urinary tract infections in infants and children. *Pediatr Infect Dis J* 8:552–555, 1989.
28. Stamey TA, Bragonje J: Resistance to nalidixic acid. A misconception due to underdosage. *JAMA* 236:1857–1860, 1976.
29. Ronold AR, Turek M, Petersdorf RG: A critical evaluation of nalidixic acid in urinary tract infections. *N Engl J Med* 275:1081–1089, 1966.
30. Veasy GL, Wiedmeier SE, Orsmond GS, et al: Resurgence of acute rheumatic fever in the intermountain area of the United States. *N Engl J Med* 316:421–427, 1987.
31. Dajani AS: Prevention of rheumatic fever. *Infect Med* 5:190–192, 1989.
32. WHO programme for the Prevention of Rheumatic Fever/Rheumatic Heart Disease in 16 Developing Countries: Report from Phase I (1986–90). WHO Cardiovascular Diseases Unit and principal investigators. *Bull World Health Organ* 70:213–218, 1992.

33. AHA Scientific Council: Prevention of rheumatic fever. Special report. *Circulation* 78:1082–1086, 1988.
34. Majeed HA, Batnager S, Yousof AM, et al: Acute rheumatic fever and the evolution of rheumatic heart disease: A prospective 12 year follow-up report. *J Clin Epidemiol* 45:871–875, 1992.
35. Massell BF, Chute CG, Walker AM, et al: Penicillin and the marked decrease in morbidity and mortality from rheumatic fever in the United States. *N Engl J Med* 318:280–286, 1988.
36. Ayoub EM: Prophylaxis in patients with rheumatic fever: Every three or every four weeks? *J Pediatr* 115:89–91, 1989.
37. Kaplan EL, Berrios X, Speth J, et al: Pharmacokinetics of benzathine penicillin G: Serum levels during the 28 days after intramuscular injection of 1,200,000 units. *J Pediatr* 115:146–150, 1989.
38. Thamlikitkul V, Kobwanthanakun S, Pruksachatvathi S, et al: Pharmacokinetics of rheumatic fever prophylaxis regimens. *J Int Med Res* 20:20–26, 1992.
39. Pugno Vanoni MC, Sticca M, Grasso E: Rheumatic fever from 1960s to 1990s. Case records in 2 hospitals of the Lombardian area. *Pediatr Med Chir* 14:415–420, 1992.
40. Castagna PC, Frattini C, Vignati G, et al: The follow-up in adulthood of subjects with progressive rheumatic disease in childhood. Considerations of secondary prevention. *Minerva Pediatr* 42:543–546, 1990.
41. Berrios X, del Campo E, Guzman B, et al: Discontinuing rheumatic fever prophylaxis in selected adolescents and young adults. *Ann Intern Med* 118:401–406, 1993.
42. International Rheumatic Fever Study Group: Allergic reactions to long-term benzathine penicillin prophylaxis for rheumatic fever. *Lancet* 337:1308–1310, 1991.
43. Dajani AS, Bisno AL, Chung KJ, et al: Prevention of bacterial endocarditis: Recommendations by the American Heart Association. *JAMA* 264:2919–2922, 1990.
44. American Academy of Pediatrics. Report of the Committee on Infectious Disease: *1994 Red Book*, ed 23. Elk Grove Village, Ill, American Academy of Pediatrics, 1994.
45. Lerner PI: Endocarditis prophylaxis: The new guidelines. *Cleve Clin J Med* 59:216–218, 1992.
46. Endocarditis Working Party of the British Society for Antimicrobial Chemotherapy: Antibiotic prophylaxis of infective endocarditis. *Lancet* 335:88–89, 1990.
47. Prevention of bacterial endocarditis: *Med Lett Drugs Ther* 31:112, 1989.
48. Clemens JD, Ransohoff DF: Quantitative assessment of pre-dental antibiotic prophylaxis for patients with mitral valve prolapse. *J Chronic Dis* 37:531–544, 1984.
49. Baddour LM, Bisno AL: Infective endocarditis complicating mitral

valve prolapse: Epidemiologic, clinical and microbiologic aspects. *Rev Infect Dis* 8:117–137, 1986.
50. Sorentino MJ: Mitral valve prolapse. Avoiding complications of a progressive disease. *Postgrad Med* 93:63–70, 79, 1993.
51. Simmons NA: Recommendations for endocarditis prophylaxis. The Endocarditis Working Party for Antimicrobial Chemotherapy. *J Antimicrob Chemother* 31:437–438, 1993.
52. Imperiale TF, Horwitz RI: Does prophylaxis prevent post dental infective endocarditis? *Am J Med* 88:131–136, 1990.
53. Bisno AL, Dismukes WE, Durack DT, et al: Antimicrobial treatment of infective endocarditis due to viridans streptococci, enterococci, and staphylococci. *JAMA* 261:1471–1477, 1989.
54. Durak DT: Prophylaxis for infective endocarditis, in Mandell GL, Douglas RG Jr, Bennett JE: *Principles and Practice of Infectious Diseases*, ed 3. New York, Churchill Livingstone, 1990, pp 716–721.
55. Everett ED, Hirschmann JU: Transient bacteremia and endocarditis prophylaxis. A review. *Medicine (Baltimore)* 56:61–77, 1977.
56. Karl T, Wensley D, Stark J, et al: Infective endocarditis in children with congenital heart disease: Comparison of selected features in patients with surgical correction or palliation and those without. *Br Heart J* 58:57–65, 1987.
57. Karchmer AW, Archer GL, Dismukes WE: Staphylococcus epidermidis causing prosthetic valve endocarditis: Microbiologic and clinical observations as guides to therapy. *Ann Intern Med* 98:447–455, 1983.
58. Tuppurainen N, Hallman M: Prevention of neonatal group B streptococcal disease: Intrapartum detection and chemoprophylaxis of heavily colonized parturients. *Obstet Gynecol* 73:583–587, 1989.
59. Boyer KM, Gotoff SP: Prevention of early-onset neonatal group B streptococcal disease with selective intrapartum chemoprophylaxis. *N Engl J Med* 314:1665–1669, 1986.
60. Yow MD, Mason EO, Leeds LJ, et al: Ampicillin prevents intrapartum transmission of group B streptococcus. *JAMA* 241:1245–1247, 1979.
61. Allardice JG, Baskett TF, Seshia MM, et al: Perinatal group B streptococcal colonization and infection. *Am J Obstet Gynecol* 142:617–620, 1982.
62. Minkoff H, Mead P: An obstetric approach to the prevention of early-onset group B beta-hemolytic streptococcal sepsis. *Am J Obstet Gynecol* 154:973–977, 1986.
63. Morales WJ, Lim D: Reduction of group B streptococcal maternal and neonatal infections in preterm pregnancies with premature rupture of membranes through a rapid identification test. *Am J Obstet Gynecol* 157:13–16, 1987.
64. Lim DV, Morales WJ, Walsh AF, et al: Group B strep broth and co-

agglutination for rapid identification of Group B streptococci in preterm pregnant women. *J Clin Microbiol* 5:452–453, 1987.
65. Franciosi RA, Knostman JD, Zimmerman RA: Group B streptococcal neonatal and infant infections. *J Pediatr* 82:707–718, 1973.
66. Committee on Infectious Diseases and Committee on Fetus and Newborn: Guidelines for prevention of group B streptococcal (GBS) infection by chemoprophylaxis. *Pediatrics* 90:775–778, 1992.
67. American College of Obstetricians and Gynecologists: *Group B Streptococcal Infections in Pregnancy*. Washington, DC, *ACOG Technical Bulletin* No 170, July 1992.
68. Larsen JW, Dooley SL: Group B streptococcal infections: An obstetrical viewpoint. *Pediatrics* 91:148–149, 1993.
69. Torres RA, Franke-Ruta G, Barr MR: Future therapies in the management of critically ill AIDS patients. *Crit Care Clin* 9:153–176, 1993.
70. Jewett JF, Hecht FM: Preventive health care for adults with HIV infection. *JAMA* 269:1144–1153, 1993.
71. Jimenez E, Carrer MT, Perez Dieppa I, et al: Experience with the use of immune intravenous immunoglobulin in symptomatic children with human immunodeficiency virus infection. *Bol Asoc Med P R* 83:538–542, 1991.
72. Mofenson L, Bethel J, Moye J, et al: Effect of intravenous immunoglobulin (IVIG) on $CD4^+$ lymphocyte decline in HIV-infected children in a clinical trial of IVIG infection prophylaxis. *J Acquir Immune Defic Syndr* 6:1103–1113, 1993.
73. Aronstam A, Congard B, Evans DI, et al: HIV infection in haemophilia—a European cohort. *Arch Dis Child* 68:521–524, 1993.
74. Fischl MA, Dickinson GM, LaVoie L: Safety and efficacy of sulfamethoxazole and trimethoprim chemoprophylaxis for Pneumocystis carinii pneumonia in AIDS. *JAMA* 259:1185–1189, 1988.
75. Ruskin J, La Riviere M: Low dose cotrimoxazole for prevention of Pneumocystis carinii pneumonia in human immunodeficiency virus disease. *Lancet* 337:468–471, 1991.
76. Carr A, Tindall B, Penny R, et al: Trimethoprim-sulfamethoxazole appears more effective than aerosolized pentamidine as secondary prophylaxis against Pneumocystis carinii pneumonia in patients with AIDS. *AIDS* 6:165–171, 1992.
77. Chaisson RE, Keruly J, Richman DD, et al: Pneumocystis prophylaxis and survival in patients with advanced human immunodeficiency virus infection treated with zidovudine. The Zidovudine Epidemiology Group. *Arch Intern Med* 152:2009–2013, 1992.
78. Martin MA, Cox PH, Beck K, et al: A comparison of the effectiveness of three regimens in the prevention of Pneumocystis carinii pneumonia in human immunodeficiency virus–infected patients. *Arch Intern Med* 152:523–528, 1992.
79. Girard PM, Landman R, Gaudebout C, et al: Dapsone-pyrimethamine vs aerosolized pentamidine for primary prophylaxis of pneumocys-

tosis and neurotoxoplasmosis (abstract 1017). Presented at the *Eighth International Conference on AIDS,* Amsterdam, 1992.
80. Von Reyn CF, Clements CJ, Mann JM: Human immunodeficiency virus infections and routine childhood immunization. *Lancet* 2:669–672, 1987.
81. Besnard M, Sauvion S, Offredo C, et al: Bacillus Calmette-Guérin infection after vaccination of human immunodeficiency virus–infected children. *Pediatr Infect Dis J* 12:993–997, 1993.
82. Carr A, Penny R, Cooper D: Prophylaxis of opportunistic infections in patients with HIV infection. *J Acquir Immune Defic Syndr* 6(suppl):56–60, 1993.
83. Centers for Disease Control and Prevention: Recommendations on prophylaxis and therapy for disseminated Mycobacterium avium complex for adults and adolescents infected with human immunodeficiency virus. *MMWR* 42:17–19, 1993.
84. Lazard T, Perronne C, Cohen Y, et al: Efficacy of granulocyte colony-stimulating factor and RU-40555 in combination with clarithromycin against Mycobacterium avium complex infection of C57BL/6 mice. *Antimicrob Agents Chemother* 37:692–695, 1993.
85. Viviani MA: Opportunistic fungal infections in patients with acquired immune deficiency syndrome. *Chemotherapy* 38:35–42, 1992.
86. Carr A, Tindall B, Brew BJ, et al: Low-dose trimethoprim-sulfamethoxazole prophylaxis for toxoplasmic encephalitis in patients with AIDS. *Ann Intern Med* 117:106–111, 1992.
87. Jacobson MA, Besch CL, Child C, et al: Toxicity of clindamycin as prophylaxis for AIDS-associated toxoplasmic encephalitis. Community Programs for Clinical Research on AIDS. *Lancet* 339:333–334, 1992.
88. Cooper DA, Pederson C, Aiuti F, et al: The efficacy and safety of zidovudine with or without acyclovir in the treatment of patients with AIDS-related complex. *AIDS* 5:933–943, 1991.
89. Powderly WG: Therapy for cryptococcal meningitis in patients with AIDS. *Clin Infect Dis* 1:554–559, 1992.
90. Henderson DK, Gerberding JL: Prophylactic zidovudine after occupational exposure to the human immunodeficiency virus: An interim analysis. *J Infect Dis* 160:321–327, 1989.
91. Ramsey SD, Nettleman MD: Cost-effectiveness of prophylactic AZT following needlestick injury in health care workers. *Med Decis Making* 12:142–148, 1992.
92. Robinson EN Jr: Arguments against the chemoprophylaxis use of Zidovudine following occupational exposure to the human immunodeficiency virus. *Clin Infect Dis* 16:357–360, 1993.
93. Shapiro ED: Prophylaxis for contacts of patients with meningococcal or Haemophilus influenzae type b disease. *Pediatr Infect Dis* 1:132–138, 1982.

94. Shapiro ED: Infections caused by Haemophilus influenzae type b: The beginning of the end? *JAMA* 269:264–266, 1993.
95. Meningococcal Disease Surveillance Group: Meningococcal disease secondary attack rate and chemoprophylaxis in the United States. *JAMA* 235:261–265, 1976.
96. Hadler SC: Public health considerations of infectious diseases in child day care centers. *J Pediatr* 105:683–701, 1984.
97. Munford RS, Taumay AE, Morais JS, et al: Spread of meningococcal infection within households. *Lancet* 1:1275, 1974.
98. Schwartz B, Al-Tobaiqi A, Al-Ruwais A, et al: Comparative efficacy of ceftriaxone and rifampin in eradicating pharyngeal carriage of group A Neisseria meningitides. *Lancet* 1:1239–1242, 1988.
99. Cuevas LE, HArt CA: Chemoprophylaxis of bacterial meningitis. *J Antimicrob Chemother* 31(suppl B):79–91, 1993.
100. Gaunt PN, Lambert BE: Single dose ciprofloxacin for the eradication of pharyngeal carriage of Neisseria meningitidis. *J Antimicrob Chemother* 21:489–496, 1988.
101. Murphy TV, Clements JF, Breedlove JA, et al: Risk of subsequent disease among day-care contacts of patients with systemic Haemophilus influenzae type b disease. *N Engl J Med* 316:5–10, 1987.
102. Osterholm MT, Pierson LM, White KE, et al: The risk of subsequent transmission of Haemophilus influenza type b disease among children in day care: Results of a two-year statewide prospective surveillance and contact survey. *N Engl J Med* 316:1–5, 1987.
103. Band JD, Fraser JW, Ajello MA: Prevention of Haemophilus influenzae type b disease. *JAMA* 251:2381–2386, 1984.
104. Francke EL, New HC: Post splenectomy infection. *Surg Clin North Am* 61:135–155, 1981.
105. Wong WY, Overturf GD, Powars DR: Infection caused by *Streptococcus pneumoniae* in children with sickle cell disease: Epidemiology, immunologic mechanisms, prophylaxis, and vaccination. *Clin Infect Dis* 14:1124–1136, 1992.
106. Zorrabi MH, Rosner F: Serious infections in adults following splenectomy for trauma. *Arch Intern Med* 144:1421–1424, 1984.
107. Dickerman JD: Splenectomy and sepsis: A warning. *Pediatrics* 64:938–940, 1979.
108. Gonzaga RAF: Fatal post-splenectomy pneumococcal sepsis despite prophylaxis. *Lancet* 2:694–695, 1984.
109. Buchanan GR, Smith SJ: Pneumococcal septicemia despite pneumococcal vaccine and prescription of penicillin prophylaxis in children with sickle cell anemia. *Am J Dis Child* 140:428–432, 1986.
110. Murdoch IA, Anjos RD, Mitchell A: Fatal pneumococcal septicoemia associated with asplenia and isomerism of the right atrial appendage. *Br Heart J* 65:102–103, 1991.
111. Chattopodhyay B: Splenectomy, pneumococcal vaccination and antibiotic prophylaxis. *Br J Hosp Med* 41:172–174, 1989.

112. Zarrobi MH, Rosner F: Rarity of failure of penicillin prophylaxis to prevent post splenectomy sepsis. *Arch Intern Med* 146:1207–1208, 1986.
113. Moyon White RT: Pneumococcal vaccine. *Thorax* 43:345–348, 1988.
114. Advisory Committee on Immunization Practices: Use of vaccines and immune globulins in persons with altered immunocompetence. *MMWR* 42(RR-4):1–18, 1993.
115. Di Padori F, Durig M, Wadstrom J, et al: Role of spleen in immune response to polyvalent pneumococcal vaccine. *BMJ* 287:1829–1832, 1983.
116. Comstock GW, Baum C, Snider DE Jr: Isoniazid prophylaxis among Alaskan Eskimos: Final report of the Bethel isoniazid studies. *Am Rev Respir Dis* 119:827–830, 1979.
117. Hsu KH: Thirty years after isoniazid: Its impact on tuberculosis in children and adolescents. *JAMA* 251:1283–1285, 1984.
118. International Union against Tuberculosis. Committee on Prophylaxis: Efficacy of various durations of isoniazid preventive therapy of tuberculosis: Five years of follow up on the IUAT trial. *Bull WHO* 60:555–564, 1982.
119. Committee on Infectious Diseases, American Academy of Pediatrics: Chemotherapy for tuberculosis in infants and children. *Pediatrics* 89:161–165, 1992.
120. American Thoracic Society: Diagnostic standards and classification of tuberculosis. *Am Rev Respir Dis* 142:725–735, 1990.
121. Barnes PF, Barrows SA: Tuberculosis in the 1990s. *Ann Intern Med* 119:400–410, 1993.
122. Altarac D, Raucher B, Beck S, et al: A reevaluation of PPD testing in a high risk cohort (abstract 1357). Presented at the 33rd Interscience Conference on Antimicrobial Agents and Chemotherapy, New Orleans, 1993.
123. Snider DE Jr, Cara GJ, Kaplan JP: Preventive therapy with isoniazid. Cost-effectiveness of different durations of therapy. *JAMA* 255:1579–1583, 1986.
124. Snider DE Jr, Rieder HL, Combs D, et al: Tuberculosis in children. *Pediatr Infect Dis J* 7:271–278, 1988.
125. Cohn DL, Iseman MD: Treatment and prevention of multidrug-resistant tuberculosis. *Res Microbiol* 144:150–153, 1993.
126. Hill DR, Pearson RD: Health advice for international travel. *Ann Intern Med* 108:839–852, 1988.
127. Murray BE: Increasing resistance to trimethoprim/sulfamethoxazole among isolates of Escherichia coli in developing countries. *J Infect Dis* 253:2700–2704, 1985.
128. Sack RB: Antimicrobial prophylaxis of traveler's diarrhea. A selected summary. *Rev Infect Dis* 8(suppl 2):160–166, 1986.
129. Wistrom J, Norrby R: Antibiotic prophylaxis of travellers' diarrhea. *Scand J Infect Dis Suppl* 70:111–129, 1990.

130. Dupont HL, Ericsson CD: Prevention and treatment of traveller's diarrhea. *N Engl J Med* 328:1821–1827, 1993.
131. Nahlen BL, Parsonnet J, Preblud SR, et al: International travel and the child younger than two years: Recommendations for prevention of traveler's diarrhea and malaria chemoprophylaxis. *Pediatr Infect Dis J* 8:735–739, 1989.
132. Liu LX: Travel medicine. Part II: Malaria, traveler's diarrhea, and other problems. *Infect Med* 10:24–28, 58, 1993.
133. Miller KD, Lobel HO, Papaivanou M, et al: Failures of combined chloroquine and Fansidar prophylaxis in American travellers to East Africa. *J Infect Dis* 154:689–691, 1986.
134. Centers for Disease Control and Prevention: Recommendations for the prevention of malaria among travelers. *MMWR* 39(RR-3):1–10, 1990.
135. Centers for Disease Control and Prevention: Change of dosing regimen for malaria prophylaxis with mefloquine. *MMWR* 40:72–73, 1991.
136. Betts RF: Amantadine and rimantidine for the prevention of influenza A. *Semin Respir Dis* 4:304–310, 1989.
137. Centers for Disease Control: Prevention and control of influenza: Recommendations of the Immunization Practices Advisory Committee (ACIP). *MMWR* 39(RR-7):1–15, 1990.
138. Payler DK, Purdhom PA: Influenza A prophylaxis with amantadine in a boarding school. *Lancet* 1:502–504, 1984.
139. Immunization Practices Advisory Committee (ACIP): Diphtheria, tetanus, and pertussis: Recommendations for vaccine use and other preventive measures. *MMWR* 40(RR-10):1–28, 1991.
140. Bass JW: Pertussis: Current status of prevention and treatment. *Pediatr Infect Dis* 4:614–619, 1985.
141. Mortimer EA Jr: Pertussis vaccine, in Plotkin SA, Mortimer EA Jr: *Vaccines*. Philadelphia, WB Saunders, 1988, pp 74–97.
142. Centers for Disease Control and Prevention: Pertussis outbreaks. *MMWR* 42:197–200, 1993.
143. Sprauer MA, Cochi SL, Zell ER, et al: Prevention of secondary transmission of pertussis in households with early use of erythromycin. *Am J Dis Child* 146:177–181, 1992.
144. Guglielmo BJ, Hohn DC, Koo PJ, et al: Antibiotic prophylaxis in surgical procedures: A critical analysis of the literature. *Arch Surg* 118:943–955, 1983.
145. Kaiser AB: Antimicrobial prophylaxis in surgery. *N Engl J Med* 315:1129–1138, 1986.
146. Classen DC, Evans RS, Restotnik SL, et al: The timing of prophylactic administration of antibiotic and the risk of surgical-wound infection. *N Engl J Med* 326:281–286, 1992.
147. Bergquist EJ, Murphy SA: Prophylactic antibiotics for surgery. *Med Clin North Am* 71:357–368, 1987.

148. Wenzel RP: Preoperative antibiotic prophylaxis. *N Engl J Med* 326:337–339, 1992.
149. Kaiser AB: Postoperative infections and antimicrobial prophylaxis, in Mandell GL, Douglas RG Jr, Bennett JE: *Principles and Practice of Infectious Diseases*, ed 3. New York, Churchill Livingstone, 1990, pp 2245–2257.
150. Antimicrobial prophylaxis in surgery. *Med Lett Drugs Ther* 34:5–8, 1992.
151. Currier JS, Campbell H, Platt R, et al: Perioperative antimicrobial prophylaxis in middle Tennessee, 1989–1990. *Rev Infect Dis* 13(suppl 10):874–878, 1991.
152. Feigin RD, Matson DO: The compromised host, in Feigin RD, Cherry JD: *Textbook of Pedatric Infectious Diseases*, ed 3. Philadelphia, WB Saunders, 1992, pp 963–964, 980, 1992.
153. Ranaboldo CJ, Karran SE, Bailey IS, et al: Antimicrobial prophylaxis in "clean" surgery: Hernia repair. *J Antimicrob Chemother* 31(suppl B):35–41, 1993.
154. Weitehamp MR, Caputo GM: Antibiotic prophylaxis: Update on common clinical uses. *Am Fam Physician* 48:597–604, 1993.
155. Pifer LL, Hughes WT, Stagno S, et al: Pneumocystis carinii infection: Evidence for high prevalence in normal and immunosuppressed children. *Pediatrics* 61:35–41, 1978.
156. Gurwith MJ, Brunston JL, Lank BA, et al: A perspective controlled investigation of prophylactic trimethoprim-sulfamethoxazole in hospitalized granulocytopenic patients. *Am J Med* 66:248–256, 1979.
157. Hughes WT, Rivera GK, Schell MJ, et al: Successful intermittent chemoprophylaxis for Pneumocystis carinii pneumonitis. *N Engl J Med* 316:1627–1632, 1987.
158. Green M, Michaels MG: Infectious complications of solid organ transplantation in children, in Aronoff SC, Hughes WT, Kohl S, et al: *Advances in Pedictric Infectious Diseases*, vol 7. St Louis, Mosby, 1992, pp 181–204.

Control of Sexually Transmitted Diseases in Adolescents: The Clinician's Role*

Carol A. Ford, M.D.
Fellow, Division of Adolescent Medicine, Department of Pediatrics, University of California, San Francisco School of Medicine, San Francisco, California

Anna-Barbara Moscicki, M.D.
Associate Professor of Pediatrics, Department of Pediatrics, University of California, San Francisco School of Medicine, San Francisco, California

Rates of sexually transmitted diseases (STDs) and STD complications in the United States demonstrate the magnitude of problems associated with these infectious agents and the enormity of the task of control of STDs.[1–4] Adolescents remain one of the principal groups in which there is continued failure to control STDs.[1–3]

Although the control of STD rates is dependent on highly complex interactions among sociocultural-environmental issues,[5] access to health care, and characteristics of the health care system, the primary care clinician remains critical to achieving this ambitious goal. However, many clinicians lack specific skills related to prevention, diagnosis, and treatment of STDs, especially with adolescent patients.[6, 7] These skills include the ability to do the following:

1. Address issues regarding adolescent sexuality.
2. Identify risk-associated sexual behavior and proceed with specific risk-reduction counseling.

*Supported by funds provided by the Maternal and Child Health Bureau, Department of Health and Human Services, Grant No. MCJ 000978, and the National Institutes of Health, National Cancer Institute, Grant No. CA-51323

3. Perform appropriate STD screening in asymptomatic adolescents.
4. Evaluate symptomatic patients.
5. Manage STDs.

The goal of this review is to enhance health professionals' competency and comfort when addressing STD-related issues with adolescents in the clinical setting.

EPIDEMIOLOGY OF SEXUALLY TRANSMITTED DISEASE

A review of the estimated frequency of bacterial STDs among adolescents reveals alarming rates. Trends in *Neisseria gonorrhoeae* infection rates are most reflective of general STD patterns. In 1991, gonorrhea rates among 15- to 19-year-old male and female adolescents were higher than in any other age group.[1, 2] Like gonorrhea, rates of *Chlamydia trachomatis* infection appear to be highest among adolescents, with chlamydia being two to three times more common than gonorrhea.[1, 2, 8] From 1981 to 1991, 10% to 12% of reported primary and secondary *Treponema pallidum* cases were in adolescents. During this time there was a 41% increase in rates among 15- to 19-year-old males and an approximate 110% increase among 10- to 19-year-old females.[1] In addition, chancroid, a bacterial STD caused by *Haemophilus ducreyi*, has re-emerged in the United States during the last decade. Although the incidence of this infection appears to be quite low, focal outbreaks continue to occur, with true rates of *H. ducreyi* infection being underestimated because available culture techniques are inadequate.[9]

Similar to bacterial STDs, rates of viral infection appear to show increasing trends. The number of 15- to 19-year-old females visiting an office-based practice for genital human papillomavirus (HPV) or herpes simplex virus (HSV) infections increased sixfold and eightfold respectively between 1966 and 1988.[2] However, as diagnostic methods for both of these infections have improved, it has become clear that prevalence estimates based on office visits are misleadingly low. Seroprevalence studies of HSV-2 suggest that up to 17% of certain subgroups of adolescents have had exposure to HSV-2.[10] Estimates of the prevalence of genital HPV infection by molecular techniques including polymerase chain reaction (PCR) are even higher than those for HSV-2, which makes this currently the most common sexually transmitted infection detected in adolescents.[11]

Hepatitis B virus (HBV) and human immunodeficiency virus (HIV) infections can be transmitted through sexual as well as nonsexual routes. Most HBV infections (up to 60%) in adolescents are not associated with an identifiable source of infection. However, among cases in which a source of HBV infection can be identified, 50% will have been acquired by sexual transmission or other person-to-person contact.[12] Similarly, 36% of male and 54% of female adolescents with acquired immunodeficiency syndrome (AIDS) contract the disease from sexually acquired HIV infection.[13] Because of the average 11-year latency period between initial HIV infection and an AIDS-defining illness, it is suspected that a substantial portion of individuals in whom AIDS was diagnosed in their twenties (63,718 cases, or 19% of all AIDS cases) were infected during adolescence through sexual transmission.[13, 14] Table 1 summarizes the current data available on the frequency of STDs among adolescents.

In addition to variation in STD trends by the type of infection and gender, different patterns of reported STD rates have been observed according to sociodemographic characteristics such as race, ethnicity, and geographic region.[1, 5, 10, 13] However, because of limitations in existing sociodemographic data, interpretation of these differences should be cautious since they may reflect social, economic, behavioral, or other factors that have not been measured.[22]

In summary, the epidemiologic data underscore the magnitude of the problem that clinicians face in achieving STD control among adolescents. In addition, the wide variation in STD rates by the type of infection, gender, race/ethnicity, and region requires that clinicians obtain information about STD prevalence within their local community in order to develop appropriate evaluation and treatment strategies.

COMPLICATIONS AND SEQUELAE OF SEXUALLY TRANSMITTED DISEASES

Significant complications and long-term sequelae are associated with many STDs (Table 2). Chlamydia- and/or gonorrhea-related pelvic inflammatory disease (PID) is the most common complication in adolescents and is one of the most costly by any measure.[4] In addition to the acute morbidity associated with PID, it has become increasingly clear that postinfectious tubal damage causes long-term sequelae. Westrom found that 9% of patients in whom one episode of PID was diagnosed were infertile and 52% were infertile after three or more episodes of PID.[26] The risk of ectopic pregnancy is also increased sevenfold to tenfold over baseline in

TABLE 1.
Estimated Frequency of Sexually Transmitted Diseases in Adolescents and Young Adults

STD*	Data Source	Estimates of Frequency†			
Neisseria gonorrhoeae	CDC	*Rates‡ of gonorrhea by sex and age group (yr) in 1991*[1]			
			10–14	15–19	20–29
		Males	32.4	882.6	779.6
		Females	99.2	1,043.6	595.0
Chlamydia trachomatis	Physician visits	*Range of chlamydia prevalence reported in adolescent populations*			
		Males	9%–32%[15]		
	Sentinel surveillance	Females	8%–40%[2, 15]		
Treponema pallidum	CDC	*Rates‡ of primary/secondary syphilis by sex and age group (yr) in 1991*[1]			
			10–14	15–19	20–29
		Males	0.4	18.1	44.8
		Females	2.5	35.0	46.4

Haemophilus ducreyi	CDC	*Total number of reported U.S. cases*[9]		
		1987	5,035	
	Sentinel surveillance	1990	4,223	
HSV	Physician visits	*Range of HSV-2 seroprevalence by population studied*		
		6.9% of all aged 15–29 (17% among select groups by age 20)[10]		
	Seroprevalence studies	6%–34% of all aged 20–24[16]		
HPV	Physician visits	*Prevalence in sexually active population by diagnostic technique*[17]		
		Diagnostic technique		HPV prevalence
	Surveillance projects	External inspection for visible genital warts		1%
		Cervical cytology		1%–10%
		Colposcopy		10%–27%
		Polymerase chain reaction		46%–80%
HBV	CDC	*Total reported hepatitis B infections by age group (yr) in 1992*[18]		
		10–14	15–19	20–24
		211	1,105	2,295

(continued)

TABLE 1 (continued).

HIV	HIV: seroprevalence in selected populations	*Range of HIV seroprevalence by population studied* 0.03% of U.S. military recruits (0.1% of select groups)[19] 0.36% of Job Corp applicants (2.4% among select groups)[20]
	AIDS: CDC	5.3% among 15–20-year-old runaway and homeless youth[21] *Total reported AIDS cases by sex and age (yr) at diagnosis through 9/93 in the United States*[13]

	13–19	20–24	25–29
Males	977	10,071	43,576
Females	435	2,641	7,430

*STD = sexually transmitted disease; CDC = Centers for Disease Control and Prevention; HPV = human papillomavirus; HBV = hepatitis B virus; HIV = human immunodeficiency virus; AIDS = acquired immunodeficiency syndrome.
†Available data may be reported as prevalence of disease or incidence of disease and are not directly comparable.
‡Incidence per 100,000 population.

TABLE 2.
Sexually Transmitted Disease Complications and Sequelae*

STD†	Complications	Vertical Transmission	Long-Term Sequelae
Neisseria gonorrhoeae (GC)	Pelvic inflammatory disease Tubo-ovarian abscess Perihepatitis Epididymitis Disseminated GC GC conjunctivitis Bartholinitis	Ophthalmia neonatorum Neonatal disseminated GC	Pelvic adhesions Chronic pelvic pain Ectopic pregnancy Infertility
Treponema pallidum	Secondary syphilis Neurosyphilis Syphilitic eye disease Tertiary syphilis	Congenital syphilis	Gumma Cardiovascular disease Neurologic disease
Chlamydia trachomatis	Pelvic inflammatory disease Tubo-ovarian abscess Perihepatitis Epididymitis Reiter syndrome Conjunctivitis Bartholinitis	Ophthalmia neonatorum Chlamydial pneumonia	Pelvic adhesions Chronic pelvic pain Ectopic pregnancy Infertility

(continued)

TABLE 2 (continued).

HSV	Secondary infection of lesions Disseminated HSV infection	Neonatal HSV	Neurologic dysfunction
HPV	Anogenital dysplasia	Laryngeal papillomatosis	Anogenital carcinoma
HBV	Chronic carrier state Chronic active hepatitis	HBV infection	Cirrhosis of the liver Hepatocellular carcinoma
HIV	AIDS	HIV infection	Opportunistic infections Increased risk of anogenital cancer, Kaposi sarcoma, and lymphomas

*Data from references 3, 23, 24, and 25.

†STD = sexually transmitted disease; GC = gonorrhea; HSV = herpes simplex virus; HPV = human papillomavirus; HBV = hepatitis B virus; HIV = human immunodeficiency virus; AIDS = acquired immunodeficiency syndrome.

patients with a history of PID.[26] The total economic costs for PID and PID-associated ectopic pregnancy/infertility in the United States are projected to be over $9 billion in the year 2000.[4]

Although most persons infected with HBV will have transient self-limited hepatitis, approximately 3% of patients with acute HBV will require hospitalization, and 0.1% will die of fulminant disease.[27] Of adults acutely infected with HBV, 6% to 10% will become chronic HBV carriers and remain potentially infectious as well as at increased risk for the development of chronic hepatitis, hepatic cirrhosis, and hepatocarcinoma. An estimated 5,000 deaths per year in the United States are caused by complications of hepatitis B.[3]

Recent epidemiologic and laboratory data have strongly linked specific types of HPV (including types 16, 18, 31, 33, 45, and 56) with the development of anogenital cancers.[28, 29] However, the high prevalence of HPV infection in combination with observation that few HPV-infected females progress to cancer suggests that HPV is necessary but not sufficient for the development of invasive cancer. Among adolescents with HPV infection, the prevalence of dysplasia (squamous intraepithelial lesions) on cervical cytology has been found to be as high as 20%.[30] Although few dysplastic lesions progress, prediction of progression of disease remains difficult. Therefore, high prevalence rates have resulted in huge societal costs and burdens for evaluation of abnormal cytology.

A description of HIV complications and sequelae is beyond the scope of this article, although appropriate references have been noted.[14, 24, 31] The emotional, medical, and economic costs of HIV will continue to escalate as this infection affects larger numbers of adolescents and young adults.

Certainly, prevention of initial STD infections is the most effective method to influence the frequency of these complications and sequelae. Prevention of viral STD complications and sequelae largely depends on avoidance of the primary infection. For curable STDs (e.g., gonorrhea, chlamydia, syphilis, and chancroid), early identification of uncomplicated STDs with effective treatment of both patients and their partners is necessary to decrease rates of STD complications and long-term sequelae.

RISK FACTORS FOR TRANSMISSION OF SEXUALLY TRANSMITTED DISEASE

Risk factors associated with the acquisition of STDs include a complex interaction among sexual behaviors, condom use, and substance use. Sexual intercourse among U.S. adolescents is common, with 54% to 78% of students in grades 9 to 12 reporting current sexual activity.[32] Although most clinicians equate sexual intercourse with vaginal intercourse, oral and anal intercourse is common practice among adolescents, with 73% of adolescents reporting oral intercourse and 21% reporting a history of heterosexual anal intercourse.[33] Clarification of the type of sexual intercourse is important because specific types of unprotected sex are associated with different levels of risk and STD syndromes. For example, anal intercourse, particularly for the receptive partner, is associated with a higher risk of HIV transmission and STD proctitis than are other types of intercourse.[34] Additionally, almost all STDs may be transmitted through oral-genital or oral-anal contact.[35] Sexual contact with a partner at risk of having STDs or contact with multiple partners (whether defined by nonmonogamous relationships or serial monogamy) increases an individual's risk of STDs, as does inconsistent condom use.[36] Unfortunately, inconsistent condom use is reported by 70% to 93% of adolescents.[33, 37]

Substance use has both direct and indirect associations with STDs. Sharing of unsterile needles during injection drug use is directly associated with a risk of HIV and HBV infection. All substance use (alcohol, noninjection drugs, or injection drugs) is thought to be indirectly associated with a risk of acquiring an STD related to impaired decision making regarding sexual behavior.

In addition to behavioral risk factors, biological factors most likely play a significant role in STD acquisition in adolescents. It appears that the risk for STD infection in females is inversely related to the age of initial sexual intercourse (sexual debut) even when the number of sexual partners has been taken into account, which suggests that maturational or immunologic factors may be important. Specific attention has been given to the biological immaturity of the adolescent cervix, defined by the predominance of both columnar and metaplastic epithelium as compared with the squamous epithelium of a mature cervix. Several STDs have been shown to preferentially adhere and infect this immature epithelium.[2, 38]

CONTROL OF SEXUALLY TRANSMITTED DISEASES: THE CLINICIAN'S ROLE

The role of the clinician in STD control among adolescents includes the following:

- Routine STD risk assessment in all adolescents
- Appropriate STD screening in asymptomatic adolescents at risk of infection

- Recognition and evaluation of adolescents with symptoms of STDs
- Appropriate management of STDs
- Primary and secondary prevention counseling

RISK ASSESSMENT: THE SEXUAL HISTORY

Identification of adolescents who are at risk of having an STD requires a thorough sexual history. However, incorporation of a sexual history into a practice setting has often been identified as difficult by many practitioners.[39] Addressing sexual issues during routine adolescent health care in a systematic and organized manner may assist in overcoming these difficulties.

Anticipatory guidance regarding normal sexual development should begin in early childhood.[40] As a child approaches adolescence, time spent talking with the patient privately should be incorporated into routine visits and policies regarding confidentiality made explicitly clear to adolescents as well as their parents. The confidentiality of adolescent discussions with a physician regarding issues related to sexual behavior is protected by professional standards and legal statutes.[41] In acute care settings where continuity of care is lacking, a routine description of these policies at the initiation of all adolescent visits is helpful.

Since most adolescents make the transition from virginal to nonvirginal status during the adolescent years, it is recommended that adolescents (aged 11 to 21) receive annual health guidance to promote a better understanding of their sexual growth and psychosocial/psychosexual development. This should include health guidance regarding sexual behaviors and screening for involvement in sexual behaviors that may result in unintended pregnancy and/or STDs.[41, 42] This could occur within the context of a yearly routine visit or visits required for sports, camp, or school participation. Adolescents seen for problem-oriented visits unrelated to STDs and who have not discussed sexual issues with a health care professional within the past year should be encouraged to schedule a routine visit. If a return visit is unlikely, general assessment of sexual development and issues may be appropriate within the context of an acute visit after an explanation of the clinician's decision to address these topics. If issues associated with risky sexual behavior are identified but time prohibits adequate attention, it is appropriate to schedule a follow-up appointment.

Sexual histories should be obtained in a manner that is adjusted to the adolescent's level of biological, cognitive, and social development. Explicit dialogue and visual materials are often required to avoid miscommunication. Equally important when obtaining a sexual history is a nonjudgmental attitude and avoidance of assumptions, particularly those regarding types of sexual behavior or sexual orientation. Figure 1 demonstrates a format for obtaining a sexual history during an adolescent visit. Identification of an adolescent's range of sexual experience will assist with ap-

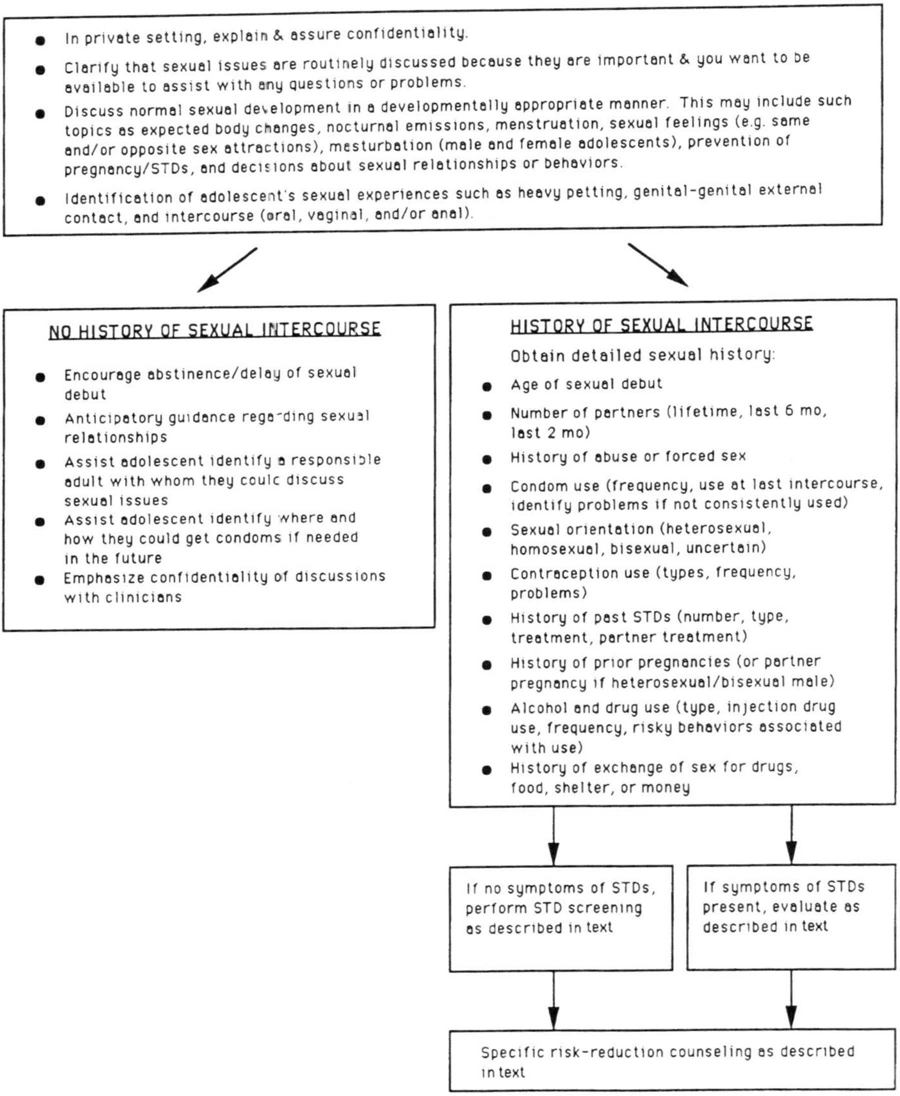

FIGURE 1.
Format for incorporation of sexual history into adolescent visit.

propriate anticipatory guidance and provide information for a focused discussion of past, present, and future sexual decision making. The most critical component of the sexual history is determining whether an adolescent has ever had sexual intercourse (oral, vaginal, or anal) either volitionally or nonvolitionally.[15] When adolescents who have had sexual intercourse are identified, specific attention should be focused on a history of effective condom and contraception use. A substance use history is included because of the potential for nonsexual transmission of HBV and HIV through injection drug use, as well as for assessing the influence of substance use on sexual behavior.

ASYMPTOMATIC ADOLESCENTS AT RISK FOR SEXUALLY TRANSMITTED DISEASES

The majority of adolescents infected with an STD do not report symptoms (Table 3). Therefore, routine screening for STDs is recommended for all asymptomatic sexually active adolescents (Table 4).[42] This should include adolescents who report close nonpenetrative as well as penetrative genital-genital, anal-genital, oral-genital, or oral-anal contact. Although theoretically adolescents who report consistent condom use are at low risk of infection, for purposes of screening, these adolescents are considered at risk of acquiring an STD because of concerns about reliable reporting of condom use and because condom use does not completely protect from the acquisition of all STDs.[36]

Yearly screening should include testing for gonorrhea, chlamydia, and HPV. In females, an annual pelvic examination should include visual inspection for genital warts, testing for both *N. gonorrhoeae* and *C. trachomatis* (see Cervicitis), and cervical cytology. In males, an annual genital examination should include a visual inspection for genital warts and a urine dipstick test for leukocyte esterase (LET) in a first-void urine specimen (collected from the first portion of the urinary stream). If LET is positive (LET $\geq$ trace +), urethral or urine testing for *N. gonorrhoeae* and *C. trachomatis* should follow (see Urethritis).[42, 52] If signs of infection are found on examination, evaluation for a specific diagnosis is indicated as discussed in the following section on STD clinical syndromes. Male and female adolescents who engage in regular anal intercourse should have rectal screening for *N. gonorrhoeae* as well as inspection for anal warts.[51] The cost-effectiveness of rectal screening for *C. trachomatis* in asymptomatic patients remains to be determined.[51] Pharyngeal screening for gonorrhea in asymptomatic adolescents who engage in oral intercourse is not recommended.

Persons identified to be at high risk of having STDs are those having more than one sexual partner within the last 6 months, having a history of an STD, men who have had sex with other men, women who have had sex with male bisexual partners, having exchanged sex for drugs or money, using injection drugs, having sex with a person living in an area endemic for infection, and having had a sexual partner who is at risk for infection. Any person in whom one STD is diagnosed is at high risk of having other STDs.[42] In these high-risk adolescents, increased frequency of STD screening should be considered, and the following should be performed: (1) nontreponemal test for *T. pallidum*, (2) confidential HIV testing, and (3) HBV vaccination.[42] A presumptive diagnosis of latent syphilis in an asymptomatic adolescent can be made by a reactive nontreponemal test confirmed by a treponemal test in a person with no history of syphilis or, in a person with a history of syphilis, at

TABLE 3.
Frequency of Asymptomatic Sexually Transmitted Diseases

STD*	Percentage of Those Infected Who Are Asymptomatic
Neisseria gonorrhoeae	10% of males[43] 80% of females[44]
Treponema pallidum	12% had no symptoms of primary or secondary syphilis in a small study of male and female adolescents[45]
Chlamydia trachomatis	25% of males[43] 70% of females[46]
HSV	54%–81% of males[47] 61%–90% of females[47, 48]
HPV	>90% (no evidence of HPV by unaided visual inspection)[17]
HBV	75%[27]
HIV	30%–50% with primary HIV infection do not have clinically recognizable acute symptoms[49] It is suspected that the majority of those infected with HIV are asymptomatic[50]

*STD = sexually transmitted disease; HSV = herpes simplex virus; HPV = human papillomavirus; HBV = hepatitis B virus; HIV = human immunodeficiency virus.

TABLE 4.
Guidelines for Adolescent Preventive Services Screening Recommendations for Asymptomatic Sexually Active Adolescents*

STD†	Screening Method	Frequency
Neisseria gonorrhoeae‡	Female: cervical culture Male: urine leukocyte esterase (if positive, do urethral culture)	Yearly§
Chlamydia trachomatis	Female: immunologic or culture test of cervical fluid Male: urine leukocyte esterase (if positive, immunologic test or culture of urethra)	Yearly§
HPV	Female: visual inspection and Papanicolaou test of cervix Male: Visual inspection	Yearly§
Treponema pallidum	Serologic test	High-risk categories¶
HIV	Offer confidential serologic screening with ELISA and confirmatory test; performed only in conjunction with pretest and posttest counseling	High-risk categories¶

*Data from Elster AB, Kuznets NJ: *AMA Guidelines for Adolescent Preventive Services (GAPS): Recommendations and Rationale.* Baltimore, Williams & Wilkins, 1994.
‡Although not addressed in GAPS, some experts recommend that persons engaging in regular anal intercourse be screened for *N. gonorrhoeae*[51]
†STD = sexually transmitted disease; HPV = human papillomavirus; HIV = human immunodeficiency virus; ELISA = enzyme-linked immunosorbent assay.
§The frequency of screening for STDs depends on the sexual practices of the individual and history of STDs.
¶High-risk category: more than one sexual partner in the last 6 months, the presence or history of other STDs, a male who has engaged in sex with other males, intravenous drug use, having exchanged sex for drugs, having lived in an area endemic for infection, having had a sexual partner who is at high risk.

least a fourfold increase in titer of a quantitative nontreponemal test.[3] Early latent syphilis is defined by positive serology for syphilis in an asymptomatic patient when the infection was acquired within the preceding year. The acquisition of infection is documented by seroconversion from negative to positive serology or at least a fourfold increase in titer of a nontreponemal serologic test within the past 12 months. Late latent syphilis is defined as latent infection acquired more than 12 months before diagnosis.[3] Late latent infection is presumed if there is no prior serologic documentation. Testing for HIV should only be performed after informed consent has been obtained from the adolescent and in conjunction with both pretest and posttest counseling.[3, 42, 53]

Special attention to HBV infection is indicated because this is most commonly asymptomatic and is the only STD that is preventable by vaccination. Although universal HBV vaccination of adolescents is the most effective strategy to rapidly have an effect on the prevalence of this disease, it has been decided that universal immunization of infants is more cost-effective. However, widespread HBV immunization of all adolescents is recommended if resources permit. At minimum, all high-risk adolescents should be immunized.[42, 54, 55] Serologic screening for prior immunity to HBV from either HBV infection or immunization before vaccinating adolescents may be cost-effective in high-risk groups.[3, 42] Immunity can be assessed by screening for antibody to hepatitis B surface antigen (anti-HBs) and anti-HB core (total). If anti-HBs is used alone, HBV carriers will be missed.[3]

Although not covered in this review, STD screening in pregnant adolescents is essential to decrease vertical transmission of STDs. All pregnant women should be tested for *N. gonorrhoeae*, *C. trachomatis*, HBV carrier status (hepatitis B surface antigen), and *T. pallidum*.[3] Although universal HIV testing of pregnant females is controversial, pregnant adolescents with risk factors for HIV should be offered HIV testing.[3]

Specimens collected for medicolegal evaluation of rape or sexual abuse are often obtained from patients without STD symptoms and may require specific methods of testing, which should be discussed with the laboratory processing the specimens.[3, 23]

SYMPTOMATIC ADOLESCENTS: UNCOMPLICATED SEXUALLY TRANSMITTED DISEASE SYNDROMES

Most adolescents with symptoms and/or signs suggestive of STD syndromes can be recognized during a thorough history and physical examination that includes a pelvic examination in females and a genital examination in males.[56, 57] Recognition of a syndrome is followed by testing to clarify the cause of the clinical syndrome since determination of an organism-specific diagnosis is often needed to direct treatment and may improve patient compliance, management of sexual partners, and effectiveness of risk-reduction counseling. Additionally, organism-specific diagnoses are important for public health reporting. Guidelines for laboratory testing are described in the following sections. Although available methods of testing may vary in a specific clinical setting and will influence strategies chosen for STD evaluation, the clinician must be aware of the potential limitations of any testing method performed.[23, 58–60]

Vaginitis

Symptoms suggestive of vaginitis include vaginal discharge, dysuria, vaginal odor, or vulvar itching. Signs of vaginitis include an abnormal vaginal discharge and inflammation of the vulvar or vaginal epithelium. Sexually active females with vaginitis should be evaluated for *Trichomonas vaginalis*, bacterial vaginosis (BV), and candidiasis. *Trichomonas vaginalis* is usually transmitted sexually. Bacterial vaginosis is associated with sexual activity and having multiple partners but is not considered exclusively an STD. Candidiasis is not usually sexually acquired or transmitted, but it is common among females with vaginitis complaints.[3]

The cause of the vaginitis can usually be determined by microscopic evaluation of fresh samples of vaginal discharge as described in Table 5. The normal saline (NS) wet mount is examined for white blood cells (WBCs), *T. vaginalis*, clue cells, lack of lactobacilli, and *Candida albicans* (budding cells or pseudohyphae). KOH is also helpful for identification of *C. albicans*. All sexually active adolescents evaluated for vaginitis should also have endocervical testing for *N. gonorrhoeae* and *C. trachomatis* because cervicitis caused by either of these organisms may cause a vaginal discharge (see Cervicitis).

Cervicitis

Although cervicitis is often asymptomatic, symptoms may include vaginal discharge, abnormal vaginal bleeding (e.g., postcoital, prolonged, irregular, or heavy bleeding), or symptoms of an associated urethritis such as dysuria.[3] The clinical diagnosis of mucopurulent cervicitis (MPC) is based on the presence of yellow mucopurulent endocervical exudate or detection of WBCs (definitions vary from ≥5 to ≥30 WBCs per oil immersion field)[44, 61] on microscopic examination of a Gram-stained endocervical specimen.[44] Cervical friability may or may not be present. However, MPC has not been found to be a sensitive predictor of STD infection, and organism-specific testing is indicated in sexually active adolescents with any symptoms or signs suggestive of cervicitis (Table 6).[3] Although new diagnostic tests have been introduced for *N. gonorrhoeae* screening, culture remains the most sensitive and cost-effective method

TABLE 5.
Evaluation of Vaginitis*

Organisms	Laboratory Tests	Diagnosis
Trichomonas vaginalis Bacterial vaginosis† *Candida albicans*	Obtain specimen of vaginal discharge for 0.9% NS‡ wet mount 10% KOH wet mount "Whiff" test (KOH amine odor test) Determination of pH (range, 4.5–8.0) Obtain endocervical specimens for *N. gonorrhoeae* culture *C. trachomatis* testing (see Table 6)	*Trichomoniasis:* suggested if profuse yellow-green, frothy vaginal discharge with pH > 4.5 and NS‡ wet mount with white blood cells but no clue cells (which are epithelial cells appearing granular because of adherent bacteria); diagnosed if motile *T. vaginalis* on NS‡ wet mount (viability of organisms on wet mount dependent on fresh specimen being examined within 1–2 min) *Bacterial vaginosis:* diagnosed by clinical criteria if three of the following present: A homogenous discharge (usually white or gray) that adheres to vaginal walls Clue cells present on microscopy of NS wet mount (with lack of lactobacilli) pH of vaginal fluid > 4.5 Positive "whiff" test (fishy odor before or after addition of 10% KOH) *Acute vulvovaginal candidiasis:* suggested if white, clumped vaginal discharge with pH < 4.5; diagnosed if typical yeast (budding cells) or pseudohyphae on microscopy of KOH or NS wet mount

*Data from Centers for Disease Control and Prevention: *MMWR* 42(RR-14):1–102, 1993; Centers for Disease Control: *Sexually Transmitted Disease: Clinical Practice Guidelines, May 1991*. Atlanta, US Department of Health and Human Services, 1991.
†Disorder characterized by a change in the vaginal microbial flora, including an increase in *Gardnerella vaginalis, Bacteroides* spp., *Mobiluncus* spp., and *Mycoplasma hominis* and a decrease in lactobacilli.
‡NS = normal saline.

TABLE 6.
Evaluation of Cervicitis*

Organisms	Laboratory Tests	Diagnosis
Neisseria gonorrhoeae† *Chlamydia trachomatis*† HSV	Obtain vaginal specimens for evaluation of vaginal infection (Table 5) Obtain endocervical specimen for Culture for *N. gonorrhoeae* Test for *C. trachomatis* Consider Gram stain Consider HSV testing if severe cervicitis, ulcerative cervicitis, or testing for *N. gonorrhoeae* and *C. trachomatis* negative Obtain serology for *T. pallidum* if testing results positive	Since Gram-stained smears of the endocervix are only 50%–70% sensitive for detection of GNID‡ in infected females, the absence of GNID does not exclude gonorrhea Some experts suggest that the presumptive diagnosis of mucopurulent cervicitis can be made on the basis of increased white blood cells on a Gram-stained smear of endocervical exudate, although this is not a sensitive predictor of STD infection Diagnosis should be made on the basis of organism-specific test results If likelihood of infection is high or the patient is unlikely to return for treatment and initiation of treatment is based on presumptive diagnoses, it must include therapy for both *N. gonorrhoeae* and *C. trachomatis*

*Data from Centers for Disease Control and Prevention: *MMWR* 42(RR-14):1–102 1993; Centers for Disease Control: *Sexually Transmitted Diseases: Clinical Practice Guidelines, May 1991*. Atlanta, US Department of Health and Human Services, 1991.
†Most common organisms.
‡GNID = gram-negative intracellular diplococci; HSV = herpes simplex virus; STD = sexually transmitted disease.

available.[59] Specimen collections for *C. trachomatis* require special techniques because these organisms are obligate intracellular organisms that infect columnar epithelial cells.[23] Culture isolation of *C. trachomatis* has a 70% to 95% sensitivity and approximately 100% specificity for detection of infection but is technically difficult. Multiple nonculture tests are available as alternative methods of testing in adolescents, such as Chlamydiazyme enzyme immunoassay (EIA) and Micro Trak direct fluorescent antibody (DFA).[23] Advantages of these methods are lower cost, technical ease, and shorter development time. Disadvantages include a slightly decreased sensitivity as compared with culture, especially in low-prevalence populations. Whether a culture or nonculture technique is used, the objective of specimen collection is to obtain columnar epithelial cells from the endocervix. Specimen collection is with either an endocervical swab or brush and will be determined by which chlamydia test is being performed. To obtain the specimen, a swab or brush should be inserted 1 to 2 cm into the endocervical canal (once cervical secretions and exudate have been wiped from the os) and rotated several times against the wall of the endocervical canal.[23]

Patients with severe cervicitis, ulcerative cervicitis, or cervicitis with negative gonorrhea and chlamydia testing should be tested for HSV since this organism has been found in 10% to 20% of cases of cervicitis. In addition, *T. vaginalis* and *C. albicans* may cause an ectocervicitis, but they are typically associated with signs of vaginitis.

Proctitis

Proctitis is associated with receptive anal intercourse and may cause symptoms of anorectal pain, tenesmus, and rectal discharge. Diarrhea and abdominal cramps may be present but are not common in uncomplicated proctitis. Anoscopy or sigmoidoscopy examination reveals inflammation limited to the distal rectum. The evaluation of persons with symptoms of uncomplicated acute proctitis is described in Table 7. It should be emphasized that culture is the preferred method for detecting *C. trachomatis* in rectal specimens because nonculture methods have low specificity from this site.[23]

Urethritis

Symptoms from inflammation of the urethra may include dysuria, urethral itching, or mucoid to purulent urethral discharge. This STD syndrome occurs in both male and female adolescents, al-

TABLE 7.
Evaluation of Proctitis*

Organisms	Laboratory Tests	Diagnosis
Neisseria gonorrhoeae† *Chlamydia trachomatis*† (including LGV‡ serovars) Herpes simplex virus† *Treponema pallidum*	Perform anoscopy and obtain specimens for Culture for *N. gonorrhoeae* Culture for *C. trachomatis* HSV testing Gram stain Evaluate for *T. pallidum*	If anorectal pus or if polymorphonuclear leukocytes on Gram-stained smear of anorectal secretions, may empirically treat for *N. gonorrhoeae* and *C. trachomatis* while awaiting test results Definitive diagnosis should be made on the basis of organism-specific test results

*Data from Centers for Disease Control and Prevention: *MMWR* 42(RR-14):1–102, 1993.
†Most common organisms.
‡LGV = lymphogranuloma venereum.

though the evaluation differs and will therefore be treated separately.

Evaluation of sexually active female adolescents with symptoms of urethritis should include analysis of a midstream clean-catch urine specimen as well as evaluation for vaginitis and cervicitis (Table 8).

Urethral symptoms in male adolescents are most commonly caused by *N. gonorrhoeae*, *C. trachomatis*, or *Ureaplasma urealyticum*. Evaluation includes examination of a Gram-stained urethral smear, urethral culture for *N. gonorrhoeae*, and urethral testing for *C. trachomatis*.[44] Although EIA and DFA testing for chlamydia in first-voided urine is available, the urethra currently remains the preferred site for chlamydia testing in symptomatic male patients.[3, 23, 52] Urethral specimens for chlamydia testing are best obtained by gently inserting the urogenital swab 2 to 4 cm into the urethra and rotating in one direction for several revolutions.[23] Testing for *U. urealyticum* is not routinely available.

Based on Gram-stain results, a presumptive diagnosis of gonococcal or nongonococcal urethritis (NGU) can usually be made during the initial clinic visit in male patients with symptomatic urethritis (see Table 8). Although immediate treatment of symptomatic male patients with urethritis may be based on presumptive diagnoses, confirmatory organism-specific testing for gonorrhea and chlamydia should be performed in most clinical settings.[3] Empirical treatment of NGU is directed at *C. trachomatis*, which will also eradicate *U. urealyticum* (see Table 10). If patients do not respond to initial treatment for NGU, a wet mount examination for *T. vaginalis* and culture of an intraurethral swab specimen for *T. vaginalis* and HSV should be performed.[3]

Genital Ulcers

The symptoms caused by genital ulcers and the characteristics of ulcers found on examination vary widely.[62] The spectrum of clini cal manifestations of sexually transmitted genital ulcer syndromes

TABLE 8.
Evaluation of Urethritis*

Organisms	Laboratory Tests	Diagnosis
Neisseria gonorrhoeae† *Chlamydia trachomatis*† *Ureaplasma urealyticum*† *Trichomonas vaginalis* Herpes simplex virus Uncharacterized	Female Obtain urine specimen for UA‡ Consider urethral specimens for *N. gonorrhoeae* and *C. trachomatis* testing if bacterial UTI is not suspected or confirmed. However, because of the low sensitivity of urethral testing, endocervical testing for *N. gonorrhoeae* and *C. trachomatis* must also be performed	Female If pyuria and bacteriuria present, further evaluate for bacterial UTI‡ If STD‡ urethritis suspected Evaluate for vaginitis (Table 5) Evaluate for cervicitis (Table 6) If no evidence of vaginitis or clinically detectable cervicitis, consider empirical treatment for presumptive diagnosis of *C. trachomatis* while awaiting endocervical test results

Male Obtain urethral exudate§ or intraurethral swab specimen for Gram stain Culture for *N. gonorrhoeae* Test for *C. trachomatis*	Male A presumptive diagnosis of gonococcal urethritis can be made if typical gram-negative intracellular diplococci are found on a Gram-stained smear of urethral exudate A presumptive diagnosis of NGU‡ can be made if ≥5 polymorphonuclear leukocytes per oil immersion suggestive of *N. gonorrhoeae* are identified If treatment is initiated based on a presumptive diagnosis, it must include therapy for both *N. gonorrhoeae* and *C. trachomatis*

*Data from Centers for Disease Control and Prevention: *MMWR* 42(RR-14):1–102, 1993; Holmes KK, Mardh PA, Sterling PF, et al: *Sexually Transmitted Diseases*, ed 2. New York, McGraw-Hill, 1990.
†Most common organisms.
‡UA = urinalysis; UTI = urinary tract infection; STD = sexually transmitted disease; NGU = nongonococcal urethritis.
§If exudate is not visible, it may be expressed by "milking" or stripping the urethra by applying pressure from the proximal bulbous urethra toward the meatus.

is such that even experienced clinicians fail to achieve a correct clinical diagnosis in many cases.[63] To make the diagnosis even more complex, 3% to 10% of patients with genital ulcers may be infected with more than one organism.[3] For these reasons, diagnosis based on history and examination alone is often inaccurate and specific testing is necessary (Table 9). Even with complete testing, at least 25% of patients with genital ulcer syndromes have no laboratory-confirmed diagnosis.[3]

All patients with genital ulcers should be evaluated with at least a serologic test for syphilis[3]; most experts also recommend culturing for HSV. The most common cause of genital ulcers in the United States is HSV, although *H. ducreyi* and *T. pallidum* are also common in many areas of this country.[1, 3, 9] Because of the clinical difficulty in differentiating causes of ulcers and excluding coinfection, specific testing for HSV is recommended even when a pa-

TABLE 9.
Genital Ulcers*

Organisms	Laboratory Tests	Diagnosis
Herpes simplex virus† HSV type 1 HSV type 2 *Treponema pallidum*† *Haemophilus ducreyi*† *Chlamydia trachomatis* serovars L1, L2, L3 (lymphogranuloma venereum from *C. trachomatis* is a rare cause of genital ulcers in the United States)	Use of the following tests may be influenced by test availability and clinical or epidemiologic suspicion: Darkfield examination or direct immunofluorescence of ulcer exudate for *T. pallidum* Culture or antigen test for HSV Culture for *H. ducreyi* All patients should have serologic testing for *T. pallidum*. A nontreponemal test should be obtained, and if positive, a treponemal test should be performed	HSV SDx‡:multiple painful or itching ulcers and associated vesicles; may have a history of past episodes if recurrent HSV; may have consitutional symptoms and inguinal lymphadenopathy PDx: typical lesions and multinucleated giant cells on Tzanck smear of lesion scrapings DDx: detection of HSV by culture or nonculture test of vesicular fluid or lesion scraping Primary Syphilis SDx: lesion typical of chancre (usually 1 painless, sharply demarcated, indurated ulcer) and sexual contact with person known to have syphilis PDx: if typical chancre and either (1) reactive nontreponemal test (which is confirmed by a treponemal test) in a patient without a history of syphilis or (2) at least a fourfold increase in

	Nontreponemal tests VDRL (Venereal Disease Research Laboratory) RPR (rapid plasma reagin card test) Treponemal tests FTA-ABS (fluorescent treponemal antibody adsorbed) MHA-TP (microhemagglutination assay for antibody to *T. pallidum*)	titer on a quantitative nontreponemal test in a patient with a history of syphilis and a reactive treponemal test DDx: *T. pallidum* identified from a chancre or aspirate of regional lymph node by either darkfield microscopy or direct fluoroscopy antibody test
Chancroid		SDx: painful ulcers (typically multiple soft excavated ulcers with violaceous, undermined borders, and purulent, hemorrhagic secretions) with tender inguinal adenopathy (suppurative adenopathy is almost pathognomonic) PDx: 1 or more painful ulcers and (1) no evidence of *T. pallidum* by darkfield examination of exudate or by serologic test for syphilis done at least 10 days after onset of the ulcer and (2) ulcers are atypical for HSV or HSV testing negative DDx: *H. ducreyi* in culture

*Data from references 3, 44, and 62.
†Most common organisms.
‡SDx = suggestive diagnosis; PDx = presumptive diagnosis; DDx = definitive diagnosis.

TABLE 10.
Recommended Treatment Regimens for Uncomplicated Infections*

Organism	Treatment	Management Considerations†
Bacterial vaginosis	Metronidazole, 500 mg po bid × 7 days *or* Clindamycin, 2% cream 5 g intravaginally qhs × 7 days *or* Metronidazole, 0.75% gel 5 g intravaginally bid × 5 days	Avoid alcohol with metronidazole Metronidazole contraindicated during first trimester of pregnancy, during which time intravaginal clindamycin is the preferred treatment‡ No partner treatment
Candida albicans	Multiple intravaginal formulations are available and recommended (e.g., clotrimazole 1% cream 5 g intravaginally for 7–14 days, or terconazole 0.8% cream 5 g intravaginally for 3 days)	No partner treatment
Trichomonas vaginalis	Metronidazole, 2 g po × 1 dose	Avoid alcohol Metronidazole contraindicated during first trimester of pregnancy Treat partner(s)

Chlamydia trachomatis	*Urethritis or cervicitis* Doxycycline, 100 mg po bid × 7 days *or* Azithromycin, 1 g po × 1 dose *Proctitis* Doxycycline, 100 mg po bid × 7 days	Doxycycline contraindicated during pregnancy Safety and efficacy of azithromycin during pregnancy not established *Ureaplasma urealyticum* also eradicated If repeat testing performed, must be 3 wks after treatment Partner(s) should be evaluated and treated
Neisseria gonorrhoeae	Ceftriaxone, 125 mg IM × 1 dose *or* Cefixime, 400 mg po × 1 dose *or* Ciprofloxacin, 500 mg po × 1 dose *or* Ofloxacin, 400 mg po × 1 dose *plus* treatment for possible *C. trachomatis* If pharyngeal infection is a concern, ceftriaxone or ciprofloxacin should be used	Quinolones should not be used during pregnancy Partner(s) should be evaluated and treated for both, *N. gonorrhoeae* and *C. trachomatis*
Herpes simplex virus	*Genital ulcers* First episode: acyclovir, 200 mg po 5 times a day for 7–10 days or until clinical resolution Recurrent episodes: usually no treatment Suppressive therapy: acyclovir, 400 mg po bid *Proctitis* Acyclovir, 400 mg po 5 times a day for 10 days or until clinical resolution	The safety of systemic acyclovir during pregnancy has not been established Discuss the natural history of HSV infection and risk of neonatal HSV infection Partner(s) may benefit from evaluation and counseling

(continued)

TABLE 10 (continued).

Haemophilus ducreyi	Azithromycin, 1 g po × 1 dose *or* Ceftriaxone, 250 mg IM × 1 dose *or* Erythromycin base, 500 mg po qid × 7 days	Safety and efficacy of azithromycin during pregnancy not established Partner(s) with contact within 10 days of onset of symptoms should be evaluated and treated, even if asymptomatic
Treponema pallidum	*Primary, secondary, and early latent syphilis* Benzathine penicillin G, 2.4 million units IM × 1 dose *Late latent syphilis or latent syphilis of unknown duration* Benzathine penicillin G, 7.2 million units total, administered as 3 doses of 2.4 million units IM each at 1-wk intervals *Neurosyphilis* 12–24 million units of aqueous crystalline penicillin G daily given as 2–4 million units IV q4h for 10–14 days	Re-evaluate at 3 and 6 mo (clinically and by serology) to assess treatment response Partner(s) exposed within preceding 90 days: evaluate and presumptively treat. If partner(s) exposed >90 days: evaluate and treat based on test results, although presumptively treat if delay in serologic tests or compliance with follow-up is uncertain

Human papillomavirus	*External genital/perianal warts* Cryotherapy with liquid nitrogen or cryoprobe *or* Podophyllin, 10%–25% in a compound of tincture of benzoin applied to warts weekly *or* Trichloroacetic acid, 80%–90% applied to warts weekly *or* Electrodesiccation or electrocautery *or* Podofilox, 0.5% solution for self-treatment (apply to warts bid for 3 days, followed by 4 days of no therapy, and may be repeated for 4 cycles) (Caution should be used with home treatment in adolescents)	Podophyllin is contraindicated during pregnancy Annual Papanicolaou smear Refer if vaginal, cervical, or anal lesions Refer if warts refractory to treatment Examination of partner(s) recommended

*From Centers for Disease Control and Prevention: *MMWR* 42(RR-14):1–102, 1993.

†All adolescents in whom one STD has been diagnosed should be evaluated for other STDs, including gonorrhea, chlamydia, syphilis, and HPV. HIV testing should be recommended.

Among patients with diagnoses of syphilis or chancroid who have an initial HIV test that is negative, the CDC recommends repeat HIV testing in 3 months.

‡Alternative regimens and guidelines for treatment in special circumstances such as pregnancy or HIV infection may be found in reference 3.

tient has the typical symptoms and signs of HSV infection. Certainly, specific testing for HSV is indicated when clinical signs and symptoms are atypical.

If primary syphilis is suspected, an immediate definitive diagnosis should be sought by direct examination of the ulcer exudate for *T. pallidum*. If no organism is found or direct testing for *T. pallidum* is not available, the diagnosis can be determined by serology. Although a nontreponemal test is the initial screening test recommended, this test may be nonreactive if the ulcer has been present for less than 10 days (70% to 75% sensitivity) and should be repeated at least 10 days after the ulcer appeared in patients in whom the index of suspicion for syphilis is high and direct examination for *T. pallidum* has not been diagnostic.[3, 44]

The ability to make a definitive diagnosis of chancroid is compromised by the lack of commercially available testing for *H. ducreyi*. Even with the use of organism-specific culture media in optimal settings, the sensitivity is no higher than 80% and is usually lower.[3] When chancroid is suspected for clinical or epidemiologic reasons (e.g., clinical evidence suggestive, known presence of *H. ducreyi* infection in the community, or partner with a high risk of *H. ducreyi* infection), the threshold for making a presumptive diagnosis of chancroid and empirically treating should be low.

All patients with genital ulcers should be seen in follow-up for assessment of the clinical course and response to treatment. If the patient fails to respond to initial therapy, then organism-specific testing for HSV, *T. pallidum* (by direct examination of ulcer exudate and serology), and *H. ducreyi* must be performed. Empirical treatment for chancroid should be considered in this situation.

Exophytic Lesions

Exophytic genital lesions are usually asymptomatic. Although minor symptoms and discomfort are occasionally reported, most are cosmetic complaints. The differential diagnoses include HPV-related lesions such as condyloma acuminata, condyloma lata associated with secondary syphilis, and molluscum contagiosum. Condyloma acuminata lesions usually appear as painless exophytic growths located in the anogenital area and may involve the perineum, penis, urethra, vagina, cervix, anus, or perianal area. When on squamous epithelium, these lesions often have the appearance of a polyploid mass with a keratotic, fissured, and irregular surface. When located on mucosal surfaces, these lesions often appear soft, pink, and sessile.[11] Other HPV-related lesions such as flat condyloma may be present in conjunction with condyloma acuminata, but they usually require the application of acetic acid and colposcopy for visualization. Since HPV infections, particularly those of the cervix, are associated with the development of dysplasia and malignancy, all adolescents with genital warts require cervical cytology at the time of diagnosis. Since cytology has known limitations in sensitivity and specificity, some experts suggest that colposcopic evaluation be performed in addition to cytology and that colposcopy or cytology be repeated every 3 months in these patients.[64] If no abnormalities are found on cervical cytology, these patients should minimally receive annual Papanicolaou smears (as is recommended for all sexually active females). The presence of atypical genital lesions or cervical cytology suggestive of dysplasia (low- or high-grade squamous intraepithelial lesion [SIL] or its equivalent) should result in referral for appropriate evaluation and management that includes colposcopy and biopsy. Management of patients with cervical cytology revealing atypical cells of undetermined significance remains controversial. However, most suggest that cytology should be repeated in 3 to 4 months. Persistent abnormalities or progression is an indication for referral.

Molluscum contagiosum lesions, which are caused by a poxvirus, can usually be presumptively diagnosed by their typical appearance of smooth, spherical papules with umbilicated centers. Condyloma lata lesions of secondary syphilis are usually moist papules in the anogenital region and can be diagnosed by identification of *T. pallidum* in the lesions or syphilis serology consistent with infection. A description of the signs and symptoms of secondary syphilis are beyond the scope of this review but can be found elsewhere.[25]

MANAGEMENT OF SEXUALLY TRANSMITTED DISEASES

Treatment

Although treatment based on the results of organism-specific testing is preferred in adolescents, in certain circumstances treatment may be prescribed empirically for a presumptive diagnosis, i.e., when symptoms and signs suggestive of STDs are present. These treatment decisions are influenced by the likelihood of infection and the impact of withholding treatment until a more definitive diagnosis is made. Assessment of the likelihood of infection is determined by a combination of clinical evidence of disease and risk of infection. Risk of infection is related to the prevalence of infection within the community as well as risk-associated sexual behaviors. Adolescents who practice risky sexual behaviors within a community with high rates of STDs are more likely to be treated empirically based on presumptive diagnoses, especially if the likelihood of the patient returning for treatment after test results are known is low. It is emphasized that organism-specific tests should be obtained even when adolescents are empirically treated in order to confirm the presumptive diagnoses.

All patients in whom one STD has been diagnosed and treated should be evaluated for the presence of other STDs, including screening for *N. gonorrhoeae*, *C. trachomatis*, and *T. pallidum*, as well as consideration of HIV testing. The presence of genital ulcers has been associated with an increased risk of HIV infection, and therefore HIV testing should be particularly considered in all adolescents with genital ulcers, especially those with syphilis or chancroid.[3]

Treatment of most patients with vaginitis is based on a definitive diagnosis and started at the initial clinical visit. Therapy for BV, trichomoniasis, and candidiasis is outlined in Table 10. Although multiple treatment options exist for candidiasis therapy, preference should be given to preparations that are not oil based and therefore do not weaken condoms or diaphragms. Strong consideration should be given to the use of 3-day treatment regimens for candidiasis to enhance compliance.

Neisseria gonorrhoeae and *C. trachomatis* are the most common sexually transmitted organisms associated with cervicitis, urethritis, and proctitis. All patients who are given presumptive or definitive diagnoses of *N. gonorrhoeae*–related syndromes should receive treatment for both *N. gonorrhoeae* and *C. trachomatis* since coinfection is common (occurs in up to 50% cases of cervicitis and 30% of male gonococcal urethritis) and the sensitivity of available chlamydia tests is insufficient to exclude the presence of infection (see Table 10).[23] Azithromycin may be the preferred regimen for adolescents with chlamydial urethritis and cervicitis because of improved compliance associated with single-dose therapy. However, it is not currently recommended for the treatment of proctitis.[3]

Initiation of treatment of genital ulcers is often based on suspected diagnoses (see Table 10). If genital HSV is suspected, an attempt should be made to assess whether this is an initial HSV episode or a recurrent episode based on the clinical history. Acyclovir treatment shortens the duration and decreases the severity of signs and symptoms during initial HSV episodes. However, treatment of the initial episode does not eradicate latent infection or influence recurrences of HSV symptoms. Acyclovir is not usually recommended for recurrent HSV symptoms in most immunocompetent patients.[3] In patients with frequently recurring HSV symptoms, suppressive therapy may be helpful since it reduces the frequency of recurrences by at least 75% among patients with six or more episodes per year. Suppression therapy should be discontinued after 9 to 12 months to assess patients' rate of recurrent episodes. It is recommended that empirical treatment for *H. ducreyi* be initiated when a presumptive or suggestive diagnosis of chancroid is made because of the insensitive tests currently available for identification of this organism (see Table 9).[3] Fluctuant lymphadenopathy associated with *H. ducreyi* may require needle aspiration, even with effective antimicrobial therapy.[3] All patients with ulcerative disease, whether treated or not, should be re-examined within 3 to 7 days of initiation of therapy to document improvement and within 3 weeks to document complete resolution.

Treatment for infection with *T. pallidum* varies depending on the stage and extent of disease (see Table 10). Patients with latent infection of unknown duration (no previously documented serology) should be managed as though they have late latent syphilis.[3] Neurosyphilis can occur during any stage of syphilis. If symptoms or signs of neurologic or ophthalmic disease are present, the patient must have an evaluation for neurosyphilis (including cerebrospinal fluid [CSF] analysis for VDRL or rapid plasma reagin [RPR]) and syphilitic eye disease (including ocular slit-lamp evaluation).

The current rationale for treatment of visible genital warts includes (1) amelioration of signs and symptoms, (2) reduction of the risk of wart proliferation and friability, and (3) potential reduction of the risk of transmission of HPV infection. However, spontaneous clearance of clinical lesions without treatment occurs in 20% to 30% of patients within 3 months, and the recurrence rates of treated lesions are at least 25% within 3 months. In addition, no pharmacologic therapy has been shown to effectively eradicate HPV.[3] Therefore, many suggest that treatment is optional and decisions should be guided by patient preference. Multiple regimens exist for treatment of HPV warts at specific sites and usually require 6 to 8 weeks of therapy (see Table 10). Although external genital and perianal warts may be treated by primary care clinicians, management of vaginal, cervical, and rectal warts should occur in consultation with an expert. Patients with abnormal cervical cytology should be referred for evaluation and treatment.

Partner Notification and Treatment

Control of diseases transmitted by sexual activity requires that the sexual partners of infected patients be referred for evaluation regardless of symptoms. The time periods designated as the exposure interval for partner notification guidelines are somewhat arbitrary and differ according to the type of STD.[3] For *N. gonorrhoeae* and *C. trachomatis*, all partners of symptomatic patients should be evaluated and treated if their last sexual contact with the patient was within 30 days of the onset of symptoms. If the patient is asymptomatic, all partners who have had sexual contact with the patient within the past 60 days should be evaluated and treated. If the patient's last sexual intercourse preceded these time intervals, the most recent partner should be treated.[3] Exposure interval guidelines developed by the Centers for Disease Control and Prevention (CDC) for use in partner notification for other STDs can be found in Table 10.

Notification of partners can be done by either the patient or the health department staff. It is the clinician's responsibility to assist in this process. If the adolescent prefers to notify the partner(s), instructions regarding notification should be explicit and supplemented with written materials. The clinician should assess the adolescent's plan of action and assist with problem solving if indicated. If the adolescent is unwilling or unable to notify partners, the clinician should offer assistance with notification or refer the case to a local or state health department. The privacy of patients is protected during all partner notifications performed by health departments, and patients may prefer this because of the advantage of confidentiality. Special guidelines apply to partner notification regarding HIV infection and can be found in the CDC "1993 Sexually Transmitted Diseases Treatment Guidelines."[3]

Partners of adolescents in whom an STD has been diagnosed should be evaluated for the disease of known exposure as well as for other STDs and receive appropriate counseling. If effective therapy exists for the infection(s) of known exposure, partners should be treated with medication before the results of specific testing are available. This is important to prevent wider transmission of infection as well as prevent reinfection of an index case.

Public Health Notification Responsibilities

Sexually transmitted diseases, HIV infection, and AIDS cases should be reported in accordance with local statutory requirements and in a timely manner. Syphilis, gonorrhea, and AIDS are reportable diseases in every state, and *Chlamydia* infection is reportable in most states.[1] Clinicians should become familiar with local STD reporting requirements, which are available from local health departments or state STD programs. Sexually transmitted disease and

HIV reports are confidential and in many jurisdictions are protected by statute from subpoena.[3]

Assessment of Treatment Efficacy

All adolescents in whom an STD has been diagnosed should be seen for a follow-up visit. In symptomatic patients the resolution of symptoms, compliance with medication, and partner treatment should be confirmed. Routine repeat testing to confirm treatment efficacy may not be indicated for uncomplicated STDs if recommended treatment regimens were prescribed, the patient was compliant with medication, all symptoms resolve, and there is no risk of reinfection. However, some experts believe that all adolescents should have repeat testing to document clearance of treatable STDs since rates of compliance with treatment and abstinence during treatment are often low. Repeat testing must be performed to document resolution of infection if alternative treatment regimens were used, medication compliance was suboptimal, symptoms persist, or there is any risk of reinfection. Repeat testing is always indicated after treatment for syphilis. The patient should be reexamined clinically and serologically (nontreponemal test titer) at 3 and 6 months to document the response to treatment. Repeat testing is also indicated after any treatment of complications of STD infections (e.g., PID).

COUNSELING

Primary Prevention Counseling

Counseling focused on prevention of acquisition of STDs in adolescents ultimately has the goal of influencing adolescent sexual behavior. Despite the need for better definition of effective strategies to optimally influence sexual behavior,[65] experts in health promotion do agree that communication of clear, consistent, and repetitive messages from multiple sources will be required.[66] Although adolescents receive information about STDs including HIV and AIDS through media, school, and community-wide programs, clinicians are in a unique position to reinforce these messages and assist the adolescent in translating prevention messages into decisions regarding personal sexual behavior. For clinical purposes, the focus of primary prevention counseling appropriate to adolescents includes the following:

1. Delay of sexual debut in virginal adolescents
2. Support for choice of abstinence in adolescents with a history of sexual intercourse
3. Education and encouragement of sexual behaviors associated

with little or no risk of STD acquisition in adolescents who choose to continue sexual activities (e.g., nonpenetrative sexual behaviors such as kissing, hugging, massage, self or partner masturbation)
4. Consistent and correct condom use in adolescents who choose to have oral, vaginal, and/or anal intercourse
5. Limiting the number of sexual partners

Adolescents who have not had sexual intercourse should receive reinforcement of their decision to delay sexual debut. A discussion regarding normal sexual development and anticipatory guidance regarding sexual feelings, partner relationships, choice of sexual behaviors, as well as STD and pregnancy prevention is also recommended. In a recent study of 16- to 18-year-old females, virginal adolescents perceived physicians as an appropriate source of counseling regarding issues such as partner relationships, decisions regarding sexual debut, and how to refuse sex.[67]

Adolescents with a history of sexual intercourse should receive counseling that includes discussions of responsible sexual decision making. Behaviors such as abstinence, nonpenetrative sexual activities, consistent condom use, and limiting the number of partners must be supported and reinforced. When behaviors associated with a risk of STD acquisition are identified, the adolescent must receive clear information about the risk of these behaviors, education regarding ways to decrease this risk, assistance with developing strategies to decrease risky sexual behaviors, and focused problem solving regarding anticipated barriers to implementation. Counseling regarding condom use should include condom demonstrations (preferably on a simulated model) and distribution of adequate, renewable supplies of condoms (Table 11). Risk-reduction counseling is strengthened by interactive dialogue with adolescents, which may be enhanced by role playing, health education games, audiovisual programs, and/or discussion of written materials. Return appointments are important to assess the effectiveness of counseling in reducing risk-associated behaviors and provide reinforcement for safer sexual practices. Depending on the clinical setting, this counseling may be performed by physicians, nurse practitioners, nurses, health educators, or social workers.

Secondary Prevention Counseling

Secondary prevention counseling refers to discussions with a patient in whom an STD has been diagnosed and is focused on ensuring compliance with treatment, prevention of transmission, and avoidance of reinfection. An adolescent may be particularly receptive to counseling when an STD has been diagnosed. Consequently, the opportunity to address issues related to the current infection, sexual decision making, and the need for risk reduction must not be missed.

Adolescents in whom a treatable STD is diagnosed should receive clear instructions regarding medications and education about the importance of medication compliance. Compliance is most likely enhanced by the use of single-dose or short-course therapies when these are an option. Adolescents should be advised to abstain from sexual activity until both they and their partners are cured. In the absence of a specific "test of cure," cure is assumed when medication is completed for both patient and partner(s) and all symptoms or signs have resolved.[3]

Patients with HSV should be advised that no effective cure for this infection is currently available. Additionally, they should be aware of the potential for recurrent HSV episodes and the risk of transmission during both symptomatic and asymptomatic periods. Patients should also be advised that the risk of transmission may be decreased by consistent condom use as well as abstinence dur-

TABLE 11.
Recommendations for Proper Condom Use*

Use a new latex condom with each act of intercourse
Carefully handle the condom to avoid damaging it with fingernails, teeth, or other sharp objects
Put condom on after the penis is erect and before any genital contact with the partner
Ensure that no air is trapped in the tip of the condom (e.g., by holding the tip of the condom when putting it on)
Ensure that there is adequate lubrication during intercourse, possibly requiring the use of exogenous lubricants
Use only water-based lubricants (e.g., K-Y Jelly or glycerine) with latex condoms
Oil-based lubricants (e.g., petroleum jelly, shortening, mineral oil, massage oils, body lotions, or cooking oil) may weaken the latex condom and should never be used
Hold the condom rim firmly against the base of the penis during withdrawal, and withdraw the penis when it is still erect to prevent slippage

*Data from Centers for Disease Control and Prevention: *MMWR* 42(RR-14):1–102, 1993.

ing recurrent episodes. It is important to discuss the risk of neonatal HSV infection with both male and female patients and recommend reporting this infection to clinicians providing prenatal care. Patients with HPV should be advised that experts believe that this infection may persist throughout life in a dormant or latent state in some individuals and that spontaneous reactivation of the virus may occur. The infectivity associated with latent states is unknown but presumed to be low. Consistent condom use must be encouraged in patients with HSV and HPV because viral shedding and sexual transmission may occur even when no visible lesions are present.[3]

Patients with HBV infection (acute and chronic) or HIV infection must be clearly informed that infection may be transmitted through sharing of needles during activities such as intravenous drug use, tattoos, body piercing, skin popping, or injecting steroids/hormones as well as through sexual contact.

Acquisition of any STD is an indication of risky behavior. Counseling focused on reduction of identified specific risk behavior should occur at the time of initial evaluation and diagnosis, as well as at follow-up visits.[68] The guidelines for this counseling are similar to those described for primary prevention counseling. However, in this situation it is clear that current behavior is placing the adolescent at risk of acquiring STDs. Once specific behaviors associated with a risk of infection have been identified, attention should be focused on perceived barriers to safer behaviors and ways to address these barriers. In addition to counseling about choices regarding abstinence or the number of partners, all discussions should include reinforcement of existing knowledge about condom use, problem solving regarding inconsistent condom use, and condom distribution to both female and male adolescents. If needle use is reported by the adolescent, counseling should address issues of substance use, needle sharing, and education on proper cleaning of needles.[14]

SUMMARY

Sexually transmitted diseases common in the adolescent population are associated with significant acute morbidity, complications, and long-term sequelae. Clinicians have the opportunity to play a unique and important role in the control of STD rates among adolescents. Not only are clinicians in a position to routinely discuss healthy sexual development, decision making, and primary STD prevention, they are also in a position to effectively diagnose and manage STDs among both asymptomatic and symptomatic adolescents. Addressing issues related to sexuality and STDs in a consistent and repetitive manner during routine visits will likely increase physician proficiency in this important area of clinical care of adolescents, as well as increase adolescents' recognition of the clinician as a valuable resource.

REFERENCES

1. Webster LA, Berman SM, Greenspan JR: Surveillance for gonorrhea and primary and secondary syphilis among adolescents—United States, 1981–1991, in CDC Surveillance Summaries, August 13, 1993. *MMWR* 42(SS-3):1–11, 1993.
2. Cates W Jr: The epidemiology and control of sexually transmitted diseases in adolescents, in Schydlower M, Shafer MA: *Adolescent Medicine: State of the Art Reviews: AIDS and Other Sexually Transmitted Diseases*. Philadelphia, Hanley & Belfus, 1990, pp 409–427.
3. Centers for Disease Control and Prevention: 1993 Sexually transmitted diseases treatment guidelines. *MMWR* 42(RR-14):1–102, 1993.
4. Washington AE, Katz P: Cost of and payment source for pelvic inflammatory disease: Trends and projections, 1983 through 2000. *JAMA* 266:2565–2569, 1991.
5. Boyer CB: Psychosocial, behavioral, and educational factors in preventing sexually transmitted diseases, in Schydlower M, Shafer MA: *Adolescent Medicine: State of the Art Reviews: AIDS and Other Sexually Transmitted Diseases*. Philadelphia, Hanley & Belfus, 1990, pp 597–613.
6. Centers for Disease Control and Prevention: HIV prevention practices of primary-case physicians—United States, 1992. *MMWR* 42:988–992, 1994.
7. Nussbaum MP, Shenker IR, Feldman JG: Attitudes versus performance in providing gynecologic care to adolescents by pediatricians. *J Adolesc Health Care* 10:203–208, 1989.
8. Schydlower M, Shafer MA: *Chlamydia trachomatis* infections in adolescents, in Schydlower M, Shafer MA: *Adolescent Medicine: State of the Art Reviews: AIDS and Other Sexually Transmitted Diseases* Philadelphia, Hanley & Belfus, 1990, pp 615–628.
9. Centers for Disease Control: Chancroid—United States, 1981–1990: Evidence for underreporting of cases, in CDC Surveillance Summaries, May 29, 1992. *MMWR* 42(SS-3):57–61, 1992.
10. Johnson RE, Nahmias AJ, Magder LS, et al: A seroepidemiologic survey of the prevalence of herpes simplex virus type 2 infection in the United States. *N Engl J Med* 321:7–12, 1989.
11. Ellen JM, Moscicki, AB, Shafer MA: Genital herpes simplex virus and human papillomavirus infection. *Adv Pediatr Infect Dis* 9:97–124, 1994.

12. Margolis HS, Alter MJ, Hadler SC: Hepatitis B: Evolving epidemiology and implications for control. *Semin Liver Dis* 11:84–92, 1991.
13. Centers for Disease Control and Prevention: *HIV/AIDS Surveillance Report* 5:1–19, 1993.
14. Kunins H, Hein K, Futterman D, et al: Guide to adolescent HIV/AIDS program development. *J Adolesc Health* 14(suppl 5):4–140, 1993.
15. Shafer MA: Sexually transmitted disease syndromes, in McAnarney ER, Kreipe RE, Orr DP, et al: *Textbook of Adolescent Medicine*. Philadelphia, WB Saunders, 1992, pp 696–710.
16. Siegel D, Golden E, Washington AE, et al: Prevalence and correlates of herpes simplex infections: The population-based AIDS in multiethnic neighborhoods study. *JAMA* 268:1702–1708, 1992.
17. Moscicki AB: Genital human papillomavirus infections, in Schydlower M, Shafer MA: *Adolescent Medicine: State of the Art Reviews: AIDS and Other Sexually Transmitted Diseases*. Philadelphia, Hanley & Belfus, 1990, pp 451–469.
18. Center for Disease Control and Prevention: Summary of notifiable diseases, United States, 1992. *MMWR* 41:1–12, 1992.
19. Burke DS, Brundage JF, Goldenbaum M, et al: Human immunodeficiency virus infections in teenagers. *JAMA* 263:2074–2077, 1990.
20. St Louis ME, Conway GA, Hayman CR, et al: Human immunodeficiency virus infection in disadvantaged adolescents: Findings from the US job corps. *JAMA* 266:2387–2391, 1991.
21. Stricof RL, Kennedy JT, Nattell TC, et al: IX. HIV seroprevalence in a facility for runaway and homeless adolescents: Findings from the US job corps. *JAMA* 266:2387–2391, 1991.
22. Toomey KE, Moran JS, Rafferty MP, et al: Epidemiological considerations of sexually transmitted diseases in underserved populations. *Infect Dis Clin North Am* 4:739–752, 1993.
23. Centers for Disease Control and Prevention: Recommendations for the prevention and management of *Chlamydia trachomatis* infections, 1993. *MMWR* 42(RR-12):1–39, 1993.
24. Centers for Disease Control and Prevention: 1993 Revised classification system for HIV infection and expanded surveillance case definition for AIDS among adolescents and adults. *MMWR* 41(RR-17):1–19, 1992.
25. Holmes KK, Mardh PA, Sparling PF, et al: *Sexually Transmitted Diseases*, ed 2. New York, McGraw-Hill, 1990.
26. Westrom L: Incidence, prevalence, and trends of acute pelvic inflammatory disease and its consequences in industrialized countries. *Am J Obstet Gynecol* 138:880–892, 1980.
27. Centers for Disease Control: Protection against viral hepatitis: Recommendations of the immunization practices advisory committee (ACIP). *MMWR* 39(S-2):1–26, 1990.
28. Muñoz N, Bosch FX, Shah KV, et al: *The epidemiology of human papillomavirus and cervical cancer*. Lyon, France, International Agency for Research on Cancer, 1992.

29. Moscicki AB, Broering J, Powell K, et al: Comparisons between colposcopic, cytologic, and histologic findings in women positive and negative for human papillomavirus DNA. *J Adolesc Health Care* 14:74–79, 1993.
30. Moscicki AB, Palefsky JM, Gonzales J, et al: Colposcopic and histologic findings and HPV DNA test variability in young women positive for HPV DNA. *J Infect Dis* 166:951–957, 1992.
31. American Medical Association: HIV early intervention, in *Physician Guidelines,* ed 2. Chicago, American Medical Association, 1994.
32. Center for Disease Control and Prevention: Selected behaviors that increase risk for HIV infection, other STDs, and unintended pregnancy among high school students—United States, 1991. *MMWR* 41:945–950, 1992.
33. Moscicki AB, Millstein SG, Broering J, et al: Risks of human immunodeficiency virus infection among adolescents attending three diverse clinics. *J Pediatr* 122:813–820, 1993.
34. Parra W, Drotman DP, Siegel K, et al: Patient counseling and behavior modification, in Holmes KK, Mardh PA, Sparling PF, et al: *Sexually Transmitted Diseases,* ed 2. New York, McGraw-Hill, 1990, pp 1057–1068.
35. Ostrow, OG: Homosexual behavior and sexually transmitted diseases, in Holmes KK, Mardh PA, Sparling PF, et al: *Sexually Transmitted Diseases,* ed 2. New York, McGraw-Hill, 1990, pp 61–69.
36. Stratton P, Alexander NJ: Prevention of sexually transmitted infections: Physical and chemical barrier methods. *Infect Dis Clin North Am* 7:841–859, 1993.
37. Hingson RW, Strunin L, Berlin BM, et al: Beliefs about AIDS, use of alcohol and drugs, and unprotected sex among Massachusetts adolescents. *Am J Public Health* 80:295–299, 1990.
38. Moscicki AB, Winkler B, Irwin CE, et al: Differences in biologic maturation, sexual behavior, and sexually transmitted disease between adolescents with and without cervical intraepithelial neoplasia. *J Pediatr* 115:487–493, 1989.
39. Igra V, Millstein SG: *Physician attitudes towards delivering STD and HIV-related preventive services to teens.* Presented at The Society for Adolescent Medicine Conference, Los Angeles, March 1994.
40. American Academy of Pediatrics: *Guidelines for Health Supervision II.* Elk Grove Village, Ill, American Academy of Pediatrics, 1988.
41. Council on Scientific Affairs, American Medical Association: Confidential health services for adolescents. *JAMA* 269:1420–1424, 1993.
42. Elster AB, Kuznets NJ: *AMA Guidelines for Adolescent Preventive Services (GAPS): Recommendations and Rationale.* Baltimore, Williams & Wilkins, 1994.
43. Stamm WE, Koutsky LA, Benedetti JK, et al: Chlamydia trachomatis urethral infections in men: Prevalence, risk factors, and clinical manifestations. *Ann Intern Med* 100:47–51, 1984.

44. Centers for Disease Control: *Sexually Transmitted Diseases: Clinical Practice Guidelines, May 1991*. Atlanta, US Department of Health and Human Services, 1991.
45. Silber TJ, Niland NF: The clinical spectrum of syphilis in adolescence. *J Adolesc Health Care* 5:112–116, 1984.
46. Schachter J, Stoner E, Moncada J: Screening for chlamydial infections in women attending family planning clinics: Evaluation of presumptive indicators for therapy. *West J Med* 138:375–379, 1983.
47. Mertz GJ: Epidemiology of genital herpes infections. *Infect Dis Clin North Am* 7:825–839, 1993.
48. Koutsky LA, Stevens CE, Holmes KK, et al: Underdiagnosis of genital herpes by current clinical and viral-isolation procedures. *N Engl J Med* 326:1533–1539, 1992.
49. Pantaleo G, Graziosi C, Fauci AS: Mechanisms of disease: The immunopathogenesis of human immunodeficiency virus infection. *N Engl J Med* 328:327–335, 1993.
50. Centers for Disease Control and Prevention: Projections of the number of persons diagnosed with AIDS and the number of immunosuppressed HIV-infected persons, United States, 1992–1994. *MMWR* 41(RR-18):1–29, 1992.
51. Remafedi R: Sexually transmitted diseases in homosexual youth, in Schydlower M, Shafer MA: *Adolescent Medicine: State of the Art Reviews: AIDS and Other Sexually Transmitted Diseases*. Philadelphia, Hanley & Belfus, 1990, pp 565–581.
52. Shafer MA, Schachter J, Moncada J, et al: Evaluation of urine-based screening strategies to detect *Chlamydia trachomatis* among sexually active asymptomatic young males. *JAMA* 270:2065–2070, 1993.
53. Centers for Disease Control and Prevention: Recommendations for HIV testing services for inpatients and outpatients in acute-care hospital settings; and technical guidance on HIV counseling. *MMWR* 42(RR-2):11–17, 1993.
54. Centers for Disease Control: Hepatitis B virus: A comprehensive strategy for eliminating transmission in the United States through universal childhood vaccination: Recommendations of the immunization practices advisory committee (ACIP). *MMWR* 40(RR-13):1–25, 1991.
55. American Academy of Pediatrics Committee on Infectious Diseases: Universal hepatitis B immunization. *Pediatrics* 89:795–800, 1992.
56. Wilson MD, Joffe A: Step-by-step through the pelvic exam. *Cont Pediatr* 5:92–104, 1988.
57. Kapphahn C, Schlossberger N: Male reproductive health: Part 1, in *Adolesc Health Update*, vol 4., Elk Grove Village, Ill, American Academy of Pediatrics 1992, pp 1–8.
58. Gilchrist MJR, Rauh JL: Office microscopic examination for sexually transmitted diseases: A tool to lower costs. *J Adolesc Health Care* 6:311–320, 1985.
59. Schachter J: Office and laboratory testing for STDs: Present and fu-

ture, in Schydlower M, Shafer MA: *Adolescent Medicine: State of the Art Reviews: AIDS and Other Sexually Transmitted Diseases.* Philadelphia, Hanley & Belfus, 1990, pp 583–595.

60. Thomas DL, Quinn TC: Serologic testing for sexually transmitted diseases. *Infect Dis Clin North Am* 7:793–824, 1993.
61. Moscicki AB, Shafer MA, Millstein SG, et al: The use and limitations of endocervical Gram stains and mucopurulent cervicitis as predictors for *Chlamydia trachomatis* in female adolescents. *Am J Obstet Gynecol* 157:65–71, 1987.
62. Piot P, Plummer FA: Genital ulcer adenopathy syndrome, in Holmes KK, Mardh PA, Sparling PF, et al: *Sexually Transmitted Diseases,* ed 2. New York, McGraw-Hill, 1990, pp 711–716.
63. Dangor Y, Ballard RC, Exposto FL, et al: Accuracy of clinical diagnosis of genital ulcer disease. *Sex Transm Dis* 17:184–189, 1990.
64. Moscicki AB, Palefsky JM, Gonzales J, et al: The association between human papillomavirus deoxyribonucleic acid status and the results of cytologic rescreening tests in young, sexually active women. *Am J Obstet Gynecol* 165:67–71, 1991.
65. Aral SO, Peterman TA: Defining behavioral methods to prevent sexually transmitted diseases through intervention research. *Infect Dis Clin North Am* 7:861–873, 1993.
66. Millstein SG, Petersen AC, Nightingale EO (eds): *Promoting the Health of Adolescents: New Directions for the Twenty-First Century.* New York, Oxford University, 1993.
67. Ford CA, Millstein SG, Irwin CE Jr: *Discussing sexual relationships: Virginal adolescents' perceptions of the physician's role* (abstract). *Pediatr Res* 35:5A, 1994.
68. Stiffman AR, Earls F: Behavioral risks for human immunodeficiency virus infection in adolescent medical patients. *Pediatrics* 85:303–310, 1990.

Antibiotic Allergy in Children

Nevin W. Wilson, M.D.
West Virginia University, Department of Pediatrics, Section of Allergy and Immunology, Robert S. Byrd Health Science Center, Morgantown, West Virginia

Adverse reactions to antibiotics are a common and serious complication in pediatric practice. An adverse reaction may be defined as any unwanted response that occurs at an appropriate dose of an agent during or following a course of therapy. An adverse reaction may be due to a pharmacologic or an immunologic mechanism. A variety of pharmacologic mechanisms may produce an adverse reaction. Intolerance is an excessive response to a normal drug dose. Side effects are known, unavoidable, and undesirable effects of a drug. Idiosyncratic reactions are reactions unrelated to the known pharmacologic properties of the drug. Adverse reactions caused by proven or suspected immunologic mechanisms are referred to as allergic reactions.

The approach to an infected child with a history of allergic reactions to one or more antibiotics is often far from clear. Many patients who claim to be allergic to an antibiotic will not react when challenged. This may be due to the patient or the patient's family confusing a side effect of the drug, toxicity from an overdose of the drug, or a drug interaction with an allergy. Some infections caused by viruses may produce apparent urticarial rashes that may be blamed on coincident antibiotic therapy.[1] Unfortunately, some allergic reactions can lead to devastating consequences such as anaphylaxis or toxic epidermal necrolysis. The risk of this occurring, although small, usually precludes future use of the antibiotic in those with a history that suggests a possible allergy.

All too often, these medications have been repeatedly prescribed to children with antibiotic allergies for inappropriate conditions such as viral upper respiratory infections. Many parents have come to expect and demand antibiotics for such infections; however, if an allergic reaction prevents appropriate use of the antibiotic at some future time when a serious bacterial infection threatens the child, then that child has been done a significant disservice. Education of both parents and physicians concerning the appropriate use of antibiotics would greatly decrease the incidence of antibiotic allergy.

It is important to realize that most of what is known about antibiotic allergy is from studies of penicillin. Much less is known about the immunochemistry of cephalosporin allergy and almost nothing about allergy to the non–β-lactam antibiotics. It is misleading and dangerous to extrapolate what is known about penicillin to the other antibiotics.

This chapter reviews the immunologic mechanisms of antibiotic allergy and discusses the methods of diagnosis and management of patients with likely antibiotic allergy. Special problems such as antibiotic allergy in patients with cystic fibrosis and those infected with human immunodeficiency virus (HIV) will be considered.

INCIDENCE AND CLASSIFICATION OF ANTIBIOTIC ALLERGY

Complete information on the incidence of allergic reactions to antibiotics is not available. The numbers available probably represent an underestimation inasmuch as many reactions go unrecognized. Estimates of the overall chance of any allergic reaction during a course of β-lactam therapy have ranged from 1% to 10%,[2] with more recent estimates around 1% to 2% for penicillin and 2% to 3% for cephalosporins.[3]

Earlier literature estimated that penicillin caused about 400 to 800 deaths per year.[4] More recent information suggests a much lower death rate. Between 1964 and 1983, only 22 deaths were attributed to penicillin allergy in the United Kingdom.[5] In 1981, 16 deaths were attributed to penicillin in the United States.[6] This decrease probably reflects various factors, including underreporting of deaths and the fact that penicillin was contaminated with haptenated biological conjugates 20 years ago.[7] In addition, these preparations have been largely replaced in the United States by various cephalosporins.

Antibiotic allergies may be categorized by the Gell and Coombs classification or as to the time of onset.[8, 9] Under the Gell and Coombs classification, type I reactions are IgE mediated, type II are cytotoxic antibody mediated, type III are immune complex mediated, and type IV are mediated by sensitized lymphocytes. Classification of antibiotic allergies according to the time of onset divides reactions into immediate, accelerated, and delayed. Table 1 outlines the classification of antibiotic allergy.

TABLE 1.
Classification of Antibiotic Allergy

Allergic Reaction	Mechanism
Immediate allergic Reactions (<1 hr)	
Urticaria	Type I
Angioedema	
Acute asthma	
Laryngeal edema	
Vomiting and diarrhea	
Anaphylatic shock	
Accelerated reactions (1–72 hr)	
Urticaria	Type I
Pruritus	
Acute asthma	
Angioedema	
Nonurticarial, maculopapular skin rashes	Type III?, type IV?
Late reactions (>72 hr)	
Serum sickness–like reactions	Type III
Urticaria	Type I, type III
Vasculitis	Type III
Erythema multiforme	
Stevens-Johnson syndrome	Type IV?
Toxic epidermal necrolysis	
Autoimmune hemolytic anemia	Type II
Autoimmune neutropenia	
Autoimmune thrombocytopenia	
Acute interstitial nephritis	Type II?, type IV?
Pulmonary infiltrates with eosinophilia	?

IMMEDIATE ALLERGIC REACTIONS

Immediate reactions to antibiotics include urticaria, angioedema, and anaphylaxis. These reactions occur within 60 minutes of administration of the antibiotic and are responsible for much of the morbidity and mortality of antibiotic allergy.

Immediate allergic reactions are due to type I hypersensitivity and occur because specific IgE antibodies on the surface of mast cells and basophils interact with the antibiotic causing the cells to release mediators such as histamine. These mediators cause vasodilatation and subsequent hypotension and tissue edema. Anaphylaxis, shock, bronchospasm, laryngeal edema, rhinitis, urticaria, angioedema, as well as gastrointestinal symptoms such as nausea, vomiting, and cramping may occur alone or in various combinations.

Anaphylactic reactions to penicillin occur at a frequency of 0.04%[10] and are much less common with third-generation cephalosporins. Although anaphylactic reactions occur primarily in adults, full anaphylaxis has been documented even in young infants.[11] It is clear, however, that true anaphylaxis to penicillin is a vary rare event in children less than 12 years of age.[12]

ACCELERATED REACTIONS

Reactions that occur between 1 and 72 hours after administration of the drug are classified as accelerated reactions. These are usually characterized by dermatitis. Many of these reactions are urticarial and represent type I reactions due to specific IgE. In addition to urticaria, pruritus, bronchospasm, or angioedema may occur. Death, however, is an extremely rare event.[8]

Nonurticarial skin rashes such as the typical maculopapular rashes may also occur during this period. These may occur as early as 24 hours after starting to take the antibiotic or as late as 28 days after administration. The maculopapular skin rash is probably the most common manifestation of antibiotic allergy and is very difficult to distinguish from a viral exanthem. This rash complicates 5% to 10% of ampicillin or amoxicillin courses[13, 14] as compared with about 2% to 3% for other β-lactam antibiotics.[15] Both a type III immune complex–mediated reaction and a type IV cell-mediated reaction have been suggested as the cause of maculopapular antibiotic rashes, but the actual mechanism is unknown.[3] Occasionally, continued administration can lead to generalized erythroderma and/or scaling.

LATE REACTIONS

Reactions that occur after 72 hours are known as late or delayed reactions. Although simple morbilliform or maculopapular skin rashes may appear, immune complex (type III)-mediated serum sickness–like reactions are the most common late reactions to antibiotics. In reactions to penicillin, antibodies of the IgG and IgM class are typically found, although IgE also may be present. These reactions are similar to classic serum sickness caused by foreign protein injection. Symptoms usually occur 7 days after the antibiotic is started and consist of fever, malaise, myalgia, arthralgia, arthritis, splenomegaly, and lymphadenopathy. Rashes may be either urticarial or maculopapular. Urticarial rashes may be due to IgE or may be complement mediated.[8] Renal abnormalities may follow deposition of immune complexes in the glomeruli. Penicillin, amoxicillin, cefaclor, cefalexin, and trimethoprim-sulfamethoxazole have all been associated with this type of reaction.[16]

Erythema multiforme caused by antibiotics also occurs during this period. With this skin disorder, lesions vary in size and shape and may resemble urticarial lesions. Classically, there is central clearing or even a central spot producing a target lesion. The lesions of erythema multiforme may become bullous. Systemic symptoms such as fever, malaise, arthralgia, and nausea also often occur. Stevens-Johnson syndrome is a bullous severe extension of this disorder involving the mucous membranes. Ocular injury may also occur. Both sulfa drugs and penicillins have been implicated in Stevens-Johnson syndrome. Toxic epidermal necrolysis is a severe and sometimes fatal variant of erythema multiforme and consists of extensive desquamation of the skin and mucous membranes.[17]

Autoimmune hemolytic anemia, neutropenia, or thrombocytopenia may occur during a course of antibiotic therapy. These responses are usually due to a type II, cytotoxic antibody–mediated mechanism. In most cases the antibiotic binds to the cell membrane and an IgG antibody directed against the antibiotic leads to cell destruction. A positive antiglobulin Coombs' test will develop in about 3% of patients receiving intravenous penicillin or a cephalosporin in large doses.[18, 19] The development of hemolytic anemia through this mechanism appears to be quite rare.[20] Neutropenia and leukopenia have long been attributed to certain antibiotics. The actual mechanism is unknown, and both immunologic and toxic mechanisms have been held responsible. An antineutrophil antibody capable of opsonizing normal neutrophils has been found in the serum of patients taking semisynthetic penicillins.[21] Drug-associated neutropenia appears to be both dose and time related. An incidence of neutropenia of 0.1% with a short course of penicillin or cephalosporin increases to 5% to 15% when high doses are given for longer than 10 days.[22]

Acute interstitial nephritis leading occasionally to renal failure has been associated with the use of methicillin and other penicillin analogues. Renal injury occurs most often in patients receiving the antibiotic for a prolonged period of time.[23] In addition to gross or microscopic hematuria, pyuria, and proteinuria, acute interstitial nephritis may be accompanied by fever, rash, arthralgias, and eosinophilia.[24, 25] As with many delayed reactions to antibiotics, the actual mechanism is uncertain. Both humoral and type IV cell-mediated mechanisms have been implicated in this disorder. The penicilloyl group has been found bound to the renal tubular basement membrane along with immunoglobulin and complement.[26, 27] Cell-mediated mechanisms have been implicated because of positive delayed-type hypersensitivity, skin test reactions in these patients,[26] and *in vitro* lymphocyte reactivity to methicillin.[25] Mononuclear infiltration is also usually found on renal biopsy.[28]

In general, all of the reactions described in this section can occur with any of the penicillins or cephalosporins. The newer penicillins such as the semisynthetic penicillins and the aminopenicillins as well as the newer third-generation cephalosporins tend to have much fewer reactions when compared with the older antibiotics, except for some antibiotics mentioned earlier in this section.[8] Table 2 lists the frequency of immediate hypersensitivity-like reactions to non–β-lactam antibiotics. Mechanisms are unknown for most of these reactions.

TABLE 2.
Immediate Hypersensitivity-like Reactions to non–β-Lactam Antimicrobial Drugs*

Frequent
Acedapsone
Clindamycin
Dapsone
Gentamicin
Isoniazid
Micronazole
Nitrofurantoin
Streptomycin
Sulfonamides
Trimethoprim-sulfamethoxazole
Occasional
Amantadine
Amikacin
p-Aminosalicylic acid
Chloramphenicol
Ethambutol
Ethionamide
Furazolidone
Griseofulvin

Ketoconazole
Lincomycin
Methenamine hippurate
Methisazone
Nalidixic acid
Nystatin
Rifampin
Trimethoprim

Rare

Amphotericin B
Capreomycin
Erythromycin
Kanamycin
Miconazole
Pentamidine†
Polymyxins
Tetracyclines
Trifluridine
Troleandomycin
Vancomycin

*Adapted from Sullivan TJ: *J Allergy Clin Immunol* 74:594, 1984.
†Possibly more common in HIV infection.

Adverse reactions to trimethoprim-sulfamethoxazole usually consist of skin lesions. The most common is toxic erythema, but other reactions such as erythema multiforme, Stevens-Johnson syndrome, and toxic epidermal necrolysis can occur.[29] Urticarial reactions appear to be very rare.[30] Acute interstitial nephritis has also been reported after trimethoprim-sulfamethoxazole administration.

Erythromycin and other macrolide antibiotics are among the least toxic antibiotics prescribed.[31] The rate of skin reactions to erythromycin ranges from 0.5% to 2.3%,[32] and both the maculopapular and urticarial types have been described. Anaphylaxis has been described but is very rare.[33]

Aminoglycosides such as gentamicin or tobramycin can on very rare occasions induce an IgE-mediated allergy, although the actual immunochemistry of such reactions is almost completely unknown.[34] Urticaria appears to be the main symptom. A type IV hypersensitivity contact dermatitis can also occur with topical use.[35]

RISK FACTORS

Although slightly controversial, it is generally accepted that being an atopic individual or having a family history of atopy does not put a person at higher risk for reacting to penicillin.[36] Most deaths from penicillin have occurred in patients with no previous history of allergy.[2] It is clear that a history of a reaction to another drug does put a patient at higher risk of reacting to an antibiotic. In one study, patients who have reacted to an unrelated drug were three times more likely to react to penicillin.[37] Conversely, patients allergic to the mold *Penicillium* are at no higher risk of allergy to penicillin.[38]

Allergic reactions may occur at any age but are most common between the ages of 20 and 49 years.[8] Depending on the study, both males and females have been found to be at higher risk for reacting to antibiotics.[39, 40] There is no relationship between HLA type and penicillin allergy, and race does not appear to be a factor.[41]

Parenteral administration appears to be a risk factor. The vast majority of reported deaths from penicillin reactions have followed intravenous infusion,[11] although deaths from oral administration have been reported.[42, 43] Whether this is due to a difference in dosage or some inherent dissimilarity in handling and absorption of antigen is unclear.[38]

It is generally thought that the cumulative exposure to antibiotics over time increases the risk of a reaction. Allergy to β-lactam or aminoglycoside antibiotics is a frequent problem in children with cystic fibrosis as a result of their frequent exposure to these drugs.[34] Allergic reactions to drugs, particularly trimethoprim-sulfamethoxazole, occur at a higher rate in individuals with HIV infection.[44] This increase in allergic reactions may in part be due to altered T-lymphocyte regulation of IgE synthesis.[45]

IMMUNOLOGY AND CROSS-REACTIVITY

Penicillin is a low–molecular-weight substance and by itself is not immunogenic. Its metabolic products, however, are haptens and must form multivalent drug-protein complexes to become immunogenic.

The basic structure of penicillins consists of a β-lactam ring bound to a thiazolidine ring to form the 6-aminopenicillanic acid nucleus (Fig 1). For cephalosporins, the β-lactam ring is joined to a dihydrothiazine ring to form the 7-aminocephalosporanic acid nucleus. Metabolism of penicillin occurs at the β-lactam ring, and about 95% of penicillin is metabolized to penicilloyl. This antigen

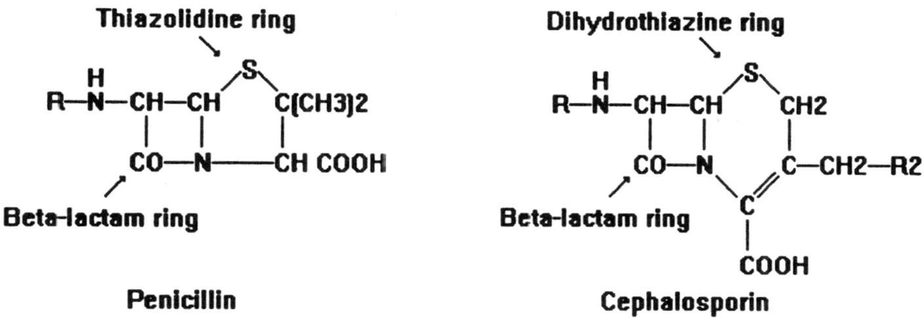

FIGURE 1.
Basic structure of penicillins and cephalosporins.

is responsible for the majority of accelerated IgE-mediated reactions to penicillin[8] and is generally referred to as the major determinant of penicillin.[9] The remainder is metabolized to penicilloate, penilloate, penicilloylamine, and other incompletely understood products. These degradation products are known collectively as the minor determinants. The minor determinants are responsible for the majority of cases of immediate IgE-mediated anaphylaxis and deaths. The structure of the major determinant and some of the minor determinants is shown in Figure 2. Similar antigens are probably formed from the β-lactam ring of other penicillin derivatives.[46] The cephalosporin major-determinant equivalent of penicilloyl, cephaloyl, may be formed in vitro,[47] although it not clear that minor-determinant equivalents exist in cephalosporin allergy.[48]

Cross-reactivity occurs between all members of the penicillin class,[49] although this cross-reactivity is clinically variable. Furthermore, it is apparent that allergic reactions may occur to one or more drugs of this class without reacting to all penicillins. Specific IgE antibody to the side chains of some of the semisynthetic penicillins has been identified,[50, 51] and patients in whom anaphylaxis has developed from amoxicillin but who can tolerate penicillin and cephalosporins have been described.[52] In general, if a person reports a history of an allergy to any of the penicillins, it should be assumed that they are allergic to all of the drugs in the penicillin class.[53]

The issue of cross-reactivity between cephalosporins and penicillins has been discussed since shortly after introduction of the cephalosporins. Cephalosporins share the β-lactam ring with the penicillins (see Fig 1); however, they also have different side chains that are potentially immunogenic. Animal anticephalosporin antibodies strongly cross-react with the penicilloyl group of penicillin.[54] In humans, similar *in vitro* cross-reactivity is well established.[18] Fortunately, *in vivo*, clinically relevant cross-reactivity is very low. Of 171 patients with a history of allergy to penicillin, 2 of 151 with negative penicillin skin test responses reacted to a cephalosporin whereas none with positive skin test responses reacted to challenge.[46] In a large study, 8.1% of patients with a history of penicillin allergy reacted to a cephalosporin as compared with 1.9% of non–penicillin-allergic patients.[55] Overall, the reaction rate to cephalosporins appears to be between 3% and 7% in patients with a positive history of penicillin allergy.[56] Second- and third-generation cephalosporins such as cefotaxime, ceftizoxime, ceftriaxone, ceftazidime, and cefixime are considerably less cross-reactive than earlier antibiotics of this class. The reasons for this are unclear, but it has been suggested that the bulky side chains on these antibiotics block access to the β-lactam ring.[57] Acute IgE-mediated anaphylaxis to cephalosporins is exceptionally rare as

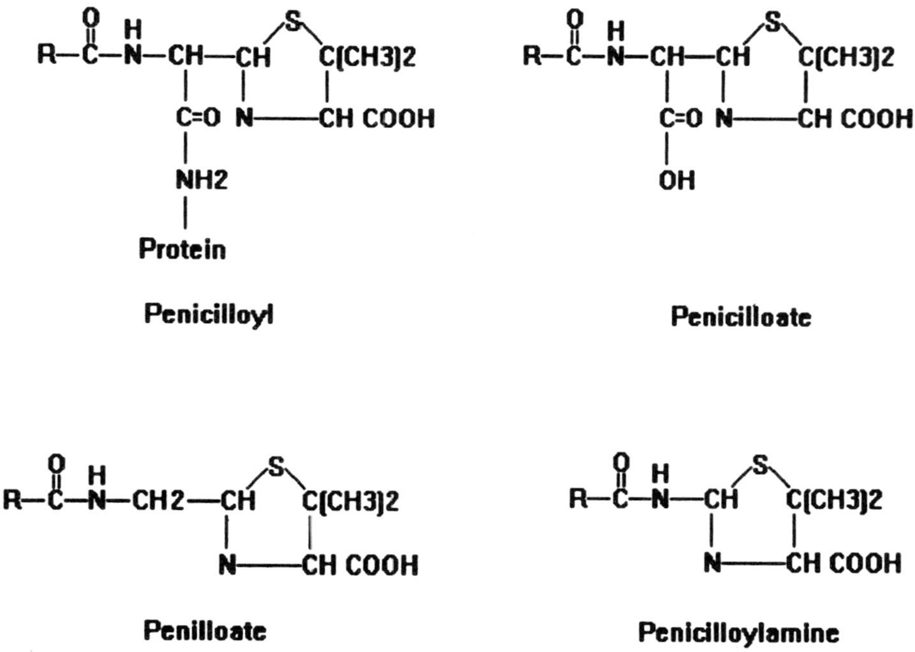

FIGURE 2.
Structure of the major and some of the minor determinants of penicillin.

compared with penicillins.[58] Allergy to cephalosporins without sensitivity to penicillin can occur but is also extremely rare.[59]

Aztreonam, a monobactam, appears to have no cross-reactivity with other cephalosporins or penicillin, which makes it suitable for use in penicillin-allergic patients.[60] The only available carbapenem, imipenem, however, is significantly cross-reactive with penicillins and should be used with extreme caution in penicillin-allergic patients.[61]

Cross-reactivity between structurally similar drugs in the aminoglycoside, sulfonamide, macrolide, and tetracycline groups is common[62] and usually precludes further use of any drugs in that group after a reaction to any of them.

DIAGNOSIS

HISTORY

Since diagnostic tests for evaluation of the majority of allergic reactions to antibiotics are either nonexistent or poorly specific, the most important clinical tool is a careful history.

This history should include a detailed description of all the clinical manifestations of the suspected antibiotic reaction. A detailed list should be compiled of all medications including prescription, nonprescription, and illicit drugs that were taken within a month of the suspected allergy. This list should include dosage, onset, route of administration, and duration of therapy for each of the medications. No drug should be considered harmless or incapable of causing the suspected reaction.

The exact temporal relationship between antibiotic administration and the symptoms should be obtained and a history of prior exposure sought for each medication. Such a history may not be available because of lack of recall or because the previous exposure was from an occult source. A history of concurrent illnesses is important because many apparent allergic reactions are due to infectious causes.

The impact of discontinuation or previous rechallenge, if performed, should be assessed. If the symptoms resolved shortly after use of the antibiotic was discontinued or resumed when the drug was restarted, this would strongly suggest that the antibiotic is the cause, and this history is usually sufficient for clinical purposes. Suppressive medications such as antihistamines or steroids could significantly mask the true nature of a reaction.

After this history has been obtained, any available physical findings such as rashes, angioedema, or wheezing should be included in the analysis. The final analysis should lead to a complete characterization of the reaction, along with a classification of the probable immunologic mechanism.

If the clinical manifestations of the reaction subside shortly after treatment with the antibiotic is discontinued, they are consistent with a known immunologic mechanism, and no other explanation is found, then for most clinical situations, a diagnosis of antibiotic allergy can be made, and the antibiotic should be avoided in the future. However, direct rechallenge with a test dose remains the only absolute method of confirming a causal relationship between most antibiotics and clinical symptoms.[8]

IMMUNOLOGIC TESTING FOR ANTIBIOTIC ALLERGY

Direct rechallenge involves the potential risk of a serious or even fatal reaction. Thus a variety of *in vivo* and *in vitro* tests have been developed to attempt confirmation of the diagnosis of antibiotic allergy. Most antibiotics are relatively simple substances and are not immunogenic themselves, but are metabolized and attached to carrier proteins that are antigenic. Therefore studies that use the drug itself are often not testing the real antigens responsible for the reaction.

Although *in vivo* and *in vitro* tests have been developed for a variety of different antibiotics, reliable data about their usefulness and predictive value are lacking for almost every antibiotic except for *in vivo* testing with penicillin and its metabolites.

In Vivo Tests

Immediate hypersensitivity skin tests involve the placement of small amounts of antigen on or under the skin to cause mediator release by mast cells sensitized by specific IgE on the surface of the cells. The mediator released is primarily histamine and causes a wheal-and-flair response that is easily read in 15 to 20 minutes. The triggering of the mast cells requires cross-linking of two IgE molecules on the surface of the cell by a multivalent antigen—an antigen having two or more determinants per molecule. This is why most drugs by themselves do not trigger a response but must become multivalent after conjugating with proteins or polymerizing. Immediate skin testing is only useful for those reactions that are due to type I, IgE-mediated mechanisms. This technique has no role in diagnosing type II, III, or IV antibiotic reactions.

Only after a careful history has established the likelihood of an IgE-mediated reaction due to an antibiotic and there is a rational, current indication for using that particular antibiotic should skin testing be considered. Testing should not be done to satisfy the patient's curiosity.

It has generally been thought that skin testing should be done only immediately before starting antibiotic therapy to avoid sensitization from the skin test itself. Mendelson[63] has recently suggested that elective skin testing should be used in children since children have a higher rate of losing penicillin allergy and a lower rate of severe anaphylactic reactions. In his protocol, appropriately selected children are skin-tested when they are well and not in need of antibiotics. If the skin tests are negative, they are challenged orally with up to 400,000 units of penicillin and then dosed for 10 days. To avoid missing the small number of children who might be resensitized during this time, they repeated the skin tests 4 weeks after the oral course of antibiotics was completed. Children who do not react during this protocol should not be labeled as penicillin allergic and are at no higher risk than children with no previous history of penicillin allergy. Further research will determine whether this becomes a standard for evaluating penicillin allergy in children. Use of this type of protocol will remain limited until minor-determinant mixtures become more generally available.

For successful skin testing, certain precautions are necessary. The patient must not be taking any antihistamines for at least 72 hours. Long-acting antihistamines such as astemazole, clemastine, or tricyclic antidepressants such as doxepin may interfere with skin testing for as long as 4 to 6 weeks. There must be an adequate area of skin on the arms or back that is free from rashes or scars. Dermatographism invalidates the skin test response. Positive and negative controls using histamine and saline are required. Although skin testing is a very safe procedure, equipment and facilities for treating a systemic reaction should be available. Systemic reactions during skin testing can occur,[64] but only a few deaths have been reported.[12, 65]

For evaluation of IgE-mediated allergy to penicillin, skin testing is the most rapid and sensitive method available. A variety of studies have validated the role of penicillin skin tests. In one of the earliest studies, 16,000 patients were evaluated for penicillin allergy; 40% of those with a positive history had positive skin test responses vs. 6% of those with a negative history.[66] In a cooperative study of the American Academy of Allergy,[36] 3,000 subjects were evaluated, and 3% of patients with a positive history for penicillin allergy and negative skin test responses to the major determinant of penicillin and penicillin G reacted when challenged. Using both the major and minor determinants, Sullivan et al.[67] skin-tested 740 patients with a history of penicillin allergy, and 466 reacted. Of those with negative skin tests who were challenged, only 2.4% reacted, and these reactions were delayed and mild. In a more recent study, Sogn et al.[68] evaluated 1,326 adults with skin tests to both the major- and minor-determinant penicillin derivatives. Of the 726 history-positive patients, 566 had negative skin test responses, and when challenged, only 7 had possibly IgE-mediated reactions. Among the 600 history-negative patients, 568 received penicillin and none had a reaction. Nine of the 167 positive skin test reactors received a penicillin by incremental challenge and 2 reacted.

The use of penicillin skin testing in children with both the major and minor determinants was examined by Chandra et al.[69] In this study, 48 of 300 children with histories of penicillin allergy were skin test–positive; 11 reacted to only the minor determinant. Fifty-six of the skin test–negative children were challenged, and only two had minor skin rashes.

Fresh penicillin G is probably the most important minor determinant, and skin testing with it and the commercially available major determinant (penicilloyl-polylysine, Pre-Pen, Kremers-Urban Co., Milwaukee) will detect the majority but not all penicillin-allergic patients. Estimates of the reactivity to minor determinants such as penilloate, penicilloate, and penicillamine alone range from 1% to 17%.[3] In the recent study by Sogn et al.,[68] 16% of the 167 patients with positive skin tests reacted to only the minor determinants. Fifty percent of these did not react to fresh penicillin G. Unfortunately, the minor determinants are not commercially available for skin testing. Minor-determinant mixtures can be made from published protocols.[10, 70] Substitution of 2-week-old penicillin G for the minor-determinant mixture has been recommended but may not contain adequate amounts of some minor determinants.[69] For the most part, skin testing with the benzylpenicillin major and minor determinants has been found to be predictive of reactions to the semisynthetic penicillins.[10, 46, 68] However, Silviu-Dan et al.[50] studied 112 patients with a history of allergic reactions to one of the penicillins who were skin-tested with minor-determinant mixtures of ampicillin, amoxicillin, and cloxacillin in addition to the minor and major determinants of penicillin. Of the 21 patients who reacted to the skin tests, 10 reacted only to the semisynthetic reagents.

The technique of penicillin skin testing is relatively straightforward. Reagents should include the major determinant

TABLE 3.
Skin Testing for Penicillin Allergy*

Test†	Negative Control (Buffered Saline Solution) Concentration	Positive Control (Histamine) Concentration	Benzylpenicilloyl-Polylysine (PRE-PEN) Concentration	Penicillin G (Fresh) Concentration‡	Minor Determinant Mixture (If Available) Concentration‡
Prick Skin Test (1 Drop)	N/A	1 mg/mL	6.0×10^{-5}M	10,000 units/mL	10,000 units/mL
Intradermal (0.02 mL)	N/A	0.1 mg/mL	6.0×10^{-5}M	10,000 units/mL	10,000 units/mL

*Adapted from Erffmeyer JE: *Pediatr Asthma Allergy Immunol* 6:243–253, 1992.
†Skin tests are performed on the volar surface of the forearm. Prick skin tests are performed first and interpreted 15 minutes after performance. If prick tests are negative, perform intradermal tests.
‡Usually, patients can be skin-tested safely with single-strength reagents. If a patient is thought to be especially sensitive or has experienced an anaphylactic reaction within the past 12 months, skin tests should be performed with serially diluted weaker concentrations first before proceeding with more concentrated dilutions, e.g., initially 10 units/mL or 100 units/mL if negative, followed by 1,000 units/mL or 10,000 units/mL if negative.

penicilloyl-polylysine, the minor-determinant mixture, and fresh penicillin G at a concentration of 10,000 units/mL. In those patients with a history that suggests anaphylaxis, skin tests should first be performed with diluted reagents (1:100) and the prick-puncture method. Controls should include histamine (1 mg/mL) and saline. If no response is seen after 15 minutes, then full-strength reagents should be applied, again using the prick-puncture method. If these are also negative, then intradermal skin tests are used with a 27-gauge needle. A small 0.02-mL injection of the reagents is used starting at a concentration of 100 units/mL and ending at 10,000 units/mL. A reaction is considered positive if the wheal is 4 to 5 mm with a flair present after 15 minutes.[3] If the history involves a semisynthetic penicillin or if that antibiotic is being considered for therapy, some authors will include skin tests for that particular antibiotic.[46] Skin testing for penicillin is outlined in Table 3. Before beginning the skin tests it is essential that parents completely understand the reasons for doing the skin tests and the risks and shortcomings of this diagnostic technique. Written informed consent is advisable.

Skin testing to other antibiotics is problematic because so little information is available and in many cases the actual antigens are unknown or unavailable. Some authors have recommended adding the preferred cephalosporin diluted to 3 mg/mL to the standard penicillin skin test battery.[71] In one report,[34] a patient with urticaria was found to have a positive skin test response to tobramycin intradermally whereas no response was noted in nonallergic volunteers. Skin testing with the major haptenic determinant of sulfamethoxazole, N^4-sulfamidoyl, remains experimental.[72]

Under certain circumstances, skin testing to non–β-lactam antibiotics may still be of value even though we know little about their immunochemistry. In some cases, the hapten may combine at the site with a carrier protein and trigger an IgE-mediated response. If the test response is positive, it can be concluded that the patient is at risk for a reaction if the antibiotic is administered. If it is negative, then no conclusions can be made. When skin testing is to be done with nonpenicillin antibiotics, in addition to the standard controls the drug should also be injected into normal control individuals to rule out irritant reactions resulting from the direct release of histamine or too high a concentration of drug.

In Vitro Tests

There are occasions when it is impossible to skin-test an individual with a history of a possible IgE-mediated reaction because of the ingestion of antihistamines or overwhelming skin disease. For these occasions an in vitro test would be very valuable. A radioallergosorbent test (RAST) for the major (penicilloyl) determinant was developed in 1971[73] and is commercially available. The RAST usually correlates with skin testing to penicilloyl-polylysine; however, it is less sensitive.[8] A RAST for the minor determinants of penicillin has been developed experimentally[74] but has not come into general use.[75] Testing for only the major determinant will miss some patients with penicillin allergy who have antibody to the minor determinants and in whom anaphylaxis could potentially develop. Radioallergosorbent tests for some of the cephalosporins are also available commercially. A RAST to N^4-sulfamidoyl, the major determinant of sulfamethoxazole, has also been developed. IgE specific to N^4-sulfamidoyl was found in sera from eight of ten patients with histories of urticarial reactions to sulfamethoxazole.[76]

MANAGEMENT

Immediate discontinuation of use of the suspected antibiotic is the most important part of management of most suspected antibiotic allergies. If anti-infective therapy is required, then one should switch to an antibiotic with similar therapeutic actions but no cross-reactivity. This is particularly true for immediate and accelerated IgE-mediated reactions as well as for hemolytic anemia, neutropenia, interstitial nephritis, erythema multiforme, Stevens-Johnson syndrome, and toxic epidermal necrolysis.[77] Patients should be warned that they cannot take the class of antibiotic that caused the suspected reaction without an evaluation first.

The decision to withdraw the antibiotic, however, should only be made after evaluating the immunologic classification, the intensity of the reaction, its probable outcome, its likely response to treatment, and alternative antibiotics available. In some cases such as a non–IgE-mediated, maculopapular ampicillin rash, continuation of the antibiotic, if necessary, will not lead to further deleterious responses.[78] A child in whom mild urticaria without other symptoms develops during the course of β-lactam antibiotic treatment for an infection without an alternative therapy may be cautiously continued on that antibiotic regimen in some cases.[79] The symptoms can be treated with antihistamines alone or in combination with corticosteroids. Reintroduction of an antibiotic may sometimes be more difficult than continuing the drug with suppressive therapy.

Acute symptoms such as anaphylaxis, asthma, urticaria, or angioedema should be treated according to standard clinical recommendations. For dermatologic reactions, symptomatic relief with antihistamines such as hydroxyzine is usually adequate, although corticosteroids may be required. In addition, aspirin may be useful for serum sickness–like reactions.

Patients with a history of penicillin allergy who have negative skin test reactions may receive the antibiotic cautiously if there are no other alternatives. Although no penicillin-induced anaphylaxis has been reported in skin test–negative individuals, there is a 1% chance of an accelerated urticarial reaction and about a 3% chance of other reactions.[8] It is prudent to give a small test dose (less than 5 mg) of the desired drug by the chosen route and then observe for at least an hour before administering the full therapeutic dose. These patients should be warned that despite receiving a full course of a β-lactam antibiotic, skin testing should be performed before future exposure to the antibiotic. Parker et al.[80] found that 16% of patients with histories of penicillin allergy were skin test–positive 1 to 12 months after successfully receiving β-lactam antibiotics while hospitalized.

When the minor-determinant mixture is not available for skin testing and the patient has negative skin tests to fresh penicillin and penicilloyl-polylysine, even more caution is indicated. Under these circumstances, an incremental challenge[81] should be used. With this technique, a very small dose (usually 1% of the final dose) is given via the appropriate route. If the reported reaction is severe, the initial dose may have to be diluted up to 1,000-fold. The dosage is increased in small 2-fold to 10-fold increments over a period of hours to days until the therapeutic dose is achieved. If a reaction develops, then a decision should be made as to discontinuing use of the antibiotic or proceeding with desensitization.

Patients with positive skin test responses for penicillin should be told that penicillins should not be given to them in the future without repeat skin testing. Recommendations for wearing a medical identification bracelet stating that they are allergic to penicillin should be made.

DESENSITIZATION

If the patient has positive skin test reactions to penicillin and has a life-threatening infection that requires a β-lactam antibiotic, then desensitization is required. Desensitization should be done with the particular antibiotic required to optimally treat the infection. Desensitization should only be done in an intensive care setting with emergency equipment immediately available. A physician familiar with the procedure and knowledgeable in treating anaphylaxis should supervise. The administration of β-adrenergic medications must be discontinued. If the patient has asthma, it should be under optimal control. Written informed consent is mandatory. Desensitization should be considered controlled anaphylaxis since about 30% of patients will experience allergic symptoms during the procedure.[82] Prophylactic use of antihistamines, β-adrenergic drugs, and corticosteroids is not recommended because it does not protect against anaphylaxis and may mask early symptoms that would provide warning of an impending crisis. These drugs may be used to treat symptoms once they are present.

The mechanism of antibiotic desensitization remains unclear. Levels of circulating antipenicillin IgE antibody do not change during the process,[83] but sometimes patients lose their skin test reactivity, thus suggesting that the penicillin has consumed or blocked the IgE antibody. The process is followed by a marked increase in penicillin-specific IgG antibody. It has been suggested that slow incremental increases in dose allow gradual attachment of the molecules to the IgE on the surface of the mast cells and basophils and result in the gradual release of histamine and other mediators rather than the massive release that triggers anaphylaxis.[53] Antigen-specific desensitization of tissue mast cells with loss of skin test reactivity to β-lactam antibiotics but not to other environmental antigens has been reported.[84] Of interest is that basophil histamine release *in vitro* is unaffected by desensitization.[85]

Oral, parenteral, and subcutaneous desensitization to penicillin has been used successfully. Oral desensitization is arguably safer because reactions after oral ingestion are in general less severe and far fewer deaths have been reported after oral administration. Stark et al.[82] reported 93 cases of oral desensitization with no fatal or life-threatening reactions. Others have advocated parenteral desensitization even when oral forms of the antibiotic are available because of the higher degree of control over the rate and concentration of the drug administered.[86] During subcutaneous desensitization, a reaction may be treated by placing a tourniquet on the extremity proximal to the injection site and infiltrating epinephrine locally to slow systemic absorption of the antibiotic.[53]

The basic technique of desensitization is to start with a dose that is about one ten-thousandth of a therapeutic dose and gradually administer increasing doses over a period of hours until therapeutic dosages are reached. A protocol[87] for oral desensitization is shown in Table 4. In this protocol the dose is doubled every 15 minutes. Mild reactions require the same dose to be repeated until it is tolerated without reaction. Severe reactions may require that the next dose be withheld until the symptoms are under control and then be decreased to at least one third of the dose that caused the reaction. If the patient has positive prick-puncture skin test responses or a significant reaction to less than full-strength intradermal skin tests, then lower starting doses are used.[88]

A protocol[87] for parenteral desensitization is shown in Table 5. Again, if the prick-puncture skin tests were positive, then starting at a dose as low as 0.005 mg may be required.

During the 2 to 3 days after the procedure, the patient must be followed carefully since a variety of allergic responses may occur, most of which are dermatologic in nature and transient. Hemolytic anemia, serum sickness–like reactions, and nephritis have been reported after desensitization.[82] Only one case of fatal laryngeal

TABLE 4.
Protocol for Oral Desensitization of β-Lactam Antibiotic–Allergic Patients*†

Step	β-Lactam drug (mg/mL)	Amount (mL)	Dose Given‡ (mg)	Cumulative Dose (mg)
1	0.5	0.1	.05	.05
2	0.5	0.2	.10	.15
3	0.5	0.4	.20	.35
4	0.5	0.8	.40	.75
5	0.5	1.6	.80	1.55
6	0.5	3.2	1.60	3.15
7	0.5	6.4	3.20	6.35
8	5.0	1.2	6.00	12.35
9	5.0	2.4	12.00	24.35
10	5.0	4.8	24.00	48.35
11	50.0	1.0	50.00	98.35
12	50.0	2.0	100.00	198.35
13	50.0	4.0	200.00	398.35
14	50.0	8.0	400.00	798.35
15	Observe the patient for 30 minutes and then administer 1 g of the same agent intravenously.			

*Adapted from Sullivan TJ: *Allergy Principles and Practice*, ed 4. St Louis, Mosby, 1993.
†Interval between doses: 15 minutes.
‡Drug suspension diluted in 30 mL of water for ingestion.

TABLE 5.
Protocol for Parenteral Desensitization of β-Lactam Antibiotic–Allergic Patients*†

Step	β-Lactam Drug (mg/mL)	Amount (mL)	Dose Given‡ (mg)	Cumulative Dose (mg)
1	0.1	0.1	0.01	0.01
2	0.1	0.2	0.02	0.03
3	0.1	0.4	0.04	0.07
4	0.1	0.8	0.08	0.15
5	1.0	0.16	0.10	0.31
6	1.0	0.32	0.32	0.63
7	1.0	0.64	0.64	1.27
8	10	0.12	1.20	2.47
9	10	0.24	2.40	4.87
10	10	0.48	4.80	10
11	100	0.10	10	20
12	100	0.20	20	40
13	100	0.40	40	80
14	100	0.80	80	160
15	1,000	0.16	160	320
16	1,000	0.32	320	640
17	1,000	0.64	640	1,280
18	Observe the patient for 30 minutes and then administer 1 g of the same agent intravenously			

*Adapted from Sullivan TJ: *Allergy Principles and Practice*, ed 4. St Louis, Mosby, 1993.
†Interval between doses: 15 minutes.
‡Dose administered subcutaneously (or intramuscularly or intravenously).

edema has been reported in this period.[89] If treatment with the antibiotic is discontinued for more than 2 days, then the patient is no longer desensitized and must have the procedure repeated if antibiotics are resumed.

Successful desensitization has also been achieved for some non–β-lactam antibiotics such as tobramycin[34] and trimethoprim-sulfamethoxazole.[90]

PROGNOSIS

For many patients, antibiotic allergy is a transient problem. Several studies have shown that only about 10% to 15% of patients with a history of penicillin allergy are still allergic when skin-tested. Probably many of the reactions that these patients and their physicians attribute to penicillin were actually caused by intercurrent viral infections. Many patients with true IgE-mediated allergy lose their reactivity over time. Of patients with a positive skin test response to penicillin, up to 80% percent will no longer be allergic 10 years later.[91] Children are even more likely to lose their reactivity over time.[92]

SPECIAL PROBLEMS

CYSTIC FIBROSIS

Pseudomonas aeruginosa is responsible for chronic lung infections in children with cystic fibrosis, and antipseudomonal antibiotics are widely used to treat these infections. Children with cystic fibrosis receive a much greater cumulative exposure to multiple, high-dose, intravenously administered courses of β-lactam and non–β-lactam antipseudomonal antibiotics. In addition, they have a higher rate of allergy in general.[93] Because of this, allergy to the semisynthetic penicillins is relatively common. An immediate allergic reaction during an infusion developed in 11% of patients with cystic fibrosis in a 1-year period.[94]

Because of the frequency of allergic reactions in this population, attempts to desensitize them have been common. Several papers have documented successful desensitization to both β-lactam antibiotics[94, 95] and aminoglycosides,[34] although patients with cystic fibrosis appear to be more difficult to desensitize. After acute desensitization, oral penicillin twice daily may sustain a chronic desensitized state between courses of higher-dose intravenous therapy.[82, 96] Moss et al.[94] reported that in six patients with cystic fibrosis who underwent sustained desensitization, two had a recrudescence of allergic symptoms and two had repeated allergic reactions on intravenous challenge. These authors recommend that patients with cystic fibrosis be desensitized on each admission requiring intravenous antibiotics.

HUMAN IMMUNODEFICIENCY VIRUS INFECTION

Antibiotic allergy was one of the first allergic symptoms of HIV infection described and remains the most common and significant allergic manifestation. In 1983, Mitsuyasu et al.[97] found that 69% of HIV-infected patients receiving trimethoprim-sulfamethoxazole for *Pneumocystis carinii* infection had cutaneous reactions as compared with 2.2% of controls. Pentamidine has been associated with reactions in about 20% of HIV-infected patients.[98] Allergy to a variety of other antimicrobial agents including ampicillin, amoxicillin–clavulanic acid, dapsone, sulfadiazine, and isoniazid has been shown to be more common in HIV-infected individuals.[99] For the most part, these reactions consist of fever and morbilliform reactions occurring 7 to 12 days after the start of therapy. The rash is usually erythematous, maculopapular, and pruritic—consistent with a non–IgE-mediated mechanism. Repeat exposure may lead to much more rapid and severe reactions such as Stevens-Johnson syndrome. Interestingly, IgE-mediated reactions such as anaphylaxis do not appear at increased frequency.

Why there is not more obviously IgE-mediated antibiotic allergy in these patients is unclear. Atopic diseases are associated with progressive HIV infection.[100] Atopic dermatitis is seen in up to 50% of children with HIV,[101] and asthma is found in 31% of HIV-infected adults.[102] Altered T-lymphocyte regulation of IgE and polyclonal B-cell activation appears to increase serum IgE levels with progressing disease.[103]

Although some HIV-infected patients will have positive skin test responses to these antibiotics, for the most part skin tests or *in vitro* testing is not useful. Under these circumstances, if an antibiotic is absolutely essential, then an incremental challenge[81] should be used. Challenge should not be attempted if there is a history of exfoliative dermatitis or Stevens-Johnson syndrome. Should any dermatitis appear, then the indications for using the drug should be reviewed and use of the drug discontinued or the patient desensitized. Patients with HIV infection have been successfully desensitized to trimethoprim-sulfamethoxazole, pentamidine, and sulfadiazine,[104] although in some cases long-term prednisone is required.

MULTIPLE ANTIBIOTIC ALLERGIES

Patients with allergic reactions to more than one class of antibiotic represent a difficult management challenge. Kamada et al.[105] reported on 120 children with histories of reactions to more than one class of antibiotic. Of the 337 adverse reactions reported in these children, 186 were due to β-lactam antibiotics. Eighty-six were due to sulfonamides and 32 to macrolides. Reactions to tetracyclines, vancomycin, and aminoglycosides were also reported. Twenty-two patients had reactions to three classes of antibiotics. Reactions were both of the immediate IgE-mediated type and also due to other mechanisms such as serum sickness–like reactions, erythema multiforme, Stevens-Johnson syndrome, and hepatitis. Twenty-six of 78 children who were skin-tested to penicillin had positive reactions. In adults, Sullivan et al.[106] reported that of 312 adults with penicillin allergy, 21% reacted to a second antibiotic and 7% to three or more classes of antibiotic.

The reasons for multiple antibiotic allergy remain unknown. Since many of these reactions are apparently due to non–IgE-mediated mechanisms, a genetic predisposition to make specific IgE cannot be an underlying cause. With the wide variety of different antibiotics reported to cause reactions, a genetic propensity to react to specific antigens would also not appear to be a likely explanation.

Children with allergy to more than one class of antibiotic would be the most appropriate initial candidates for elective penicillin skin testing with protocols such as those proposed by Mendelson.[63]

REFERENCES

1. Anderson JA: *Allergic Diseases of Infancy, Childhood and Adolescence*. Philadelphia, WB Saunders, 1980, p 690.
2. VanArsdel PP: Allergic reactions to penicillin. *JAMA* 191:172, 1965.
3. Shepherd GM: Allergy to β-lactam antibiotics. *Immunol Allergy Clin North Am* 11:611–633, 1992.
4. Valentine M: Allergic emergencies, in *NIAID Task Force Report: Asthma and Other Allergic Diseases*, Department of Health Education and Welfare, Public Health Service, NIH Publication 79–387, May 1979, p 501.
5. Beeley L: Allergy to penicillin. *BMJ* 288:511, 1984.
6. Berkelman RL, Finton RJ, Elsea WR: Beta adrenergic antagonists and fatal anaphylactic reactions to oral penicillin. *Ann Intern Med* 104:134, 1986.
7. Ahlstedt S: Penicillin allergy—can the incidence be reduced? *Allergy* 39:151, 1984.
8. Deswarte, RD: Drug allergy, In Patterson R: *Allergic Diseases*. Philadelphia, JB Lippincott, 1993, p 395.
9. Levine BB: Immunologic mechanisms of penicillin allergy. A haptenic model system for the study of allergic diseases of man. *N Engl J Med* 275:1115, 1966.
10. Levine BB, Zolov DM: Prediction of penicillin allergy by immunological tests. *J Allergy Clin Immunol* 43:231, 1969.
11. Matheson A, Elegant L: Penicillin reactions in children. A study of the value of the skin test in penicillin sensitization. *J Allergy* 26:425, 1955.
12. Idsoe O, Guithe T, Wilcox RR, et al: Nature and extent of penicillin side reactions, with particular reference to fatalities from anaphylactic shock. *Bull World Health Organ* 38:159, 1968.
13. Croydon EAP, Wheeler AW, Grimshaw JJ, et al: Collaborative study group: Prospective study of ampicillin rash. *BMJ* 1:7, 1973.

14. Kerns DL, Shira JE, Go S, et al: Ampicillin rash in children: Relationship to penicillin allergy, and mononucleosis. *Am J Dis Child* 125:187, 1973.
15. Shapiro S, Stone D, Siskind D, et al: Drug rash with ampicillin and other penicillins. *Lancet* 2:969–972, 1969.
16. Platt R, Dreis M, Kennedy D, et al: Serum sickness–like reactions to amoxicillin, cefaclor, cefalexin, and trimethoprim-sulfamethoxazole. *J Infect Dis* 158:474, 1988.
17. Kaplan AP: Drug induced skin disease. *J Allergy Clin Immunol* 74:573, 1984.
18. Abraham GN, Petz LD, Fudenburg HH: Immunohaematological cross-reactivity between penicillin and cephalothin in humans. *Clin Exp Immunol* 3:343, 1968.
19. Petz LD: Immunologic reactions of humans to cephalosporins. *Postgrad Med J* 47(suppl):67, 1971.
20. Garratty G, Petz LD: Drug-induced immune hemolytic anemia. *Am J Med* 58:398, 1975.
21. Weitzman SA, Stossel TP: Drug-induced immunological neutropenia. *Lancet* 1:723, 1978.
22. Neftel KA, Hauser SP, Muller MR, et al: Cephalosporin-induced neutropenia (letter). *BMJ* 62:394, 1986.
23. Appel GB: A decade of penicilin related acute interstitial nephritis—more questions than answers. *Clin Nephrol* 13:151, 1980.
24. Galpin JE, Shinaberger LH, Stanley TM, et al: Acute interstitial nephritis due to methicillin. *Am J Med* 65:756, 1978.
25. Ditlove J, Weidmann P, Bernstein M, et al: Methicillin nephritis. *Medicine (Baltimore)* 56:483, 1977.
26. Baldwin DS, Levine BB, McCluskey RT, et al: Renal failure and interstitial nephritis due to penicillin and methicillin. *N Engl J Med* 279:1245, 1968.
27. Border WA, Lehman DH, Egan JD, et al: Antitubular basement membrane antibodies in methicillin-associated interstitial nephritis. *N Engl J Med* 291:281, 1974.
28. Ooi BS, Jao W, First MR, et al: Acute interstitial nephritis. A clinical and pathologic study based on renal biopsies. *Am J Med* 59:614, 1975.
29. Lawson DH, Paice BJ: Adverse reactions to trimethoprim-sulfamethoxazole. *Rev Infect Dis* 4:429, 1982.
30. Girdwood RH: The nature of possible adverse reactions to cotrimethoxazole. *Scand J Infect Dis Suppl* 8:10, 1976.
31. Slater JE: Hypersensitivity to macrolide antibiotics. *Ann Allergy* 66:193, 1991.
32. Arndt KA, Jick H: Rates of cutaneous reactions to drugs. *JAMA* 235:918, 1976.
33. Abramav LA, Yust IC, Fierstater EM, et al: Acute respiratory distress caused by erythromycin hypersensitivity. *Arch Intern Med* 138:1156, 1978.
34. Earl HS, Sullivan TJ: Acute desensitization of a patient with cystic

fibrosis allergic to both beta-lactam and aminoglycoside antibiotics. *J Allergy Clin Immunol* 79:477, 1987.
35. Fisher AA: Topical medicaments which are common sensitizers. *Ann Allergy* 49:97, 1982.
36. Green GR, Rosenblum A: Report of the penicillin study group—American Academy of Allergy. *J Allergy Clin Immunol* 48:331, 1971.
37. Smith JW, Johnson JE, Cluff LE: Studies on the epidemiology of adverse drug reactions. II. An evaluation of penicillin allergy. *N Engl J Med* 274:998, 1966.
38. Sogn DD: Penicillin allergy. *J Allergy Clin Immunol* 74:589, 1984.
39. Miller FF: History of drug sensitivity in atopic persons. *J Allergy* 40:46, 1967.
40. Smith JW, Johnson JE, Cluff LE: Studies on the epidemiology of adverse drug reactions. *N Engl J Med* 274:988, 1966.
41. Spengler H, de Weck AL: Evaluation of genetic control of the immune response to penicillin in man. *Monogr Allergy* 11:116, 1977.
42. Levin MI, Perri L, Anthony JJ: A fatal anaphylactic reaction to oral penicillin. *J Allergy Clin Immunol* 31:487–491, 1960.
43. Delage C, Irey NS: Anaphylactic deaths: A clinicopathologic study of 43 cases. *J Forensic Sci* 17:525, 1972.
44. Gordin FM, Simon GL, Wofsy CB, et al: Adverse reactions to trimethoprim-sulfamethoxazole in patients with the acquired immunodeficiency syndrome. *Ann Intern Med* 100:495, 1984.
45. Carr A, Cooper DA, Penny R: Allergic manifestations of human immunodeficiency virus (HIV) infection. *J Clin Immunol* 11:55, 1991.
46. Solley GO, Gleich GJ, Van Dellen RG: Penicillin allergy: Clinical experience with a battery of skin test reagents. *J Allergy Clin Immunol* 69:238, 1982.
47. Batchelor FR, Dewdney JM, Gazzard D: Penicillin allergy: The formation of penicilloyl determinant. *Nature* 206:362, 1965.
48. Levine BB: Antigenicity and cross-reactivity of penicillins and cephalosporins. *J Infect Dis* 128(suppl):364, 1973.
49. Stewart GT: Cross-reactivity of penicillin G and and related substances. *Lancet* 1:509, 1962.
50. Silviu-Dan F, McPhillips S, Warrington RJ: The frequency of skin test reactions to side-chain penicillin determinants. *J Allergy Clin Immunol* 91:694, 1993.
51. Blanca M, Mayorga C, Sanchez F, et al: Difference on serum antibody to benzylpenicillin and amoxicillin measured by RAST in a group of penicillin allergic patients. *Allergy* 46:632, 1991.
52. Martin JA, Igea JM, Frai J, et al: Allergy to amoxicillin in patients who tolerated benzylpenicillin, aztreonam and ceftizidime. *Clin Infect Dis* 14:592, 1992.
53. Erffmeyer JE: Adverse reactions to penicillin, part I. *Ann Allergy* 47:288, 1981.

54. Brandriss MW, Smith JW, Steinman HG: Common antigenic determinants of penicillin G, cephalothin and 6-aminopenicillanic acid in rabbits. *J Immunol* 94:696, 1965.
55. Petz, LD: Immunologic cross-reactivity between penicillins and the cephalosporins, a review. *J Infect Dis* 137(suppl):74, 1978.
56. Saxon A, Heall GN, Rohr AS: Immediate hypersensitivity reactions to beta-lactam antibiotics. *Ann Intern Med* 107:204, 1987.
57. Adkinson NF: Immunogenicity and cross-reactivity of aztreonam. *Am J Med* 88(suppl):12, 1990.
58. Lin RY: A perspective on penicillin allergy. *Arch Intern Med* 152:930, 1992.
59. Igea JM, Fraj J, Davila I, et al: Allergy to cefazolin: Study of in vivo cross reactivity with other beta lactams. *Ann Allergy* 68:515, 1992.
60. Saxon A, Adelman DC, Swabb EA, et al: Lack of cross-reactivity between aztreonam, a monobactam antibiotic, and penicillin in penicillin allergic subjects. *J Infect Dis* 149:16, 1984.
61. Saxon A, Adelman DC, Patel A, et al: Imipenem cross-reactivity with penicillin in humans. *J Allergy Clin Immunol* 82:213, 1988.
62. Sullivan TJ: Allergic reactions to antimicrobial agents. A review of reactions to drugs not in the beta lactam antibiotic class. *J Allergy Clin Immunol* 74:594, 1984.
63. Mendelson LM: A call for elective testing in children with a history of penicillin allergy. *Curr Issues Allergy Immunol* 3:14, 1992.
64. Ettinger E, Kaye D: Systemic manifestations after a skin test with penicilloyl-polylysine. *N Engl J Med* 271:1105, 1964.
65. Dogliotti M: An instance of fatal reaction to the penicillin scratch-test. *Dermatologica* 136:489, 1963.
66. Brown BC, Price EV, Moore MB: Penicilloyl-polylysine as an intradermal test of penicillin sensitivity. *JAMA* 189:87, 1964.
67. Sullivan TJ, Wedner J, Shatz GS, et al: Skin testing to detect penicillin allergy. *J Allergy Clin Immunol* 68:171, 1981.
68. Sogn DD, Evan R, Shepherd GM, et al: Results of the National Institute of Allergy and Infectious Diseases Collaborative Clinical Trial to Test the Predictive Value of Skin Testing with Major and Minor Penicillin Derivatives in Hospitalized Adults. *Arch Intern Med* 152:1025, 1992.
69. Chandra RK, Oglekar SA, Tomas E: Penicillin allergy: Anti-penicillin IgE antibodies and immediate hypersensitivity skin reactions employing major and minor determinants of penicillin. *Arch Dis Child* 55:857, 1980.
70. Ressler C, Neag PM, Mendelson M: A liquid chromatography study of the stability of the minor determinants of penicillin allergy: A stable determinant mixture skin test preparation. *J Pharm Sci* 74:448, 1985.
71. Saxon A: Immediate hypersensitivity reactions to beta lactam antibiotics. *Rev Infect Dis* 5(suppl 2):368, 1983.

72. Gruchalla ES, Sullivan TJ: Detection of IgE to sulfamethoxazole by skin testing (abstract). *J Allergy Clin Immunol* 87:231, 1991.
73. Wide L, Juhlin L: Detection of penicillin allergy of the immediate type by radioimmunoassay of reagins (IgE) to penicilloyl conjugates. *Clin Allergy* 1:171, 1971.
74. Edwards RG, Spackman DA, Dewdney JM: Development and use of three new radioallergosorbent tests in the diagnosis of penicillin allergy. *Int Arch Allergy Appl Immunol* 68:352, 1982.
75. Gruchalla RS, Sullivan TJ: In vivo and in vitro diagnosis of drug allergy. *Immunol Allergy Clin North Am* 11:595, 1991.
76. Carrington DM, Earl HS, Sullivan TJ: Studies of human IgE to a sulfonamide determinant. *J Allergy Clin Immunol* 79:442, 1987.
77. Prendiville JS, Herbert AA, Greenwald MJ, et al: Management of Stevens-Johnson syndrome and toxic epidermal necrolysis in children. *J Pediatr* 115:881, 1989.
78. Kraemer MJ, Smith AL: Rashes with ampicillin. *Pediatr Rev* 1:197, 1980.
79. Boguniewicz M, Leung YM: Management of the patient with allergic reactions to antibiotics. *Pediatr Pulmonol* 12:113, 1992.
80. Parker PJ, Parrinello JT, Condemi JJ, et al: Penicillin resensitization among hospitalized patients. *J Allergy Clin Immunol* 88:213, 1991.
81. Patterson R, Deswarte RD, Greenberger PA, et al: Drug allergy and protocols for management of drug allergies. *Allergy Proc* 7:325, 1986.
82. Stark BJ, Earl HS, Gross GN, et al: Acute and chronic desensitization of penicillin allergic patients using oral penicillin. *J Allergy Clin Immunol* 69:275, 1982.
83. Naclerio R, Mizrahi EA, Adkinson NF Jr: Immunologic observations during desensitization and maintenance of clinical tolerance to penicillin. *J Allergy Clin Immunol* 71:294, 1983.
84. Sullivan TJ: Antigen-specific desensitization of patients allergic to penicillin. *J Allergy Clin Immunol* 69:500, 1982.
85. Pienkowski MM, Kazmier J, Adkinson NE Jr: Basophil histamine release remains unaffected by clinical desensitization to penicillin. *J Allergy Clin Immunol* 82:171, 1988.
86. Borish L, Tamir R, Rosenwasser LJ: Intravenous desensitization to beta-lactam antibiotics. *J Allergy Clin Immunol* 80:314, 1987.
87. Sullivan TJ: Drug allergy, et al: in Middleton E, Reed CE, Ellis EF, *Allergy: Principles and Practice.* St Louis, Mosby, 1988, pp 1523–1536.
88. Wendel GD, Stark BJ, Jamison RB, et al: Penicillin allergy and desensitization in serious infections during pregnancy. *N Engl J Med* 312:1229, 1985.
89. Graybill JR, Sande MA, Reinarz JA, et al: Controlled penicillin anaphylaxis leading to desensitization. *South Med J* 67:62, 1974.
90. Boxer MB, Dykewicz MS, Patterson R, et al: The management of patients with sulfonamide allergy. *Allergy Proc* 9:219, 1988.

91. Finke S, Grieco MH, Connell JT, et al: Results of comparative skin tests with penicilloyl-polylysine in patients with penicillin allergy. *Am J Med* 38:71, 1965.
92. Graff-Lonnevig V, Hedlin G, Lindfors A: Penicillin allergy—a rare pediatric condition. *Arch Dis Child* 63:1342, 1988.
93. Moss RB: Immunology of cystic fibrosis, in Lloyd-Still J: *Textbook of Cystic Fibrosis*. Boston, John Wright, 1983, p 109.
94. Moss RB, Babin S, Hsu YP, et al: Allergy to semisynthetic penicillins in cystic fibrosis. *J Pediatr* 104:460, 1984.
95. Hilman BC, Rao K: Desensitization with anti-pseudomonal penicillins after allergic reactions to ureidopenicillins in cystic fibrosis. *J Allergy Clin Immunol* 77:167, 1986.
96. Brown LA, Golbert NB, Shearer WT: Long-term ticarcillin desensitization by continuous oral administration of penicillin. *J Allergy Clin Immunol* 69:51, 1982.
97. Mituyasu R, Groopman J, Volberding PA, et al: Cutaneous reaction to trimethoprim-sulfamethoxazole in patients with AIDS and Kaposi's sarcoma. *N Engl J Med* 308:1535, 1983.
98. Gordin FM, Simon GL, Wofsy CB, et al: Adverse reactions to trimethoprim-sulfamethoxazole in patients with the acquired immunodeficiency syndrome. *Ann Intern Med* 103:738, 1985.
99. Carr A, Cooper DA, Penny R: Allergic manifestations of human immunodeficiency virus (HIV) infection. *J Clin Immunol* 11:55, 1991.
100. Webb EL: Immune dysregulation: Implication for the increased allergic manifestations associated with AIDS. *Insights Allergy* 8:2, 1993.
101. Straka BF, Whitaker DL, Morrison SH, et al: Cutaneous manifestations of the acquired immunodeficiency syndrome in children. *J Am Acad Dermatol* 18:1089, 1988.
102. O'Donnell CR, Bader MB, Zibrak JD, et al: Abnormal airway function in individuals with the acquired immunodeficiency syndrome. *Chest* 94:945, 1988.
103. Wright DN, Nelson RP, Ledford DK, et al: Serum IgE and human immunodeficiency virus (HIV) infection. *J Allergy Clin Immunol* 85:445, 1990.
104. Greenberger PA, Patterson R: Management of drug allergy in patients with acquired immunodeficiency syndrome. *J Allergy Clin Immunol* 79:484, 1987.
105. Kamada M, Twarog FJ, Leung DYM: A comparison of multiple versus single antibiotic sensitivity in pediatric patients. *Allergy Proc* 12:347, 1991.
106. Sullivan TJ, Ong RC, Gilliam LK: Studies of the multiple drug allergy syndrome (abstract) *J Allergy Clin Immunol* 83:270, 1989.

Intravenous Catheter–Related Infections

Mark B. Salzman, M.D.
Department of Pediatrics, Kaiser Foundation Hospital–West Los Angeles, Los Angeles, California

Lorry G. Rubin, M.D.
Division of Infectious Diseases, Department of Pediatrics, Schneider Children's Hospital of Long Island Jewish Medical Center, New Hyde Park, New York; Long Island Campus for the Albert Einstein College of Medicine, Long Island, New York

Vascular catheter–related infections are an important cause of mortality and morbidity in hospitalized patients. At Schneider Children's Hospital, catheter-related infections are the leading cause of nosocomial bacteremia and bacteremia in pediatric oncology patients and premature infants in the neonatal intensive care unit. Although all intravascular devices are prone to local or systemic infection, the infection rate varies with the type and location of the catheter. Infections may be local and characterized by purulence at the exit site of the catheter or inflammation overlying a catheter segment. Catheter-related sepsis is the most severe complication and is most commonly related to central venous catheters.

EPIDEMIOLOGY

The reported incidence of catheter-related infection varies widely and depends on the type of catheter, patient characteristics, and underlying diagnosis. The risk of bacteremia or fungemia is greater for patients with central than with peripheral intravenous catheters.[1] However, patients in whom central venous catheters are placed are often sicker and are more likely to have significant underlying diseases than patients with peripheral venous catheters. Additionally, central venous catheters are generally in place longer than peripheral venous catheters, and the cumulative risk of infection increases linearly with the duration of use.[2] Central venous catheters may enter the vein directly at the skin puncture site or be subcutaneously tunneled and exit skin at a site distant from the vein entry site. The reported incidence of central venous catheter–related bloodstream infection has varied between 3.5% and 48% in studies of hospitalized patients.[3–9] Because the cumulative risk of infection increases with the duration of catheter placement and the duration of catheterization varies, the preferred method of reporting infection rates is the number of catheter-related infections per 1,000 days of catheter use. Compiling the results of 21 studies of infection rates of subcutaneously tunneled central venous catheters including studies in pediatric patients, Decker and Edwards found an overall rate of 1.7 episodes of catheter-related bloodstream infections per 1,000 days of catheter use.[10] The infection rates were higher for pediatric patients, 2.4 per 1,000 days. For neonates, the rate was 3.9 per 1,000 days. In a separate study, the infection rate in neonates with birth weights less than 1,500 g was 20 per 1,000 days.[7]

The underlying diagnosis may also influence the catheter-related infection rate. Among pediatric oncology patients, Decker and Edwards[10] found that the infection rate was lower (2.2 per 1,000 catheter days) than in nononcology patients, who typically used the catheters for parenteral nutrition. Infection rates were higher in inpatients than in outpatients. This difference was most marked for the patients receiving only parenteral nutrition.

DEVICE-SPECIFIC ISSUES

Peripheral venous devices can be made of various plastics or metal. Steel needles have lower infection rates than plastic catheters when used for peripheral venous access.[11] Other risk factors for infection of peripheral catheters include placement by venous cutdown and lower extremity placement.[12] However, femoral venous catheterization was not associated with an increased infection rate in a study of critically ill children[13] or adult burn patients.[14] Infections are seldom seen in catheters in place less than 72 hours; the infection rate rises when catheters are left in place longer than 72 hours.[12]

There are several types of materials used to manufacture catheters for central venous cannulization. Plastic central venous catheters may be made of polyethylene, polypropylene, polyvinyl, or polytetrafluoroethylene (Teflon) and may have one, two, or three lumens.[10] Silicone (rubber or silastic) central venous catheters exit through the skin after being passed through a subcutaneous tunnel. Such catheters may be cuffed (e.g., Broviac and Hickman catheters) or noncuffed and may have one or two lumens. Cuffs are made of synthetic fibers such as Dacron and serve to anchor the catheter and act as a barrier to microorganisms.[15] The silicone cuffed catheter was pioneered by Broviac et al. in 1973[16] and later modified by Hickman and associates.[17] Noncuffed catheters do not have to be passed through a subcutaneous tunnel as do cuffed catheters, but they may be tunneled. Catheter tunneling helps anchor the catheter and acts as a physical barrier helping to prevent bloodstream entry by microorganisms that gain access to the external catheter surface at the skin insertion site. However, in a British study in which catheters were rigorously cared for by a nutrition nurse, the catheter infection rates of tunneled and nontunneled catheters were comparable.[18]

A noncuffed catheter can be inserted percutaneously through a peripheral vein and is referred to as a peripherally inserted central catheter (PICC).[19] Alternatively, such catheters may be advanced a shorter distance, not reach a central vein, and still function for a relatively long period of time.

Subcutaneously tunneled central venous catheters may also be totally implantable venous access devices (e.g. Mediport [Norfolk, Medina, NY], Port-A-Cath [Pharmacia Deltec, St Paul, Minn], or Infus-A-Port [Infusaid, Atlanta, Ga]).[10] The end of the catheter is advanced into a central vein, and the proximal end traverses a subcutaneous tunnel leading to a subcutaneous reservoir. This system is accessed by needle puncture through intact skin. When not accessed, these devices do not require daily flushing or disinfection of the access site and therefore require less manipulation than Broviac-type catheters. Catheter-related infection rates of totally implantable central venous catheters placed in pediatric patients (with a preponderance of oncology patients) have ranged from 0.34 to 1.89 per 1,000 catheter days.[20–25] These rates are lower than the mean rate of 2.2 episodes per 1,000 catheter days cited earlier for silicone central venous catheters that exit the skin on the chest wall.[10] Studies of implantable venous devices in adults have shown still lower infection rates.[26–31]

In a comparative study we examined the infection rate of cuffed silicone, subcutaneously tunneled central venous catheters, and totally implantable catheters in 62 pediatric oncology patients with 78 venous-access devices placed at a single center. The infection rate was 2.1 episodes per 1,000 catheter days for the silicone cuffed catheters vs. 1.4 for the totally implantable devices, a difference that did not achieve statistical significance.[32] At another institution the infection rate of cuffed silicone catheters in pediatric leukemia patients was 2.0 per 1,000 catheter days as compared with a rate of 0.5 per 1,000 catheter days with totally implantable devices.[20] The mean rate of infection in these seven pediatric studies[20–25, 32] was 1.1 per 1,000 catheter days for totally implantable devices, about half the infection rate cited earlier for externalized central venous catheters. Mirro et al. at St. Jude Children's Research Hospital also found lower infection rates in implantable venous access devices vs. externalized catheters in a nonrandomized prospective study.[33, 34] However, the difference only became significant after 400 days of catheter use. They found that the risk of infection was greatest during the first 100 days after placement, particularly for implantable venous access devices. Thus although a randomized, prospective comparison of infection rates has not been performed, totally implantable devices appear to have a lower rate of infection than do cuffed, silicone central venous catheters.

MICROBIOLOGY

Staphylococci are the predominant microorganisms causing catheter-related infections. Among staphylococci, coagulase-negative staphylococci are more common pathogens than *Staphylococcus aureus. Staphylococcus epidermidis* is the most common coagulase-negative staphylococcal species.[35] In a compilation of 16 studies documenting the causes of infections in central venous catheters placed in pediatric patients (predominantly oncology patients and gastroenterology patients receiving parenteral nutrition), 34% of the microbial isolates were coagulase-negative staphylococci and 16% were *S. aureus.*[10, 20, 24, 36] Gram-negative bacilli and fungi accounted for 29% and 7% of the isolates, respectively (Table I).

Among neonates in our intensive care unit, we found that coagulase-negative staphylococci were responsible for an even higher percentage of episodes of catheter-related bloodstream infections and accounted for 61% (17 of 28) of these episodes.[35] *Candida* spp. accounted for 5 (18%) of 28 episodes of catheter-related bloodstream infection, a disproportionately high number when compared with infections in older children. Other less frequently isolated microorganisms, including *Xanthomonas* spp.,[37] *Corynebacterium* spp.,[38] *Mycobacterium fortuitum* and *chelonae,*[39] and *Rhodotorula* spp,[40] have been associated with catheter-related infection.

TABLE 1.
Blood Culture Isolates in Episodes of Central Venous Catheter–Related Bloodstream Infection*

Microorganism	Number (%)
Gram-positive bacteria	254(64)
Coagulase-negative staphylococci	133(34)
Staphylococcus aureus	65(16)
Enterococcus species	17
Streptococcus, viridans group	8
Other streptococci	19
Bacillus species	7
Micrococcus species	2
Other	3
Gram-negative bacilli	113(29)
Klebsiella species	21
Escherichia coli	20
Pseudomonas species	18
Enterobacter species	15
Acinetobacter species	10
Other or unspecified	29
Fungi	29 (7)
Candida species	26
Malassezia furfur	3

*Compilation of 16 studies that included only pediatric patients. Data from references 10, 20, 24, and 35.

DIAGNOSIS

The diagnosis of a catheter-related infection is sometimes difficult because catheter-related bloodstream infections are frequently unaccompanied by signs of inflammation around the catheter. When an exit-site infection is present with purulence around the catheter insertion site, the diagnosis can be made by inspection. Inflammation without purulence does not always signify infection because inflammation may be due to mechanical factors or a reaction to foreign material.[41] A quantitative culture of the skin or subcutaneous catheter segment may be helpful to determine whether infection is present. Exit-site infections may occur with or without a bloodstream infection.

A tunnel infection involves spreading cellulitis overlying the tunnel tract of subcutaneously tunneled catheters. This type of catheter infection is usually diagnosed by noting signs of inflammation along the tunnel tract and by tenderness to palpation over the tunnel tract. Tunnel infections are more difficult to eradicate than exit-site infections, can be rapidly progressive, and generally require removal of the catheter.

Catheter-related bloodstream infection is suspected in a patient with an intravascular catheter and fever or multiple clinical signs of sepsis (fever, chills, leukocytosis, hypotension, etc.) and no other obvious source for the septicemia. In most cases of catheter-related bloodstream infection, infection of the catheter is not clinically evident, i.e., there is neither an exit site nor tunnel infection. An episode of sepsis is most likely to be catheter related when the bloodstream isolate is either a common skin microorganism such as coagulase-negative staphylococci, *S. aureus*, or *Candida* spp. Criteria for definite or probable catheter-related bloodstream infection are listed in Table 2. An episode of catheter-related bloodstream infection can be classified as catheter-related sepsis when the episode is accompanied by two of the following four conditions: (1) temperature over 38° C or less than 36° C; (2) tachycardia; (3) tachypnea; and (4) leukocytosis, leukopenia, or more than 10% immature (band) forms.[42]

When an isolate from a culture of the catheter tip is identical to the blood culture isolate, catheter-related bloodstream infection is often presumed. However, a nonquantitative culture of the catheter tip, often placed in broth culture, is of variable value because a culture performed in this manner frequently yields a microorganism even in the absence of catheter-related infection.[43, 44] Maki and colleagues pioneered the use of a semiquantitative culture technique in which the catheter segment was rolled several times across the surface of an agar plate.[43, 44] A positive catheter segment culture was defined as a culture yielding at least 15 colonies following incubation. In fact, most cultures of rolled catheter segments that were implicated in infection had confluent growth of colonies. Other authors have successfully used this method to diagnose catheter-related infections.[45–47] A limitation of this technique is that only microorganisms on the external surface of the catheters are sampled. Because the microorganisms may have gained access to the bloodstream via intraluminal migration through the catheter (as discussed in the section on pathogenesis), this method will fail to diagnose some cases of catheter-related bloodstream infection. One technique that is more cumbersome than the semiquantitative roll method quantitates the number of microorganisms that can be flushed through the internal surface of a catheter.[48] Other techniques involving sonication, vortexing, or centrifugation measure microorganisms arising from both the external and internal surface of the catheter.[49–51] Sonication has been found to be more sensitive than the roll-plate technique; this is probably because the roll-plate technique does not detect intraluminal colonization.[52] Recovery of 100 or more colony-forming units (CFU) is considered significant when the sonication technique is used.[52] Others have found that when greater than 1,000 microorganisms are removed from the surface of a vascular catheter by sonication there is a strong correlation with recovery of the same microorganism from a blood culture.[53] Other techniques for diagnosing catheter-related

TABLE 2.
Criteria for the Diagnosis of Catheter-Related Bloodstream Infection

Definite
Isolation of the same microorganism from percutaneous blood culture and from one of the following:
Exudate at the catheter exit site
A semiquantitative catheter segment culture (although fulfilling this criteria requires catheter removal)
A semiquantitative catheter hub swab culture (if blood had not previously been drawn back through the catheter)
Infusate
Quantitative blood culture with recovery of at least a 5-fold higher colony count from blood obtained through the catheter than from a percutaneous blood culture
Probable
Positive culture of blood obtained through the catheter (but a negative percutaneous blood culture) in the presence of clinical manifestations of infection and without another apparent source of infection
Clinical sepsis unresponsive to antibiotic therapy that resolves following catheter removal.

infection include Gram stain of the catheter segment,[54] Gram stain of impression smears of the catheter,[55] and acridine orange staining of the catheter.[56] These other methods are labor-intensive and still investigational but may be helpful in selected cases.

Unfortunately, the techniques described require removal of the catheter. In one study, only 8 of 91 (8.8%) central venous catheters removed because of suspected catheter-related bloodstream infection were found to be infected by sonication and roll-plate techniques.[41] To avoid catheter removal in cases where catheter-related infection is unproved, nontunneled central venous catheters with suspected infection can be removed over a guidewire and replaced with a new catheter in the same site. The removed catheter can then be semiquantitatively cultured. If cultures prove negative, the replaced catheter can remain in place. If cultures are positive, the new catheter almost always becomes infected and should be promptly removed.[57, 58]

Another strategy used to make a diagnosis of catheter-related bloodstream infection while the catheter remains in place is a comparison of results of simultaneously obtained quantitative blood cultures drawn through the catheter and obtained from a peripheral vein.[59] The colony count from the central venous catheter should be significantly higher than the colony count in blood from a peripheral vein if the bacteremia (or fungemia) is catheter related.[60–65] The required difference in colony counts for blood taken from the two sites that is considered significant is controversial. Blood that flows through central veins will pass through the lungs before reaching the peripheral circulation. The pulmonary circulation is a component of the reticuloendothelial system that is capable of removing bacteria from the circulation,[66] thereby lowering the bacterial concentration in the peripheral blood even in patients with non–catheter-related bacteremia. Crocker et al.[66] infected pigs with *Pseudomonas aeruginosa* and found that 60% to 80% of the bacteria were cleared from the blood in one passage through the lungs, thereby reducing the level of bacteremia 2.5- to 5-fold. Flynn et al.[62] infected rabbits with *Escherichia coli* by intraperitoneal injection and found the blood bacterial concentration to be between 1.1- and 3.5-fold (mean, 2.2-fold) higher in the superior vena cava than in the femoral vein. Based on an analysis of variance, they concluded that 99% of episodes of non–catheter-related bacteremia will have differences no greater than 5-fold. Therefore the authors proposed that a 5-fold or greater bacterial concentration difference be used as a criterion for the diagnosis of catheter-related bloodstream infection. Raucher et al.[61] proposed the use of a 10-fold difference based on findings from nine episodes in seven patients. Capdevila et al.[65] showed that among 17 patients only a four-fold increase was 100% predictive of catheter-related bloodstream infection and that a single bacterial count greater than 100 CFU/mL drawn from the catheter in the presence of a positive qualitative peripheral blood culture of the same microorganism is also highly predictive of catheter-related bloodstream infection. Included in these analyses are patients with negative percutaneously obtained blood cultures, which raises concern that the blood culture detected catheter colonization rather than a bloodstream infection. However, it is reasonable to consider such patients to have probable catheter-related bloodstream infection because blood cultures obtained through subcutaneously tunneled catheters in asymptomatic patients rarely have recovery of a high density of microorganisms.[61, 62]

PATHOGENESIS

Microorganisms causing catheter-related bloodstream infection can originate from several sources. These include contaminated intravenous fluids, hematogenous seeding of the catheter from a distant site of infection, the catheter insertion site, and the catheter hub (the female end of the junction to which the infusion tubing connects). The skin entry site is usually regarded as the most common portal of infection. There is growing evidence that the catheter hub is also an important portal of entry for tunneled and nontunneled central venous catheters.[35, 67–71]

Contamination of intravenous fluids is relatively uncommon but can occur at the time of manufacture,[72, 73] during supplementation of the fluids, or during clinical use.[74, 75] Different infusion fluids support the growth of different microorganisms. Most infusion-related bloodstream infections are due to aerobic gram-negative bacilli such as *Enterobacter*, *Citrobacter*, and *Serratia* species.[76] Lipid emulsions support bacterial growth extremely well[77, 78] and have been associated with *Malassezia* fungemia in both neonates and adults.[79] Additionally, *Candida parapsilosis* infection has been associated with contaminated parenteral nutrition solutions.[80, 81] Despite the reported outbreaks, contamination of intravenous fluids is an uncommon cause of catheter-related bloodstream infection.

Hematogenous seeding of the catheter from infection at a distant site can occur[82] but has rarely been demonstrated. In one study, central venous catheters removed from patients who had bacteremia unrelated to the catheter were examined by electron microscopy, but the authors were unable to detect seeding of the catheter.[83]

Most authorities consider the catheter insertion site to be the major portal of entry of microorganisms causing catheter-related bloodstream infection.[84] Microorganisms gain access to the catheter tip by extraluminal migration along the catheter and then enter the bloodstream. Microbial contamination around the catheter insertion site has been shown to be a significant risk factor for catheter-related bloodstream infection.[85] Studies that have shown a higher density of microbial colonization on the exterior surface of catheters than on the interior surface[54] support this view. Studies of removed catheters by electron microscopy showed that central venous catheters examined after short-term use (mean of 15 days) had equal colonization of the internal and external surfaces.[41] However, when catheters were in place for a mean duration of 109 days, the degree of colonization and biofilm on the internal surface of the catheter was at least twice that on the external surface.[41] Therefore it is possible that the catheter insertion site is the major portal of entry for microorganisms in infections of catheters, in place for a short time, but entry of microorganisms via the catheter hub may play an increasingly important role in infection of catheters used long-term.

Evidence implicating the catheter hub as an important portal of entry for microorganisms causing catheter-related bloodstream infection is available from several studies.[35, 67–71] In 12 of 13 episodes of coagulase-negative staphylococcal bacteremia occurring in adults with central venous catheters, the same coagulase-negative staphylococcal species was isolated from both the catheter hub culture and blood culture.[67] We prospectively cultured the hubs of central venous catheters in neonates and found the infecting microorganism in the catheter hub before isolation from the blood at the time of clinical sepsis in 10 (36%) of 28 cases of catheter-related bloodstream infection.[35] In an additional 10 cases we cultured the infecting microorganism from the hub at the time of evaluation for suspected sepsis. Therefore, as many as 71% (20 of 28) of the cases of catheter-related bloodstream infection may have been the result of microorganisms entering through the catheter hub. In only 1 of the 28 cases was an exit-site infection present at the time of clinical sepsis.

Additional evidence for the hub as the portal of entry was put forth in a study focusing on care of the catheter junction, the connection between the catheter hub and infusion tubing.[69] When a shield was placed around the catheter hub to prevent the hub from contacting the patient's skin, the incidence of catheter-related infections was reduced from 39% to 8%. In another study in which the metallic hubs of the catheters were heated on a daily basis, the catheter-related bloodstream infection rate was only 0.95%.[70] Delayed tubing changes may also reduce the incidence of catheter-related sepsis,[71] presumably by decreasing the access of microorganisms to the catheter hub.

Components of blood that are deposited on the surface of catheters contribute to microbial adherence.[86] The establishment of a fibrin sheath surrounding the blood-exposed portion of the catheter aids in microbial attachment. Plasma fibronectin has also been shown to be important because it has an affinity for inert plastics and contains binding sites for staphylococcal species, thus resulting in more effective bacterial adherence.[87] Other putative host-derived adhesins include laminin[88] and collagen.[89]

In addition to host-derived adhesins, certain microorganisms produce materials that facilitate adherence to catheters. Some strains of coagulase-negative staphylococci produce adhesins that aid in bacterial attachment and also produce a surface slime material (a fibrous glycocalyx) that protects the bacteria from host defenses and the action of antimicrobial agents.[90, 91] Coagulase-negative staphylococci that cause clinically significant disease are more likely to produce extracellular slime than coagulase-negative staphylococci that are resident skin flora.[92]

The catheter material has also been shown to affect adherence of microorganisms. Polyvinylchloride catheters have been shown to be colonized more frequently with microorganisms than Teflon catheters.[93] In addition, there is a higher affinity of coagulase-negative staphylococci for polyvinylchloride than Teflon.[93] Therefore, the host, the microorganism, and the catheter material all play an interactive role in the pathogenesis of catheter-related infections.

PREVENTION

Strict aseptic technique should be practiced whenever a central venous catheter is placed. The use of masks, hats, sterile gloves, gowns, and large drapes during placement have resulted in a lower catheter-related infection rate than more limited precautions consisting of sterile gloves and small drapes (0.6% catheter-related bloodstream infection rate vs. 3.6%).[94] The site of central venous catheter placement should be cleansed with an antiseptic. Maki et al. randomized 668 patients to receive povidone-iodine, 70% alcohol, and 2% aqueous chlorhexidine for skin disinfection before catheter placement in a surgical intensive care unit.[95] Chlorhexidine was associated with the lowest incidence of sepsis, with 2.3 infections per 100 catheters as compared with a rate of 7.1 per 100 catheters for alcohol and 9.3 per 100 catheters for povidone-iodine. Another study found povidone-iodine to be superior to 70% isopropylalcohol.[96]

The use of topical antimicrobials at the catheter insertion site has also been evaluated for efficacy in preventing colonization and infection of catheters. Mupirocin applied after skin disinfection with tincture of iodine was shown to reduce colonization of central venous catheters by microorganisms derived from the skin insertion site when compared with using tincture of iodine disinfection alone.[97] Polymyxin in combination with neomycin and bacitracin was shown to decrease the risk of catheter colonization with bacteria, but the risk of catheter colonization with *Candida* was increased; there was no change in the risk of sepsis.[98] In this same study iodophor ointment resulted in half the rate of infection (3.6% vs. 6.5%) when compared with the use of no topical agent. However, this difference was not statistically significant. In another study, the use of topical povidone-iodine ointment resulted in a catheter-related bloodstream infection rate of 5% vs. 18% when no ointment was used.[99]

The effect of the type of dressing used at the catheter insertion site on infection has been studied.[100–102] The use of occlusive transparent dressings allows continuous inspection of the insertion site and may help anchor the catheter, but it may also lead to accumulation of moisture at the insertion site with a resultant increase in the microbial load and an increase in the risk of catheter colonization and infection as compared with a dry gauze dressing.[100, 101] However, in another comparative study a difference in infection rate was not observed.[102]

A silver-impregnated cuff that is attached to the catheter just before insertion and resides just inside the skin entry site has been shown to decrease the risk of catheter colonization and bacteremia.[103, 104] However, this has only been shown with short-term non-tunneled central venous catheters in adults (mean duration of catheterization of less than 10 days) and has not reduced the risk of infection with catheters maintained for a longer period of time.[41]

The effect of the frequency of changing intravenous tubing on infection rates has been studied.[71, 105–109] Intervals ranging from 24 to 96 hours have been compared. None of these studies showed a significantly increased risk of infection with delayed tubing changes; the data from one study[71] suggested that delaying tubing changes may decrease the risk of infection, perhaps by minimizing contamination of the catheter hub, which may accompany an increase in manipulation. However, this study showed this effect only in relation to historical controls. A prospective study design comparing 48- and 96-hour intervals between tubing changes should be performed.

The practice of routinely replacing central venous catheters over a guidewire at regular intervals in an attempt to prevent catheter-related bloodstream infection is controversial. An Italian study found a decreased incidence of catheter-related bloodstream infection with weekly exchanges over a guidewire.[110] However, this benefit was present for only 1 month. Another study showed a benefit of guidewire exchanges every 72 hours,[111] whereas another did not.[112] Cobb et al.[113] recently reported that routine replacement of central venous catheters every 3 days (either over a guidewire or at a new site) did not decrease the incidence of catheter-associated infection. Overall, the literature does not support routine changing of central venous catheters over a guidewire as a measure to prevent catheter-related infection.

Whether the replacement of a noninfected catheter over a guidewire increases the risk of catheter-related bloodstream infection when compared with using a new site is unclear. Two studies found an increased infection rate when replacing over a guidewire[113, 114] whereas another did not.[57] Cobb et al.[113] found that the use of a new site increased the rate of mechanical complications when compared with replacing over a guidewire.

Instilling a solution containing vancomycin into the catheter has been successfully used to eradicate *S. epidermidis* from the internal surfaces of noninfused catheters.[115] A subsequent study used antibiotics for prophylaxis of catheter colonization and infection. When a relatively low concentration of vancomycin (well above the minimum inhibitory concentration for staphylococci but below the limit of detection for serum vancomycin assays) was added to heparin as a flush solution for catheters in pediatric oncology patients, there were no episodes of catheter-related bacteremia with vancomycin-susceptible bacteria.[116] Because gram-negative infections were not prevented, this same group of investigators are now assessing a vancomycin-ciprofloxacin-heparin flush solution.[117] The preservative chlorbutonol has also been added to heparin flush solution and has been found to reduce catheter colonization with *S. epidermidis*.[118] Benzalkonium chloride, a cationic surfactant with antimicrobial activity, is used to coat catheters to bind heparin; catheters treated with benzalkonium chloride may exhibit a reduced rate of catheter-related bacteremia.[119] Disodium ethylenediaminetetraacetic acid (disodium EDTA), a chelating agent that also acts as an anticoagulant,, has been shown to be bactericidal for *S. epidermidis* and has been suggested as a replacement for heparin flush solutions.[120] Flushes of central venous catheters with saline supplemented with the bacteriostatic agent benzyl alcohol (1%) have been shown to delay the onset of positive surveillance cultures drawn through the catheter when compared with saline flushes alone.[121]

Recently, catheters to which anti-infective compounds are bound have been studied to determine whether they reduce the incidence of catheter colonization and sepsis.[122, 123] Bonding of silver sulfadiazine and chlorhexidine has been shown to reduce the incidence of catheter-related bloodstream infection of central venous catheters[122]; however, the complete study has not been published. Cefazolin bonded to intravascular catheters has been effective in reducing bacterial colonization of catheters.[123] In a rabbit model, dicloxacillin, clindamycin, fusidic acid, or chlorhexidine decreased the risk of infection as compared with untreated control catheters after *S. aureus* inoculation.[124] Bonding a combination of rifampin and clindamycin provided protection against *S. epidermidis* colonization in hydrocephalus shunt catheters in an in vitro model.[125] Salicylic acid–treated catheters showed reduced adherence of a slime-producing *S. epidermidis* as compared with control catheters.[126] Iodine bonded to catheters inhibited the adherence of *S. epidermidis* in an in vitro model.[127] If further studies document the efficacy of catheters coated with anti-infective substances in reducing the incidence of catheter-related bloodstream infection and microbial resistance does not emerge, such catheters may be routinely used in the near future.

We are currently conducting a study that addresses the prevention of catheter-related bloodstream infections in neonates with central venous catheters. As discussed earlier, it appears that hub colonization is frequently involved in the pathogenesis of catheter-related bloodstream infection in this setting. We are seeking to determine whether swabbing the interior of the catheter hub three times weekly with 70% ethanol will reduce microbial colonization of the catheter by microorganisms that gain access through the hub. Using an in vitro model of catheter hub contamination, we have recently shown that 70% ethanol is effective in reducing microbial contamination of the catheter hub with both bacteria and yeast.[128]

We are studying the hypothesis that this intervention will reduce the incidence of catheter-related bloodstream infection in this patient population.

MANAGEMENT

The management of vascular catheter–related infections depends on the host characteristics, the type of catheter, the type of infection, and the pathogen. Removal of the catheter will result in resolution of most catheter-related infections but is not required in all situations. The most important aspect of management of infections of nontunneled central venous catheters or peripheral venous catheters is removal of the catheter. Antibiotic therapy is not always required but should be instituted if fever or local signs of infection fail to resolve despite removal of the catheter. In contrast, one may attempt to manage a subset of infections involving subcutaneously tunneled central venous catheters without catheter removal. This has been attempted in part because of the difficulty and expense involved in replacing such catheters, which are frequently placed under general anesthesia and may need general anesthesia for removal. One should note, however, that prompt removal of the catheter in cases of sepsis syndrome or septic shock related to an infected vascular catheter may be lifesaving. Exit-site infections can usually be treated with systemic antibiotics and local care without catheter removal. Some "pocket infections," infections of the subcutaneous access end of totally implantable venous devices, can be cured without device removal; this was successful in 7 of 12 (58%) cases in two studies.[26, 29] Infections overlying the subcutaneous tunnel are more difficult to treat and usually require both prompt catheter removal and intravenous antibiotic therapy. An attempt may be made to treat many cases of suspected catheter-related bloodstream infection without removing the catheter, as will be detailed later.

Appropriate management of central venous catheter infections in neonates is not well established. Prompt catheter removal with initiation of intravenous antibiotics is generally recommended.[10] Premature infants in neonatal intensive care units often require central venous catheters for a prolonged period of time to receive parenteral nutrition. Because preterm neonates are immunocompromised,[129] systemic infections can be rapidly fatal. We have previously documented a case in which *Serratia* gained access to the blood through the catheter hub; there was a rapid progression to septic shock and death in this previously well, premature infant.[35]

Such experiences suggest that a delay in removal of central venous catheters in neonates, at least with gram-negative bacilli, should generally be avoided. In one report one of three neonates with *S. epidermidis* catheter-related bacteremia and one neonate with *S. aureus* catheter-related bacteremia were successfully treated with the catheter remaining in place.[130]

For most older infants and children with subcutaneously tunneled catheters, an attempt can be made to treat many catheter-related bloodstream infections with the catheter in situ provided that the child is clinically stable. Antibiotics should be administered through the catheter, and if the catheter has more than one lumen, the infusion of antibiotics should be rotated through all lumens. In a review of 135 infections of Broviac-type catheters in pediatric patients, 101 (75%) were successfully treated without catheter removal.[10] Published data are limited, but treatment of catheter-related bloodstream infections of totally implantable venous access devices without device removal appears to have a cure rate similar to tunneled catheters that exit the skin.[32, 131] If despite appropriate antibiotic therapy the patient's symptoms fail to improve, the patient's condition is unstable or deteriorates, or blood cultures remain positive, the catheter must be removed.

Our initial choice of antibiotics for a nonneutropenic patient with suspected catheter-related bloodstream infection is vancomycin. If signs of sepsis are present, either an aminoglycoside or a third-generation cephalosporin is included in the regimen. In a neutropenic patient with fever, initial therapy usually consists of a broad-spectrum β-lactam and an aminoglycoside (e.g., ticarcillin/clavulanate and gentamicin), although monotherapy with either ceftazidime[132] or imipenem[133] has been used. The role of vancomycin or teicoplanin (a newer glycopeptide antibiotic with activity comparable to vancomycin but not Food and Drug Administration [FDA] approved) in the initial treatment of a patient with fever and neutropenia is controversial. Some argue that vancomycin should be included in the initial regimen because gram-positive bacteria resistant to β-lactam antibiotics are common in neutropenic patients with central venous catheters. Others argue that these bacteria are of low virulence and vancomycin can be safely withheld until blood culture results are available. In several studies there was no increase in morbidity when delaying the use of vancomycin until a positive culture was obtained.[134] We found that therapy with vancomycin was associated with colonization with vancomycin-resistant enterococci in pediatric oncology patients.[135] Vancomycin should be used for empirical therapy for patients with fever and neutropenia in institutions with a high frequency of methicillin-resistant *S. aureus*. Once blood culture results are available, antimicrobial chemotherapy can be adjusted accordingly.

As discussed previously, coagulase-negative staphylococci are the most frequent microorganisms causing catheter-related bloodstream infection. Catheter infections caused by these bacteria can frequently be treated without removing the catheter.[136, 137] Because the majority of coagulase-negative staphylococci are resistant to the antistaphylococcal penicillins, vancomycin is the treatment of choice.[41] Although a 5- to 7-day course of antibiotics has been shown to be adequate in uncomplicated cases when patients respond rapidly to therapy,[138] we generally prescribe a 10-day course. Although treatment is usually successful without removing the catheter, there is a risk of relapse. In one study there was a 20% rate of recurrence of bacteremia when the catheter was left in place as compared with a 3% risk of recurrence when the catheter was removed.[139] This risk should be considered when deciding whether the catheter should remain in place with catheter-related coagulase-negative staphylococcal bacteremia.

Catheter-related bacteremia caused by *S. aureus* is more frequently associated with a complicated course than is bacteremia caused by coagulase-negative staphylococci.[140, 141] In a retrospective study of adult patients with Hickman catheters, only 18% of patients with *S. aureus* bacteremia were cured without removing the catheter.[140] There was a higher sepsis-related mortality and rate of relapse when the catheter remained in place.[140] Good outcome was associated with low-density bacteremia (less than 1 CFU/mL of blood). In a study of adult oncology patients, 12 (23%) of 53 with catheter-related *S. aureus* bacteremia had septic thrombosis of the cannulated vein. Deep-seated infections developed in 5 of these 12 as compared with 2 of 38 without septic thrombosis.[141] It is unclear whether these data can be extrapolated to children; nevertheless, catheter removal should be more strongly considered in children with *S. aureus* bacteremia than in those with coagulase-negative staphylococci.

Staphylococcus aureus bacteremia is generally treated with either a semisynthetic penicillin, cephalosporin, clindamycin, or vancomycin, depending on the susceptibility of the infecting strain. The duration of treatment is controversial. Some authorities recommend a 10- to 14-day course for uncomplicated cases and longer courses (4 to 6 weeks) for complicated cases, especially with deep-seated infections.[141, 142] A recent meta-analysis in adults found a 6.1% late complication rate in 11 studies.[143] The overall complication and mortality rates were 24% and 15%, respectively. The authors concluded that the optimal duration of therapy is unknown but short-course (2 weeks or less) therapy should be viewed with caution because of the risk of late complications such as endocarditis. Although we generally treat uncomplicated catheter-related *S. aureus* bacteremia with 10 to 14 days of intravenous antibiotics with the catheter in place, we have a very low clinical threshold for removing the catheter and would give a prolonged course of therapy to patients with endocarditis or septic pulmonary emboli and those who respond slowly to antibiotic therapy.

Management of catheter-related bloodstream infection with gram-negative bacilli depends in part on the identity of the implicated bacteria. *Pseudomonas* species have been reported to be difficult to eradicate without catheter removal.[37] One study found that among 149 cases of septicemia caused by *Xanthomonas* and *Pseudomonas* species other than *P. aeruginosa*, 100% were cured with catheter removal as compared with only 53% when the catheter was left in place.[144] Other gram-negative bacilli are more easily treated with the catheter in place. Some authorities recommend as little as 7 days of parenteral antimicrobial therapy,[41] although we generally treat for 10 to 14 days.

Management of catheter-related candidemia is controversial. Most authorities recommend prompt catheter removal.[133, 145–148] In a review of pediatric patients with candidemia and central venous catheters, 5 of 8 children with initially retained catheters had persistent candidemia until removal of the catheter (3 patients) or death (2 patients). Only 1 patient had apparently successful treatment without removing the catheter. The other 2 patients had their catheters removed within 14 days for other reasons (1 for catheter-related bacteremia and 1 for catheter malfunction). Two of 13 patients who had prompt catheter removal had persistent candidemia, and there were no deaths.[149] In another study, 19 (46%) of 41 Hickman catheters associated with candidemia required catheter removal as compared with 41 (11%) of 367 associated with bacteremia.[150] The combined results of studies performed in adult and pediatric patients showed 11 (44%) of 25 failures, including 3 deaths in patients treated with amphotericin B without catheter removal as compared with 3 (12%) of 26 failures with 1 death in cases where the catheter was removed and amphotericin B was administered. When the catheter was removed and no antifungal therapy was given, 6 (30%) of 20 failed to resolve and there was 1 death.[151] Therefore it appears that although catheter-related candidemia can be successfully cured with retention of the catheter, the failure and complication rates are high and there is a risk of mortality. Based on these data, we recommend prompt catheter removal in most circumstances. In uncomplicated cases if the catheter is to be maintained, a 10- to 14-day course of amphotericin B may be sufficient,[41] but longer courses are required with complicated cases. Fluconazole, a systemic antifungal agent that can be administered intravenously or orally and has less adverse effects than amphotericin B, has not been adequately studied for use in cases of catheter-associated candidemia. Preterm infants with catheter-associated candidemia may have disseminated infection, and oral flucytosine may be used in conjunction with amphotericin B.[152] Whether antifungal therapy is required for treatment of immunocompetent patients when the catheter is promptly removed is controversial. Recently the trend has been to treat all patients with antifungal therapy except under rare circumstances[153]; fluconazole may prove to be an acceptable alternative to amphotericin B in immunocompetent patients.

Catheter-related bacteremia caused by *Bacillus* species has also been reported to be difficult to treat without removing the catheter.[154, 155] Five (63%) of 8 patients failed treatment without catheter removal in one study as compared with 18 (5.2%) of 343 patients with other bacteria. Vancomycin is the drug of choice.[154] *Corynebacterium* group JK has also been shown to be difficult to eradicate, and some advocate prompt catheter removal when this is the infecting microorganism.[156] Other microorganisms that have been difficult to eradicate without catheter removal include *M. chelonae* and *M. fortuitum*.[39] Exit-site infections with these microorganisms require surgical removal of the skin and subcutaneous tissue surrounding the tunnel tract and exit site.[157]

Catheter-related bloodstream infection caused by multiple microorganisms may also be difficult to eradicate without catheter removal. In one review, when multiple microorganisms were involved, there was a 60% failure rate without catheter removal.[145] However, this issue has not been addressed by other investigators, and most authorities do not list this as a reason for prompt catheter removal.

In addition to the use of antimicrobial therapy in the treatment of catheter-related infections, adjuvant therapies have been employed. Urokinase in conjunction with antimicrobial therapy has been successfully used.[158, 159] The rationale for the use of urokinase is removal of thrombi and fibrin deposits from the catheter that may provide a protected haven for microorganisms that survive despite antimicrobial therapy and result in reseeding of the bloodstream after discontinuation of antibiotic therapy. In one study of pediatric oncology patients,[158] only 3 (5.1%) of 59 septic episodes treated with urokinase and antimicrobial therapy required catheter removal because of recurrent sepsis. The combination of urokinase and antibiotics was successful in all 5 patients with candidemia and 10 of 11 with polymicrobial sepsis. Other adjuvant therapies have included hydrochloric acid[160] and sodium bisulfite.[161]

SUMMARY

Vascular catheter–related infection is an important cause of mortality and morbidity in hospitalized patients. The mean incidence of catheter-related bloodstream infection in hospitalized pediatric patients is 2.4 episodes per 1,000 days. Totally implantable central venous catheters may be associated with a lower risk of infection. Coagulase-negative staphylococci are the predominant cause and account for about one third of episodes of catheter-related bloodstream infection.

The diagnosis of catheter-related bloodstream infection is often difficult because there are frequently no signs of inflammation around the catheter. Diagnosis depends on either a positive quantitative catheter culture yielding the same microorganism recovered from the bloodstream or differential quantitative blood cultures with significantly greater colony counts from blood drawn through the catheter than from blood drawn through a peripheral vein. Alternatively, probable catheter-related sepsis can be diagnosed when clinical sepsis is refractory to antimicrobial therapy but responds to catheter removal. Often these criteria are not met but catheter-related bloodstream infection is presumed because a common skin microorganism is isolated from the blood when clinical manifestations of bloodstream infection are present and there is no other apparent source of infection.

Microorganisms causing catheter-related bloodstream infection gain access to the bloodstream predominantly from either the catheter insertion site or the catheter hub. Most catheter-related infections occurring shortly after catheter insertion probably gain access to the bloodstream by extraluminal migration along the catheter from the skin at the catheter insertion site. When catheters are in place for extended periods, especially greater than 30 days, the catheter hub probably plays a major role in microorganisms gaining access and then migrating endoluminally until reaching the bloodstream.

Recently employed strategies for the prevention of catheter-related infections include topical antibiotics or antiseptics at the catheter insertion site, flush solutions containing vancomycin, and bonding antimicrobial agents to the catheter.

Infection of peripheral and central venous catheters generally resolves after catheter removal. For tunneled silicone catheters, most episodes of catheter-related infection can be initially managed with antimicrobial therapy infused through the catheter without catheter removal. *Staphylococcus aureus* is generally more aggressive and associated with more complications than coagulase-negative staphylococci. Microorganisms that usually require catheter removal include *Candida* and *Bacillus* species. Adjunctive treatments of catheter infections include the use of urokinase.

Catheter-related infection remains an important complication of vascular access. Novel prevention and treatment strategies are currently being investigated. In the near future bonding of antibiotics or other agents to catheters may become routine. It is hoped that these advances will significantly reduce the infection-related morbidity and mortality associated with the use of vascular catheters.

REFERENCES

1. Nystrom B, Larsen SO, Dankert J, et al: Bacteremia in surgical patients with intravenous devices: A European multicentre incidence study. The European Working Party on Control of Hospital Infections. *J Hosp Infect* 4:338–349, 1983.
2. Fuchs PC, Gustafson ME, King JT, et al: Assessment of catheter-associated infection risk with the Hickman right atrial catheter. *Infect Control* 5:227–230, 1984.
3. Begala JE, Maher K, Cherry JD: Risk of infection associated with the use of Broviac and Hickman catheters. *Assoc Pract Infect Control* 10:17–23, 1981.
4. Hansell DT, Park R, Jensen R, et al: Clinical significance and etiology of infected catheters used for total parenteral nutrition. *Surg Gynecol Obstet* 163:469–474, 1986.
5. King DR, Komer M, Hoffman J, et al: Broviac catheter sepsis: The natural history of an iatrogenic infection. *J Pediatr* 20:728–733, 1985.
6. Loeff DS, Matlak ME, Black RE, et al: Insertion of a small central venous catheter in neonates and young infants. *J Pediatr Surg* 17:944–949, 1982.
7. Sadiq HF, Devaskar S, Keenan WJ, et al: Broviac catheterization in low birth weight infants: Incidence and treatment of associated complications. *Crit Care Med* 15:47–50, 1987.
8. Warner BW, Gorgone P, Schilling S, et al: Multiple purpose central

venous access in infants less than 1000 grams. *J Pediatr Surg* 22:820–822, 1987.
9. Weber TR, West KW, Grosfeld JL: Broviac central venous catheterization in infants and children. *Am J Surg* 145:202–204, 1983.
10. Decker MD, Edwards KM: Central venous catheter infections. *Pediatr Clin North Am* 35:579–612, 1988.
11. Askenazi S, Mirelman D: Adherence of bacteria to pediatric intravenous catheters and needles and its relation to phlebitis in animals. *Pediatr Res* 18:1361–1366, 1984.
12. Maki DG, Goldmann DA, Rhames FS: Infection control in intravenous therapy. *Ann Intern Med* 79:867–887, 1973.
13. Stenzel JP, Green TP, Fuhrman BP, et al: Percutaneous femoral venous catheterizations: A prospective study of complications. *J Pediatr* 114:411–415, 1989.
14. Murr MM, Roslenquist MD, Lewis RW, et al: A prospective safety study of femoral vein versus nonfemoral vein catheterization in patients with burns. *J Burn Care Rehabil* 12:576–578, 1991.
15. Frank U, Daschner FD: Infections associated with intravascular devices, in Carlson RW, Geheb MA (eds): *Principles & Practice of Medical Intensive Care*. Philadelphia, WB Saunders, 1993, pp 601–608.
16. Broviac JW, Cole JJ, Scribner BH: A silicone rubber atrial catheter for prolonged parenteral alimentation. *Surg Gynecol Obstet* 136:602–606, 1973.
17. Hickman RO, Buckner CD, Clift RA, et al: A modified right atrial catheter for access to the venous system in marrow transplant recipients. *Surg Gynecol Obstet* 148:871–875, 1979.
18. Keohane PP, Jones BJM, Attrill H, et al: Effect of catheter tunnelling and a nutrition nurse on catheter sepsis during parenteral nutrition. A controlled trial. *Lancet* 2:1388–1390, 1983.
19. Tice AD, Bonstell RP, Marsh PK, et al: Peripherally inserted central venous catheters for outpatient intravenous antibiotic therapy. *Infect Dis Clin Pract* 2:186–190, 1993.
20. Severien C, Nelson JD: Frequency of infections associated with implanted systems vs cuffed, tunnelled silastic venous catheters in patients with acute leukemia. *Am J Dis Child* 145:1433–1438, 1991.
21. Golladay ES, Mollitt DL: Percutaneous placement of a venous access port in a pediatric patient population. *J Pediatr Surg* 21:683–684, 1986.
22. Pegelow CH, Narvaez M, Toledano SR, et al: Experience with a totally implantable venous device in children. *Am J Dis Child* 140:69–71, 1986.
23. Shulman RJ, Rahman S, Mahoney D, et al: A totally implanted venous access system used in pediatric patients with cancer. *J Clin Oncol* 5:137–140, 1987.
24. Becton DL, Kletzel M, Golladay ES, et al: An experience with an im-

plantable port system in 66 children with cancer. *Cancer* 61:376–378, 1988.
25. McDowell HP, Hart CA, Martin J: Implantable subcutaneous venous catheters. *Arch Dis Child* 61:1037–1038, 1986.
26. Lokich JJ, Bothe A, Benotti P, et al: Complicatoins and management of implanted venous access catheters. *J Clin Oncol* 3:710–717, 1985.
27. Bothe A, Piccione W, Ambrosino JJ, et al: Implantable central venous access system. *Am J Surg* 147:565–569, 1984.
28. Gyves J, Ensminger W, Niederhuber J, et al: Totally implanted system for intravenous chemotherapy in patients with cancer. *Am J Med* 73:841–845, 1982.
29. Brincker H, Saeter G: Fifty-five patient years' experience with a totally implanted system for intravenous chemotherapy. *Cancer* 57:1124–1129, 1986.
30. Strum S, McDermed J, Korn A, et al: Improved methods for venous access: The Port-A-Cath, a totally implanted catheter system. *J Clin Oncol* 4:596–603, 1986.
31. Starkhammar H, Bengtsson M: Totally implanted device for venous access. Experience in tumour patients. *Acta Radiol* 24:173–176, 1985.
32. Wurzel CL, Halom K, Feldman JG, et al: Infection rates of Broviac-Hickman catheters and implantable venous devices. *Am J Dis Child* 142:536–540, 1988.
33. Mirro J, Rao BN, Stokes DC, et al: A prospective study of Hickman/Broviac catheters and implantable ports in pediatric oncology patients. *J Clin Oncol* 7:214–222, 1989.
34. Mirro J, Rao BN, Kumar M, et al: A comparison of placement techniques and complications of externalized catheters and implantable port use in children with cancer. *J Pediatr Surg* 25:120–124, 1990.
35. Salzman MB, Isenberg HD, Shapiro JF, et al: A prospective study of the catheter hub as the portal of entry for microorganisms causing catheter-related sepsis in neonates. *J Infect Dis* 167:487–490, 1993.
36. Olson TA, Fischer GW, Lupo MC, et al: Antimicrobial therapy of Broviac catheter infections in pediatric hematology oncology patients. *J Pediatr Surg* 22:839–842, 1987.
37. Elting LS, Bodey GP: Septicemia due to *Xanthomonas* species and non-aeruginosa *Pseudomonas* species: Increasing incidence of catheter-related infections. *Medicine (Baltimore)* 69;2:96–306, 1990.
38. Riebel W, Frantz N, Adelstein D, et al: *Corynebacterium* JK. A cause of nosocomial device-related infection. *Rev Infect Dis* 8:42–49, 1986.
39. Raad II, Vartivarian S, Khan A, et al: Catheter-related infections caused by the *Mycobacterium fortuitum* complex: 15 cases and review. *Rev Infect Dis* 13:1120–1125, 1991.
40. Kiehn TE, Gorey E, Brown AE, et al: Sepsis due to *Rhodotorula* related to use of indwelling central venous catheters. *Clin Infect Dis* 14:841–846, 1992.

41. Raad II, Bodey GP: Infectious complications of indwelling vascular catheters. *Clin Infect Dis* 15:197–210, 1992.
42. Bone RC, Balk RA, Cerra FB, et al: Definitions for sepsis and organ failure and guidelines for the use of innovative therapies in sepsis. *Chest* 101:1644–1655, 1992.
43. Maki DG, Jarrett F, Sarafin HW: A semiquantitative method for identification of catheter-related infection in the burn patient. *J Surg Res* 22:513–520, 1977.
44. Maki DG, Weise CE, Sarafin HW: A semiquantitative method for identifying intravenous-catheter–related infection. *N Engl J Med* 296:1305–1309, 1977.
45. Collignon PG, Soni N, Pearson IY, et al: Is semiquantitative culture of central vein catheter tips useful in the diagnosis of catheter-associated bacteremia? *J Clin Microbiol* 24:532–535, 1986.
46. Moyer MA, Edwards LD, Farley L: Comparative culture methods on 101 intravenous catheters. *Arch Intern Med* 143:66–69, 1983.
47. Snydman DR, Murray SA, Kornfeld SJ, et al: Total parenteral nutrition–related infections: Prospective epidemiologic study using semiquantitative methods. *Am J Med* 73:695–699, 1982.
48. Cleri DJ, Corrado ML, Seligman SJ: Quantitative culture of intravenous catheters and other intravascular inserts. *J Infect Dis* 141:781–786, 1980.
49. Bjornson HS, Colley R, Bower RH, et al: Association between microorganism growth at the catheter insertion site and colonization of the catheter in patients receiving total parenteral nutrition. *Surgery* 92:720–726, 1982.
50. Brun-Buisson C, Abrouk F, Legrand P, et al: Diagnosis of central venous catheter–related sepsis: Critical level of quantitative tip cultures. *Arch Intern Med* 147:873–877, 1987.
51. Sherertz RJ, Raad II, Balaini A, et al: Three-year experience with sonicated vascular catheter cultures in a clinical microbiology laboratory. *J Clin Microbiol* 28:76–82, 1990.
52. Raad I, Costerton W, Sabharwal U, et al: Ultrastructural analysis of indwelling vascular catheters: A quantitative relationship between luminal colonization and duration of placement. *J Infect Dis* 168:400–407, 1993.
53. Sheretz RJ, Belani A, Rand KH: Relationship between sonication vascular catheter cultures and same day blood cultures (abstract 1132). Presented at the 26th Interscience Conference on Antimicrobial Agents and Chemotherapy, Washington, DC, American Society for Microbiology, 1986.
54. Cooper GL, Hopkins CC: Rapid diagnosis of intravascular catheter–associated infection by direct Gram staining of catheter segments. *N Engl J Med* 312:1142–1147, 1985.
55. Collignon P, Chan R, Munro R: Rapid diagnosis of intravascular catheter–related sepsis. *Arch Intern Med* 147:1609–1612, 1987.
56. Zuffrey J, Rime B, Franciou P, et al: Simple method for rapid diag

nosis of catheter-associated infection by direct acridine orange staining of catheter tips. *J Clin Microbiol* 26:175–177, 1988.
57. Armstrong CW, Mayhall CG, Miller KB, et al: Prospective study of catheter replacement and other risk factors for infection of hyperalimentation catheters. *J Infect* 154:808–816, 1986.
58. Pettigrew RA, Lang SDR, Haydock DA, et al: Catheter-related sepsis in patients on intravenous nutrition: A prospective study of quantitative catheter cultures and guidewire changes for suspected sepsis. *Br J Surg* 72:52–55, 1985.
59. Wing EJ, Norden CW, Shadduck RK, et al: Use of quantitative bacteriologic techniques to diagnose catheter-related sepsis. *Arch Intern Med* 139:482–483, 1979.
60. Flynn PM, Shenep JL, Barret FF: Differential quantitation with a commercial blood culture tube for diagnosis of catheter-related infection. *J Clin Microbiol* 26:1045–1046, 1988.
61. Raucher HS, Hyatt AC, Barzilai A, et al: Quantitative blood cultures in the evaluation of septicemia in children with Broviac catheters. *J Pediatr* 104:29–33, 1984.
62. Flynn PM, Shenep JL, Stokes DC, et al: In situ management of confirmed central venous catheter–related bacteremia. *Pediatr Infect Dis J* 6:729–734, 1987.
63. Mosca R, Curtas S, Forbes B, et al: The benefits of isolator cultures in the management of suspected catheter sepsis. *Surgery* 102:718–723, 1987.
64. Armstrong CW, Mayhall G, Miller KB, et al: Clinical predictors of infection of central venous catheters used for total parenteral nutrition. *Infect Control Hosp Epidemiol* 11:71–78, 1990.
65. Capdevila JA, Planes AM, Palomar M, et al: Value of differential quantitative blood cultures in the diagnosis of catheter-related sepsis. *Eur J Clin Microbiol Infect Dis* 11:403–407, 1992.
66. Crocker SH, Lowery BD, Eddy DO, et al: Pulmonary clearance of blood-borne bacteria. *Surg Gynecol Obstet* 153:845–851, 1981.
67. Capell S, Linares J, Stiges-Serra A: Catheter sepsis due to coagulase-negative staphylococci in patients on total parenteral nutrition. *Eur J Clin Microbiol* 5:40–42, 1987.
68. Stiges-Serra A, Puig P, Linares J, et al: Hub colonization as the initial step in an outbreak of catheter-related sepsis due to coagulase negative staphylococci during parenteral nutrition. *JPEN J Parenter Enteral Nutr* 8:668–672, 1984.
69. Stotter AT, Ward H, Waterfield AH, et al: Junctional care: The key to prevention of catheter sepsis in intravenous feeding. *JPEN J Parenter Enteral Nutr* 11:159–162, 1987.
70. Sandstedt S, Hesselvik F, Marklund T, et al: Percutaneous, tunneled silicone elastomer central venous catheters for total parenteral nutrition: Low sepsis and thrombosis rate. A prospective study of 315 catheters. *Nutrition* 5:23–26, 1989.
71. Stiges-Serra A, Linares J, Perez JL, et al: A randomized trial on the effect of tubing changes on hub contamination and catheter sepsis

during parenteral nutrition. *JPEN J Parenter Enteral Nutr* 9:322–325, 1985.

72. Maki DG, Rhame FS, Mackel DC, et al: Nationwide epidemic of septicemia caused by contaminated intravenous products: I: Epidemiologic and clinical features. *Am J Med* 60:471–485, 1976.
73. Felts SK, Schaffner W, Melly MA, et al: Sepsis caused by contaminated intravenous fluids: Epidemiologic, clinical, and laboratory investigation of an outbreak in one hospital. *Ann Intern Med* 77:881–890, 1972.
74. Stamm WE, Collella JJ, Anderson MS, et al: Indwelling arterial catheters as a source of nosocomial bacteremia: An outbreak caused by *Flavobacterium* species. *N Engl J Med* 292:1099–1102, 1975.
75. Holmes CJ, Allwood MC: The microbial contamination of intravenous infusions during clinical use. *J Appl Bacteriol* 46:247–257, 1979.
76. Henderson DK: Bacteremia due to percutaneous intravascular devices, in Mandell GL, Douglas RG, Bennett JE: *Principles and Practice of Infectious Diseases*, ed 3. New York, Churchill Livingstone, 1990, pp 2189–2199.
77. Crocker KS, Noga R, Filibeck DG, et al: Microbial growth comparisons of five commercial parenteral lipid emulsions. *JPEN J Parenter Enteral Nutr* 8:391–395, 1984.
78. Jarvis WR, Highsmith AK: Bacterial growth and endotoxin production in lipid emulsion. *J Clin Microbiol* 19:17–20, 1984.
79. Dankner WM, Spector SA, Fierer J: *Malassezia* fungemia in neonates and adults: Complications of hyperalimentation. *Rev Infect Dis* 9:743–837, 1987.
80. Plouffe JF, Brown DG, Silva J, et al: Nosocomial outbreak of *Candida parapsilosis* fungemia related to intravenous infusions. *Arch Intern Med* 137:1686–1689, 1977.
81. Solomon SL, Khabbaz RF, Parker RH, et al: An outbreak of *Candida parapsilosis* bloodstream infections in patients receiving parenteral nutrition. *J Infect Dis* 149:98–102, 1984.
82. Kovalevich DS, Faubion WC, Bender JM, et al: Association of parenteral nutrition catheter sepsis with urinary tract infections. *JPEN J Parenter Enteral Nutr* 10:639–641, 1986.
83. Anaissie EJ, Raad I, Samonis G, et al: Universal colonization of central venous catheters (CVCs) and low risk of hematogenous seeding (abstract 1063). Presented at the 31st Interscience Conference on Antimicrobial Agents and Chemotherapy. Washington, DC, American Society for Microbiology, 1991.
84. Maki DG: Nosocomial bacteremia: An epidemiologic overview. *Am J Med* 70:719–732, 1981.
85. Bjornson HS, Colley R, Bower RH, et al: Association between microorganism growth at the catheter insertion site and colonization of the catheter in patients receiving total parenteral nutrition. *Surgery* 92:720–727, 1982.

86. Vaudaux P, Pittet D, Haeberli A, et al: Host factors selectively increase staphylococcal adherence on inserted catheters: A role for fibronectin and fibrinogen or fibrin. *J Infect Dis* 160:865–875, 1989.
87. Russell PB, Kline J, Yoder MC, et al: Staphylococcal adherence to polyvinyl chloride and heparin-bonded polyurethane catheters is species dependent and enhanced by fibronectin. *J Clin Microbiol* 25:1083–1087, 1987.
88. Lopes JD, Dos Reis M, Brentani RR: Presence of laminin receptors in *Staphylococcus aureus*. *Science* 229:275–277, 1985.
89. Holderbaum D, Spech RA, Ehrhart LA: Specific binding sites of collagen to *Staphylococcus aureus*. *Coll Relat Res* 5:261–271, 1985.
90. Goldmann DA: Coagulase-negative staphylococci: Interplay of epidemiology and bench research. *Am J Infect Control* 18:211–221, 1990.
91. Peters G, Locci R, Pulverer G: Adherence and growth of coagulase-negative staphylococci on surfaces of intravenous catheters. *J Infect Dis* 146:479–482, 1982.
92. Ishak MA, Groschel DHM, Mandell GL, et al: Association of slime with pathogenicity of coagulase-negative staphylococci causing nosocomial septicemia. *J Clin Microbiol* 22:1025–1029, 1985.
93. Sheth NK, Franson TR, Rose HD, et al: Colonization of bacteria on polyvinyl chloride and Teflon intravascular catheters in hospitalized patients. *J Clin Microbiol* 18:1061–1063, 1983.
94. Raad I, Gilbreath J, Suleiman N, et al: Maximal sterile barriers (MSB) during the insertion of central venous catheters (CVC) for the prevention of infection (abstract 22). Presented at the Third Annual Meeting of The Society for Hospital Epidemiology of America, Chicago, 1993.
95. Maki DG, Ringer M, Alvarado CJ: Prospective randomised trial of povidone-iodine, alcohol, and chlorhexidine for prevention of infection associated with central venous and arterial catheters. *Lancet* 338:339–343, 1991.
96. Jakobsen CJB, Grabe N, Damm MD: A trial of povidone-iodine for prevention of contamination of intravenous cannulae. *Acta Anaesthesiol Scand* 30:447–449, 1986.
97. Hill RLR, Fisher AP, Ware RJ, et al: Mupirocin for the reduction of colonization of internal jugular cannulae—a randomized controlled trial. *J Hosp Infect* 15:311–321, 1990.
98. Maki DG, Band JD: A comparative study of polyantibiotic and iodophor ointments in prevention of vascualr catheter–related infection. *Am J Med* 70:739–744, 1981.
99. Levin A, Mason AJ, Jindal KK, et al: The value of topical povidone-iodine (PV-I) ointment in the prevention of hemodialysis related sepsis (abstract 1078). Presented at the 29th Interscience Conference on Antimicrobial Agents and Chemotherapy. Washington, DC, American Society for Microbiology, 1989.
100. Conly JM, Grieves K, Peters B: A prospective, randomized study com-

paring transparent and dry gauze dressings for central venous catheters. *J Infect Dis* 159:310–319, 1989.
101. Craven DE, Lichtenberg DA, Kunches LM, et al: A randomized study comparing a transparent polyurethane dressing to a dry gauze dressing for peripheral intravenous catheter sites. *Infect Control* 6:361–366, 1985.
102. Maki DG, Ringer M: Evaluation of dressing regimens for prevention of infection with peripheral intravenous catheters. Gauze, a transparent polyurethane dressing, and an iodophor-transparent dressing. *JAMA* 258:2396–2403, 1987.
103. Maki DG, Cobb L, Garman JK, et al: An attachable silver-impregnated cuff for prevention of infection with central venous catheters: A prospective randomized multicenter trial. *Am J Med* 85:307–314, 1988.
104. Flowers RH III, Schwenzer KJ, Kopel RF, et al: Efficacy of an attachable subcutaneous cuff for the prevention of intravascular catheter–related infection. *JAMA* 261:878–883, 1989.
105. Josephson A, Gombert ME, Sierra MF, et al: The relationship between intravenous fluid contamination and the frequency of tubing replacement. *Infect Control* 6:367–370, 1985.
106. Buxton AE, Highsmith AK, Garner JS, et al: Contamination of intravenous infusion fluid: Effects of changing administration sets. *Ann Intern Med* 90:764–768, 1979.
107. Band JD, Maki DG: Safety of changing intravenous delivery systems at longer than 24-hour intervals. *Ann Intern Med* 91:173–178, 1979.
108. Snydman DR, Reidy MD, Perry LK, et al: Safety of changing intravenous (IV) administration sets containing burettes at longer than 48 hour intervals. *Infect Control* 8:113–116, 1987.
109. Maki DG, Boiticelli JT, LeRoy ML, et al: Prospective study of replacing administration sets for intravenous therapy at 48 vs. 72 hour intervals: 72 hours is safe and cost-effective. *JAMA* 258:1777–1781, 1987.
110. Bozzetti F, Terno G, Bonfanti G, et al: Prevention and treatment of central venous catheter sepsis by exchange via a guidewire. A prospective controlled trial. *Ann Surg* 198:48–52, 1983.
111. Gregory JA, Schiller WR: Subclavian catheter changes every third day in high risk patients. *Am Surg* 51:534–536, 1985.
112. Powell C, Kudsk KA, Kulich PA, et al: Effect of frequent guidewire changes on triple-lumen catheter sepsis. *JPEN J Parenter Enteral Nutr* 12:464–465, 1988.
113. Cobb DK, High KP, Sawyer RG, et al: A controlled trial of scheduled replacement of central venous and pulmonary-artery catheters. *N Engl J Med* 327:1062–1068, 1992.
114. Hilton E, Haslett TM, Borenstein MT, et al: Central catheter infections: Single- versus triple-lumen catheters. Influence of guide wires on infection rates when used for replacement of catheters. *Am J Med* 84:667–672, 1988.

115. Gaillard JL, Merlino R, Pajot N, et al: Conventional and nonconventional modes of vancomycin administration to decontaminate the internal surface of catheters colonized with coagulase-negative staphylococci. *JPEN J Parenter Enteral Nutr* 14:593–597, 1990.
116. Schwartz C, Hendrickson KJ, Roghmann K, et al: Prevention of bacteremia attributed to luminal colonization of tunneled central venous catheters with vancomycin-susceptible organisms. *J Clin Oncol* 8:1591–1597, 1990.
117. Hendrickson KJ, Dunne WM Jr: Modification of central venous catheter flush solution improves in vitro antimicrobial activity (letter). *J Infect Dis* 166:944–946, 1992.
118. Elliott TSJ, Curran A: Effects of heparin and chlorbutol on bacterial colonization of intravascular cannulae in an in vitro model. *J Hosp Infect* 14:193–200, 1989.
119. Mermel LA, Stolz SM, Maki DG: Surface antimicrobial activity of heparin-bonded and antiseptic-impregnated vascular catheters. *J Infect Dis* 167:920–924, 1993.
120. Root JL, McIntyre OR, Jacobs NJ, et al: Inhibitory effect of disodium EDTA upon the growth of *Staphylococcus epidermidis* in vitro: Relation to infection prophylaxis of Hickman catheters. *Antimicrob Agents Chemother* 32:1627–1631, 1988.
121. Wiernikowski JT, Elder-Thornley D, Dawson S, et al: Bacterial colonization of tunneled right atrial catheters in pediatric oncology: A comparison of sterile saline and bacteriostatic saline flush solutions. *Am J Pediatr Hematol Oncol* 13:137–140, 1991.
122. Maki DG, Wheller SJ, Stolz SM, et al: Clinical trial of a novel antiseptic central venous catheter (abstract 461). Presented at the 31st Interscience Conference on Antimicrobial Agents and Chemotherapy, Washington, DC, American Society for Microbiology, 1991.
123. Kamal GD, Pfaller MA, Rempe LE, et al: Reduced intravascular catheter infection by antibiotic bonding. A prospective, randomized, controlled trial. *JAMA* 265:2364–2368, 1991.
124. Sherertz RJ, Carruth WA, Hampton AA, et al: Efficacy of antibiotic-coated catheters in preventing subcutaneous *Staphylococcus aureus* infection in rabbits. *J Infect Dis* 167:98–106, 1993.
125. Bayston R, Grove N, Siegel J, et al: Prevention of hydrocephalus shunt catheter colonisation in vitro by impregnation with antimicrobials. *J Neurol Neurosurg Psychiatry* 52:605–609, 1989.
126. Farber BF, Wolff AG: The use of nonsteroidal antiinflammatory drugs to prevent adherence of *Staphylococcus epidermidis* to medical polymers. *J Infect Dis* 166:861–865, 1992.
127. Jansen B, Kristinsson KG, Jansen S, et al: In-vitro efficacy of a central venous catheter complexed with iodine to prevent bacterial colonization. *J Antimicrob Chemother* 30:135–139, 1992.
128. Salzman MB, Isenberg HD, Rubin LG: Use of disinfectants to reduce microbial contamination of hubs of vascular catheters. *J Clin Microbiol* 31:475–479, 1993.

129. Regelmann WE, Mills EL, Quie PG: Immunology of the newborn, in Feigen RD, Cherry JD: *Textbook of Pediatric Infectious Diseases*, ed 2. Philadelphia, WB Saunders, 1987, pp 921–939.
130. Klein JF, Shahrivar F: Use of percutaneous Silastic central venous catheters in neonates and the management of infectious complications. *Am J Perinatol* 9:261–264, 1992.
131. Ingram I, Weitzman S, Greenberg ML, et al: Complications of indwelling venous access lines in the pediatric hematology patients: A prospective comparison of external venous catheters and subcutaneous ports. *Am J Pediatr Hematol Oncol* 13:130–136, 1991.
132. Pizzo PA, Hathorn JW, Hiemenz J, et al: A randomized trial comparing combination antibiotic therapy to monotherapy in cancer patients with fever and neutropenia. *N Engl J Med* 315:552–558, 1986.
133. Huijgens PC, Ossenkoppele GJ, Weijers TF, et al: Imipenem-cilastatin for empirical therapy in neutropenic patients with fever: An open study in patients with hematologic malignancies. *Eur J Haematol* 46:42–46, 1991.
134. Pizzo PA, Rubin M, Freifeld A, et al: The child with cancer and infection. I. Empiric therapy for fever and neutropenia, and preventive strategies. *J Pediatr* 119:679–694, 1991.
135. Rubin LG, Tucci V, Cercenado E, et al: Vancomycin-resistant *Enterococcus faecium* in hospitalized children. *Infect Control Hosp Epidemiol* 13:700–705, 1992.
136. Wang EEL, Prober CG, Ford-Jones L, et al: The management of central intravenous catheter infections. *Pediatr Infect Dis J* 3:110–113, 1984.
137. Hiemenz J, Skelton J, Pizzo PA: Perspective on the management of catheter-related infections in cancer patients. *Pediatr Infect Dis J* 5:6–11, 1986.
138. Hampton AA, Sherertz RJ, et al: Vascular-access infections in hospitalized patients. *Surg Clin North Am* 68:57–71, 1988.
139. Raad I, Davis S, Khan A: Catheter removal affects recurrence of catheter-related coagulase-negative staphylococci bacteremia (CRCNSB). *Infect Control Hosp Epidemiol* 13:215–221, 1992.
140. Dugdale DC, Ramsey PG: *Staphylococcus aureus* bacteremia in patients wtih Hickman catheters. *Am J Med* 89:137–141, 1990.
141. Raad I, Narro J, Khan A, et al: Serious complications of vascular catheter–related *Staphylococcus aureus* bacteremia in cancer patients. *Eur J Clin Microbiol Infect Dis* 11:675–682, 1992.
142. Raad II, Sabbagh MF: Optimal duration of therapy for catheter-related *Staphylococcus aureus* bacteremia: A study of 55 cases and review. *Rev Infect Dis* 14:75–82, 1992.
143. Jernigan JA, Farr BM: Short-course therapy of catheter-related *Staphylococcus aureus* bacteremia: A meta-analysis. *Ann Intern Med* 119:304–311, 1993.

144. Benezra D, Kiehn TE, Gold GWM, et al: Prospective study of infections in indwelling central venous catheters using quantitative blood cultures. *Am J Med* 85:495–498, 1988.
145. Abrahm JL, Mullen JL: A prospective study of prolonged central venous access in leukemia. *JAMA* 248:2868–2873, 1982.
146. Darbyshire PJ, Weightman NC, Speller DCE: Problems associated with indwelling central venous catheters. *Arch Dis Child* 60:129–134, 1985.
147. Prince A, Heller B, Levy J, et al: Management of fever in patients with central vein catheters. *Pediatr Infect Dis* 5:20–24, 1986.
148. Shapiro ED, Wald ER, Nelson KA, et al: Broviac catheter–related bacteremia in oncology patients. *Am J Dis Child* 136:679–681, 1982.
149. Eppes SC, Troutman JL, Gutman LT, et al: Outcome of treatment of candidemia in children whose central catheters were removed or retained. *Pediatr Infect Dis J* 8:99–104, 1989.
150. Newman K, Tenney J, Reed W, et al: Infectious and non-infectious complications of Hickman catheters (abstract 345). Presented at the 27th Interscience Conference on Antimicrobial Agents and Chemotherapy, Washington, DC, American Society for Microbiology, 1987.
151. Dato VM, Dajani AS: Candidemia in children wtih central venous catheters: Role of catheter removal and amphotericin B therapy. *Pediatr Infect Dis J* 9:309–314, 1990.
152. Leibovitz E, Iuster-Reicher A, Amitai M, et al: Systemic candidal infections associated with use of peripheral venous catheters in neonates: A 9-year experience. *Clin Infect Dis* 14:485–491, 1992.
153. Edwards JE, Filler SG: Current strategies for treating invasive candidiasis: Emphasis on infections in nonneutropenic patients. *Clin Infect Dis* 14(suppl):106–110, 1992.
154. Banerjee C, Bustamante CI, Wharton R, et al: Bacillus infections in patients with cancer. *Arch Intern Med* 148:1769–1774, 1988.
155. Cotton DJ, Gill VJ, Marshall DJ, et al: Clinical features and therapeutic interventions in 17 cases of *Bacillus* bacteremia in an immunocompromised patient population. *J Clin Microbiol* 25:672–674, 1987.
156. Newman KA, Reed WP, Bustamante CI, et al: Venous access devices utilized in association with intensive cancer chemotherapy. *Eur J Cancer Clin Oncol* 25:1375–1378, 1989.
157. Flynn PM, Hooser BV, Gigliotti F: Atypical mycobacterial infections of Hickman catheter exit sites. *Pediatr Infect Dis J* 7:510–513, 1988.
158. Jones GR, Konsler GK, Dunaway RP, et al: Prospective analysis of urokinase in the treatment of catheter sepsis in pediatric hematology-oncology patients. *J Pediatr Surg* 28:350–357, 1993.
159. Fishbein JD, Friedman HS, Bennett BB, et al: Catheter-related sepsis refractory to antibiotics treated with adjunctive urokinase infusion. *Pediatr Infect Dis J* 9:676–678, 1990.
160. Worthley LIG: Treatment of central venous Silastic catheter infec-

tions using hydrochloric acid. *Anaesth Intensive Care* 10:314–318, 1982.
161. Kropec A, Huebner J, Frank U, et al: In vitro activity of sodium bisulfite and heparin against staphylococci: New strategies in the treatment of catheter-related infection. *J Infect Dis* 168:235–237, 1993.

Superantigens and Their Role in Infectious Disease

Rosana Schafer, Ph.D.
Research Instructor, Department of Microbiology and Immunology, West Virginia University School of Medicine, Morgantown, West Virginia

James M. Sheil, Ph.D.
Assistant Professor, Department of Microbiology and Immunology, West Virginia University School of Medicine, Morgantown, West Virginia

Although the term *superantigen* is a relatively recent addition to the scientific literature, these proteins have been studied unwittingly for over 20 years. Superantigens comprise a unique class of proteins characterized chiefly by their ability to (1) bind to the external distal surface of class II major histocompatibility complex (MHC) molecules and (2) interact with the T-cell receptor (TCR) via the variable portion of its β chain (TCR-V_β). The limited number of TCR-V_β domains available in humans and mice, the two principal species in which superantigens have been studied, thus results in activation of a large number of T lymphocytes—all of which express the same TCR-V_β domain. Whereas a particular conventional foreign antigen usually stimulates far less than 1% (generally ranging from $1{:}10^4$ to $1{:}10^6$) of all T cells, a superantigen protein is able to stimulate up to 20% to 30% of T cells found in an individual's peripheral T-cell repertoire.[1] It is for this reason that such proteins were originally designated "superantigens."

Our first concept of what was later to be defined as a "superantigen" originated from the curious observation in mice that cells from two individuals of histocompatible mouse strains (i.e., identical at the MHC) could elicit a rather strong T-cell response—much like that observed in the classic studies on T-cell–mediated alloreactivity in response to differences within the MHC. To distinguish the two responses, investigators attributed the former response to "minor lymphocyte stimulating" (Mls) antigens.[2] This functional Mls designation thus referred to an unknown entity on the cell surface of MHC-compatible individuals from certain mouse strains that could elicit strong T-cell–mediated responsiveness. Initially a limited focus of interest developed among several immunologists to examine this phenomenon in the context of the current immunology dogma at that time. Most other immunologists (and surely scientists from other disciplines) largely ignored or avoided their esoteric research endeavors inasmuch as it appeared that the immunology of Mls antigens became more confused as more and more research findings in this area were forthcoming. Nevertheless, certain important findings have emerged from these early studies on Mls immunology, and they have helped to lay the groundwork for our more recently derived understanding of superantigens and their relevance to human disease.

Several important characteristics of superantigens distinguish them from conventional foreign antigens that stimulate antigen-specific, MHC-restricted T lymphocytes. Although superantigens bind to MHC molecules like foreign antigen peptides, they apparently are not accommodated within the peptide-binding cleft on the distal surface of the molecule.[3] Indeed, it appears that superantigens do not need to be processed either for efficient MHC binding or for interaction with the TCR-V_β domain.[4] In addition, although superantigen binding to MHC proteins has been well substantiated for class II MHC molecules expressed only by certain specialized antigen-presenting cells, they have yet to be found in association with the class I MHC proteins expressed on the cell surface of most cells.[5] Unlike the conventional antigenic peptide/MHC complex that is important for recognition of foreign peptide antigens, a superantigen bound to a class II MHC molecule contacts the solvent-exposed surface of the TCR-V_β region,[6] thereby stimulating nearly all T lymphocytes that express the particular target TCR-V_β component. At the present time, two general classes of superantigens are known and have been well characterized: viral superantigens and bacterial superantigens.

VIRAL SUPERANTIGENS

The endogenous viral superantigens are perhaps best represented by those of the mouse mammary tumor virus (MMTV), which is found in essentially all inbred mouse strains. The MMTV superantigens are proteins encoded within the open reading frame (ORF) of the 3′ long terminal repeat (LTR) region of the integrated retroviral genome. It is now recognized that these viral superantigens are in fact responsible for the Mls-induced activation of T lymphocytes discussed previously (reviewed by Scherer et al.[7]).

Studies leading to our understanding that these endogenous viral superantigens are associated with the activation of certain subsets of T lymphocytes were advanced by the development of monoclonal antibodies specific for the variable domain on the β chain (V_β) of the TCR. These monoclonal antibodies can distinguish among approximately 20 different classes of TCRs in mice[8] based on their expression of unique TCR-V_β sequences. As discussed earlier, the murine Mls antigens were the first endogenous superantigens and are characterized by their capacity for strongly stimulating T-lymphocyte proliferation *in vitro*.[2] For many years, however, the biological basis for the strong T-cell proliferative response to Mls antigens could only be conjectured, and the presence of these antigens in mice remained an interesting phenomenon for which no counterpart in humans could be demonstrated. With the availability of a variety of murine TCR-V_β–specific monoclonal antibodies, however, the physiologic impact of these endogenous superantigens became clear.

Several groups initially demonstrated that certain TCR-V_β–bearing subsets of T lymphocytes were absent from the mature peripheral T-cell repertoire in Mls-positive murine strains. Among the earliest observations in this regard came from studies by both Kappler et al.[9] and MacDonald et al.[10] in which it was demonstrated that mice carrying the Mls-1^a gene had specifically deleted those T cells bearing V_β8.1 and V_β6 TCRs from their peripheral T-cell repertoire. This observation suggested that the Mls-1^a antigen might preferentially stimulate all T cells that expressed either the V_β8.1 or V_β6 domains on the β chain of their TCRs. Accordingly, mice that express Mls-1^a as an endogenous antigen may have become self-tolerant to this antigen through a process known as "clonal deletion," which occurs during thymocyte maturation within the thymus. To demonstrate the validity of this hypothesis it should also hold that whereas immature thymocytes would express all available TCR subsets, selection of the mature T-cell repertoire during thymocyte maturation should result in deletion of those T lymphocytes that react with the Mls-1^a self-antigen. Kappler et al.[9] demonstrated that indeed, V_β8.1-positive T lymphocytes were present among immature (CD4+, CD8+) thymocytes but were absent from mature (CD4+/CD8− and CD4−/CD8+) thymocyte populations. Thus it was determined that the induction of self-tolerance in Mls-1^a–positive mice is a consequence of the absence of T cells reactive to this antigen as a result of clonal deletion during their maturation within the thymus. Subsequent studies showed that V_β7- and V_β9-expressing T lymphocytes also interact with this endogenous superantigen.[11–13] It is now clear that a variety of Mls antigens exist in mice and their expression as endogenous superantigens results in the deletion of different V_β-expressing T-cell subsets.[14]

For nearly 20 years the term "Mls antigen" remained an ill-defined functional designation referring to some unknown entity in mice that could stimulate large numbers of T lymphocytes as measured by *in vitro* proliferation assays. Although for some time it had been suggested that the Mls loci might be genetically linked to certain proviral integrants of MMTV, firm evidence for a genetic linkage of this sort proved extremely difficult to obtain. In 1991, three groups independently solved this riddle by demonstrating that the Mls loci are genetically indistinguishable from endogenous MMTV loci, thereby proving that the functionally ascribed Mls antigens are encoded by these MMTV retroviral genes.[15–17] These studies showing a perfect genetic linkage between Mls loci and MMTV loci were further reinforced by the results of a concurrent study that demonstrated a clear association of Mls loci with endogenous MMTV protein expression.[18] These latter investigators showed that in neonatal C3H mice to which a milk-borne MMTV had been transmitted from the mother, V_β14-expressing T cells were specifically deleted in accordance with their reactivity with the MMTV superantigen. Shortly afterward it was further demonstrated that the MMTV superantigen is encoded by an ORF from the 3′ LTR segment of the MMTV genome[19] and mice made transgenic for this ORF gene clonally delete the V_β14-expressing T cells that are specific for this endogenous MMTV superantigen. Thus, taken together, these studies conclusively established that the ambiguously defined Mls antigens are identical to the MMTV superantigens encoded by the ORF region from the 3′ LTR of the integrated MMTV provirus.

All endogenous viral superantigens identified to date are derived from these MMTV provirus integrants. They are glycosylated, type II transmembrane proteins in which the carboxyl terminus is situated outside the cell as opposed to most transmembrane proteins, which are type I with the COOH terminus oriented in the cytoplasm. These viral superantigens are highly conserved except for the carboxy terminal 20 to 30 amino acids, which also accounts for the differences in $TCRV_\beta$ specificity of the various viral superantigens types. Each viral superantigen can be classified into one of five families based on the sequence similarity of this carboxy terminal region and their V_β specificity. Studies on the interaction between the viral superantigen vSAG7 and the TCR-V_β8.2 domain have identified V_β residues 17 or 18, 22, 70, and 71 as important for superantigen binding.[20, 21] Similar findings have been reported by Cazenave and coworkers[22] for $V_{\beta}17$ binding to MMTV superantigen. According to the model of TCR structure based on its similarity to immunoglobulin,[23] these residues would lie on the solvent-exposed face of the TCR, oriented away from the TCR-binding site for MHC/peptide and close to the V_{β} site used for interacting with bacterial superantigens. This suggestion is supported by a study with mutant $V_{\beta}8.2$ chains in which their inability to bind viral superantigens fails to alter their interaction with conventional antigenic peptides plus MHC.[21]

Given that these superantigens have been found in association with class II MHC molecules but not with class I MHC proteins, it was initially suspected that CD4+ T cells but not CD8+ T lymphocytes would be stimulated by them. However, it soon became clear that both CD4+/CD8− and CD4−/CD8+ T cells could interact with these superantigens, provided that the cell demonstrated TCR expression of the appropriate V_{β} domain. This suggests that the binding of superantigens to class II MHC molecules, particularly the interaction of these superantigen/class II MHC complexes with the TCR-V_{β} domains, is of sufficiently high avidity to supersede any additional requirement for the CD4 or CD8 coreceptors to bind to the class II or class I MHC molecules respectively, as is found necessary for T-cell responses to conventional peptide antigens.[24] This suggestion is supported by the findings of Kappler and coworkers[9] in which the Mls-1^{a}–responsive $V_{\beta}8.1$ T-cell subset was deleted from both mature CD4+/CD8− and CD4−/CD8+ T lymphocytes.

Other viruses have been shown to encode exogenous superantigens similar to the endogenous superantigens encoded by MMTV. These viral superantigens include the nucleocapsid protein of rabies virus[25] and the *gag* protein from Moloney murine leukemia virus.[26] It has also been proposed that in human immunodeficiency virus (HIV) infection an HIV-encoded viral superantigen may be largely responsible for the devastating effects caused by the loss of CD4+ T lymphocytes throughout the course of the disease.[27]

EXOGENOUS BACTERIAL SUPERANTIGENS

The most well-characterized bacterial sources of superantigens are from gram-positive *Streptococcus* and *Staphylococcus* species. Unlike the viral superantigens, these toxins have been well characterized and studied for quite some time. Recently the structure of staphylococcal enterotoxin B (SEB) has been resolved by x-ray crystallography.[28] The strong T-cell stimulatory capacity of these toxins has been recognized for a long time,[29, 30] but only in recent years has it been recognized that these toxins serve as superantigens by binding to class II MHC molecules on antigen-presenting cells and interacting with TCRs by binding to their V_β domain.[31, 32] *Staphylococcus aureus* is a common human pathogen that produces a variety of enterotoxins with superantigen properties designated SEA through SEE. These toxins are largely noted for their role in causing food poisoning as well as shock in humans; some strains of *S. aureus* produce toxic shock syndrome toxin 1 (TSST-1), which is associated with toxic shock syndrome (TSS), as well as exfoliative toxin (ExFT), which is involved in scalded skin syndrome. The group A streptococcus *Streptococcus pyogenes* is also well known for producing superantigen toxins. These streptococcal pyrogenic exotoxins, designated SPE-A through SPE-C, have also been referred to as streptococcal erythrogenic toxins or scarlet fever toxins and play a role in scarlet fever and severe toxic shock–like symptoms associated with group A streptococcal infections.

The overall structures of streptococcal and staphylococcal enterotoxins are similar in that they are globular, compact proteins ranging from 24 to 30 kDa; in keeping with their enteric acquisition, they are relatively resistant to digestion through proteolytic cleavage. In their role as superantigen toxins, they function largely as intact proteins, although limited proteolytic cleavage has been found to be accommodated without affecting their function.[33, 34] For example, cleavage of a prominent intrachain disulfide loop does not appear to alter the superantigen properties of SEB toxin, which corresponds to the location of this disulfide linkage on the side of the protein molecule distant from the presumed sites for binding to class II MHC molecules and TCR-V_β domains.[28]

Although many of the staphylococcal and streptococcal enterotoxins are similar in their primary amino acid sequences, other toxins show greater amino acid differences. Regardless of these differences, however, all superantigen toxins share the common properties of binding to multiple class II MHC molecules and activating T lymphocytes through their interaction with TCR-V_β domains. In general, the different V_β specificities correlate well with differences in amino acid sequences among these toxins; thus those toxins with similar V_β specificities are more closely similar in their primary amino acid sequences.[31, 35, 36]

Recent studies using point mutants of SEB have defined the regions of this superantigen that are important for binding to class II MHC molecules and for interacting with TCR-V_β domains.[37] In general, SEB residues toward the NH_2 terminus of the protein, which comprises three distinct regions, influence MHC class II binding as well as TCR-V_β interactions. The region encompassing residues 41 to 53 is important for MHC class II binding, and a two–amino acid region (residues 60 and 61) is critical for TCR-V_β interaction. Kappler and coworkers conclude in this study that a third region (from residues 9 to 23) is also important for both superantigen properties. A highly conserved asparagine residue in position 23 of this region appears to be a critical TCR-V_β–interacting residue. Out of five SEB mutants altered at this position, four were unimpeded in binding to class II HLA-DR molecules but failed to stimulate T lymphocytes of the $V_\beta7$ subset; only one mutant (containing an Asn→Ser substitution) was less effective in binding to class II HLA-DR molecules. Although the authors conclude that this indicates a predominant effect on TCR-V_β interaction, it is also possible that any change in this residue could alter the conformation of binding to HLA-DR without affecting the intensity of binding; this could be seen as an indirect effect on V_β interaction by rendering this site on the SEB protein less accessible to binding with the V_β domain. When these results are interpreted on the basis of the recently described SEB x-ray crystal structure,[28] one can easily discern two noncontiguous sites on SEB for MHC class II binding that are located on the same face of the molecule. The TCR-V_β–binding site is composed of residues, perhaps from both the NH_2 and COOH terminal regions, that form a single shallow cleft. Similar studies to assess the important residues of SEA and SEE showed roughly similar characteristics[38–40] for residues important in TCR-V_β interaction and class II MHC binding. Of interest, however, is that certain histidine residues in the carboxy terminal portion of both SEA and SEE (but not SEB) are critical for class II MHC binding. Binding of SEA and SEE also requires the participation of a zinc ion,[41] and an additional histidine residue in the HLA-DR β chain appears to be necessary for the stability of zinc binding and subsequent SEA/SEE interaction with the class II MHC molecule.[42, 43]

An important concern in considering how these bacterial superantigens might mediate their effects in disease pathogenesis focuses on their principal action of binding to specific TCR-V_β domains, thereby stimulating up to 20% to 30% of T lymphocytes expressing the same V_β domain. With this magnitude of T-cell stimulation, these activated T lymphocytes will subsequently be triggered to produce large quantities of interleukins (i.e., IL-2, IL-4, IL-6, and others), as well as other cytokines, including tumor necrosis factor α (TNF-α), interferon-γ (IFN-γ), and others. Thus it is likely that the disease pathology associated with various bacterial infections involving release of such toxins reflects the massive effects of these inflammatory mediators rather than the toxins themselves.

SUPERANTIGENS IN HUMAN DISEASE

The role of exogenous bacterial toxins in the pathology of disease has long been recognized. It is also now known that several of these toxins act as superantigens. The most common among these are staphylococcal enterotoxins and exotoxins of streptococci, which have been associated with gastrointestinal food poisoning and shock-like syndromes. More recently, with advances in understanding the mechanism of activation of specific T cells by superantigens and the subsequent cellular responses, their potential role in a number of acute and chronic diseases is being investigated.

KAWASAKI SYNDROME

Kawasaki disease is an acute multisystem vasculitis that afflicts children worldwide. It is normally a self-limited disease characterized by fever, rash, conjunctivitis, cervical lymphadenopathy, inflammation of mucous membranes, and erythema of the hands and feet.[44] However, complications such as coronary artery aneurysms and ectasia can develop in some patients, which makes Kawasaki disease a major cause of acquired heart disease in children in the United States.[44] The cause of Kawasaki disease is unknown, although because of epidemiologic factors the causative agent is believed to be an infectious agent.[44]

The effects of Kawasaki disease on the immune system have been reviewed by Leung and Abe et al.[45, 46] and include activation of T lymphocytes and macrophages with a concomitant increase in the production of a number of inflammatory cytokines including IL-1β, TNF-α, IL-2, IL-6, and IFN-γ.[45] These features of Kawasaki disease are remarkably similar to those seen after stimulation with bacterial superantigens as discussed earlier. Consequently, the expansion of particular V_β subsets of T cells and the presence of toxin-secreting bacteria have been studied in patients with Kawasaki disease.

Abe et al.[46] determined the TcR-V_β expression of T cells in the peripheral blood of patients in the acute and convalescent stages of Kawasaki disease. Using quantitative polymerase chain reaction (PCR) and immunofluorescense they found a significant increase in the expression of $V_\beta2$- and $V_\beta8.1$-bearing T cells in several patients with acute Kawasaki disease. This difference was not seen in patients in the convalescent phase of disease or in healthy controls. These results were confirmed, and it was further determined that the $V_\beta 2+$ T cells were expanded in a polyclonal manner with extensive junctional region diversity.[47] This is similar to what is seen after the stimulation of T cells with superantigens. These studies suggest a role for superantigens in T-cell activation and expansion during Kawasaki disease.

Further evidence for a bacterial superantigen in Kawasaki disease has been provided by a recent study by Leung et al.[48] in which bacteria that produced toxins were cultured from 13 of 16 patients with acute Kawasaki disease. A new clone of *S. aureus* that produced TSST-1 and group A streptococci that produced SPE-B and SPE-C were isolated. These bacterial toxins can stimulate T cells expressing $V_\beta 2$ or $V_\beta 8$, the subsets of T cells found by Abe et al.[46] to be preferentially expanded during acute Kawasaki disease.

In addition, it has been shown that early treatment of Kawasaki disease with intravenous administration of γ-globulin can decrease the incidence of coronary artery lesions.[49] Recent work by Takei et al.[50] has shown that intravenous γ-globulin contains antibodies that inhibit the activation of T cells by staphylococcal and streptococcal superantigens. Overall, these studies suggest that during the acute stage of Kawasaki disease a bacterial infection and the production of a superantigen toxin could occur. Stimulation by the superantigen could lead to the expansion and activation of T cells expressing the appropriate V_β molecules with the subsequent production of a number of inflammatory cytokines. If the pathology seen in Kawasaki disease is due to cytokines produced by T cells after stimulation with superantigen, this would explain how the toxin-neutralizing antibodies present in γ-globulin are effective in treating Kawasaki disease.

TOXIC SHOCK SYNDROME

Toxic shock syndrome was first reported in 1978 by Todd et al.[51] This disease is characterized by fever, rash, hypotension, and multisystem failure. It has been well documented that infection with strains of *S. aureus* that produce the superantigen TSST-1 is associated with this disease.[52–55] Staphylococci and streptococci that produce SEB,[56–58] SEA,[59] and SEC[56] have also been associated with TSS. Toxic shock syndrome toxin 1 can induce the production of IL-1β and TNF-α by human monocytes.[60–62] It also can stimulate the proliferation of T cells[63] and the production of IL-2 and IFN-γ.[60, 64] Staphylococcal enterotoxin B, SEC, and SEA have been shown to induce the production of TNF-α by human monocytes.[59] These toxins are also capable of stimulating human T cells to proliferate and produce IL-2.[65] This production of cytokines by monocytes and T cells is believed to play a major role in the pathologic changes seen in TSS by inducing fever and inflammation.

Further evidence for a potential role for superantigens in the pathogenesis of TSS is the finding that in patients with TSS a majority had an expansion of $V_\beta 2$-expressing T cells.[66] Five of eight patients with TSS had increased levels of $V_\beta 2$-TCR–positive cells with no significant expansion of any other V_β subset. The expansion of $V_\beta 2+$ T cells was seen with both CD4+ and CD8+ T cells. It was shown that the percentage of $V_\beta 2+$ T cells returned to normal levels from 1 to 4 months after the onset of disease.[66] Stimulation and activation of these cells could lead to the production of cytokines that could be involved in the pathogenesis of TSS. It was previously shown that mice that were deficient in T cells, nude mice, and mice treated with cyclosporine to inhibit T-cell function were resistant to shock induced by SEB, thus demonstrating that the toxicity of SEB was dependent on T cells.[67] Miethke et al.[68] demonstrated in a severe combined immunodeficiency (SCID) mouse model that TSST-1 induced a lethal shock that was dependent on T cells after stimulation with TSST-1 in the pathogenesis of TSS.

Toxic shock syndrome toxin 1 is also capable of inducing polyclonal activation and differentiation of B cells into Ig-secreting plasma cells through MHC-unrestricted cognate T/B-cell interaction.[69] These investigators showed that TSST-1 binds to class II MHC molecules on human tonsillar B cells and leads to a proliferation and differentiation of B cells that is dependent on contact with a critical number of T cells. Both the TCR and the expression of MHC class II antigens on the B cells were necessary for proliferation and differentiation.[69]

ARTHRITIS

T cells have been postulated to be major effector cells in a number of autoimmune diseases. This is based on the strong association of certain diseases such as rheumatoid arthritis (RA) with particular HLA-DR types[70] as well as the presence of large numbers of T cells at the sites of inflammation.[71–73] The selective expansion of T cells expressing particular V_β molecules in disease states led to the suggestion that superantigens may contribute to autoimmune disease by activating autoreactive T-cell populations.

One model system in which to study the role of superantigens in autoimmune disease is *Mycoplasma arthritidis*. *Mycoplasma ar-*

thritidis causes a chronic arthritic disease in rodents that closely resembles human RA. *Mycoplasma arthritidis* mitogen 1 (MAM) is an approximately 27-kDa protein produced by *M. arthritidis* that shares many features with superantigens. It acts as a potent T-cell mitogen that requires class II MHC, I-E+ antigen-presenting cells for T-cell activation.[74] Similar to other superantigens, however, MAM does not require antigen processing, nor is the response to MAM MHC restricted.[75, 76] In addition, MAM has been shown to preferentially activate T cells bearing $V_\beta8.1$, $V_\beta8.2$, $V_\beta8.3$, and $V_\beta6$ TCR in the mouse.[77] In humans the majority of MAM-reactive T cells are $V_\beta17$, which are most homologous to murine $V_\beta6$.[78] The evidence that MAM plays a role in arthritis induced by infection with *M. arthritidis* is that susceptible strains of mice express I-E[79] and that the injection of partially purified MAM can induce synovitis.[80] In addition, the effect of MAM on collagen-induced arthritis has been studied because of the similarity in V_β-TCR usage by MAM and collagen-reactive T cells.[77, 81–83] These studies found that in mice with previous collagen-induced arthritis, injection of MAM caused a recurrence of disease and an increase in anticollagen antibodies.[84] *Mycoplasma arthritidis* mitogen 1 could also trigger arthritis in animals in which arthritis had not developed after an earlier injection with porcine type II collagen.[84] An important unresolved question is whether MAM leads to increased severity of disease by activating specific T cells or through the nonspecific production of inflammatory cytokines.

Arthritis can also be induced in rat ankle joints after the injection of peptidoglycan polysaccharide polymers isolated from the cell walls of group A streptococci (PG-APS).[85–88] It was recently shown that injection of the superantigen TSST-1 can lead to a reactivation of arthritis in rats previously injected with PG-APS, although TSST-1 by itself did not lead to arthritis. The reactivation of arthritis by TSST-1 was dependent on functional T cells.[88]

In addition to studies in the mouse model, there have been a number of studies done to try to determine whether superantigens play a role in human RA. Paliard et al.[89] used PCR to examine TCR-V_β usage by T cells from the synovial fluid and peripheral blood of patients with RA and active disease. They found that the V_β repertoire in peripheral blood was similar to that previously reported for normal individuals.[35, 89, 90] The V_β repertoire in synovial fluid of patients with RA showed variation between individuals, but in all patients examined there was an increase in the frequency of $V_\beta14$+ T cells.[89] This was in contrast to the overall low numbers of $V_\beta14$+ T cells found in the peripheral blood of individuals with active RA. The authors also determined the clonotypes of the $V_\beta 14+$ T-cell population. They found in patients with RA a dominance in the synovial fluid of two clonotypes that varied among patients. This clonotypic dominance was not seen in T cells from peripheral blood.[89] These results demonstrate a specific expansion of $V_\beta 14+$ T cells in the synovial fluid of patients with RA, thus suggesting a role for these T cells in the disease process. The authors propose that patients with RA could be exposed to a microbial superantigen that leads to depletion of $V_\beta 14+$ cells in peripheral blood which is commonly seen after superantigen stimulation, and the preferential expansion of $V_\beta 14+$ T cells in synovial fluid. Because of cross-reactivity with self-antigens in the joints, the $V_\beta 14+$ cells are maintained in the synovium and may contribute to disease.[89]

Howell et al.[91] also used PCR analysis to determine the V_β repertoire of T cells from synovial tissue of five patients with RA. They focused on T cells that were IL-2 receptor–positive, a marker for T-cell activation. They found that $V_\beta 17$ and $V_\beta 3$ expression predominated in the patients studied. $V_\beta 14$ and $V_\beta 9$ were also found in a majority of their subjects.[91] Sequencing analysis showed clonal dominance.[89] In addition, $V_\beta 3$, $V_\beta 14$, and $V_\beta 17$ have similar complimentarity-determining region 4 (CDR4) regions in the TCRβ chain. This is of interest since it is this region of the TCR that binds exogenous and endogenous superantigens. This would suggest that the same superantigen could stimulate and expand the three V_β TCR subsets commonly found in the synovial fluid of patients with RA. These two studies suggest a role for superantigens in the expansion of T cells that play a pathogenic role in RA.

A second potential role for superantigens in the pathogenesis of RA was proposed in a study by Mourad et al.[92] They found that stimulation of human rheumatoid synoviocytes with SEA resulted in an increase in mRNA expression and protein secretion of IL-6 and IL-8.[92] The increase in cytokine production was dependent on the expression of MHC class II molecules on the synoviocytes. This study suggests that stimulation through the class II molecule by superantigen could lead to the production of inflammatory cytokines in the rheumatoid synovium.

HUMAN IMMUNODEFICIENCY VIRUS AND ACQUIRED IMMUNODEFICIENCY SYNDROME

As discussed earlier, a major advance in the study of the Mls loci and self-superantigens was the discovery that the Mls loci encode endogenous MMTV, a type B retrovirus (reviewed by Kotzin et al.[14]). Additional studies showed that these superantigens are involved in the deletion of specific T-cell subsets. One hallmark of acquired immunodeficiency syndrome (AIDS) that is caused by the HIV retrovirus is the depletion of T lymphocytes. The possibility that HIV may encode a superantigen that is responsible for T-cell depletion in these patients has been examined.

Studies by Imberti et al.[93] determined the V_β repertoire of peripheral lymphocytes in normal and HIV-infected individuals. They found that the V_β repertoire in HIV-positive patients was restricted with deletion of certain V_β subsets. This was in contrast to normal subjects, who expressed all of the V_β subsets randomly with no specific deletions seen. In particular, the V_β subsets $V_\beta14$, $V_\beta15$, $V_\beta16$, $V_\beta17$, $V_\beta18$, $V_\beta19$, and $V_\beta20$ were not detected in patients with AIDS but exist in the repertoire of normal individuals. In addition, it was found that the V_β-specific deletions were not caused by opportunistic infections but correlated with the pathogenesis of AIDS.[93]

A study by Bisset et al.[94] determined the V_β expression of T cells from asymptomatic HIV-infected individuals after in vitro stimulation with staphylococcal enterotoxin. They found a reduction in the ability of $V_\beta5.3+$ T cells to respond to SED and a reduction in the ability of $V_\beta5.1+$ and $V_\beta8+$ T cells from infected individuals to respond to SEE. There was an enhanced proliferation of $V_\beta12+$ T cells to SEE. These results demonstrate the decreased ability of particular V_β subsets in individuals with HIV infection to respond to stimulation with superantigens. This study suggests that superantigen stimulation during early HIV infection could lead to anergy of T cells bearing particular V_β chains. In addition, the enhanced ability of $V_\beta12+$ T cells to respond to SEE is interesting in light of work showing that HIV preferentially infects $V_\beta12+$ T cell lines and that this family of T cells is more resistant to the cytopathic effects of HIV.[94]

It has been reported in an earlier study that stimulation with staphylococcal superantigens induced cell proliferation in CD4+ peripheral blood mononuclear cells from four HIV-infected individuals.[95] In addition, HIV p24 expression was induced by staphylococcal enterotoxin in cultures of CD4+ T cells. Infection with pathogens expressing superantigens could lead to increased HIV-1 replication by activation of infected T cells, in particular, $V_\beta12+$ T cells as discussed earlier. Thus superantigens could act in the pathogenesis of AIDS by enhancing the spread of HIV in infected individuals.

It has been suggested that programmed cell death, or apoptosis, may be one mechanism of T-cell depletion in HIV-positive individuals.[96–98] Groux et al.[99] have shown that CD4+ T cells from 109 HIV-positive individuals underwent cell death by apoptosis after stimulation with SEB. In a separate study it was shown that in vitro stimulation with SEB, SEA, and MAM led to apoptosis of CD4+ T cells from the peripheral blood of HIV-infected patients but not from control individuals.[98] The authors suggest that the T cells from patients are somehow "primed" in vivo for apoptosis by antigenic activation and upon further stimulation die. Thus apoptosis could be one mechanism that contributes to T-cell depletion during AIDS either through an HIV-encoded superantigen or after infection with an opportunistic pathogen that expresses a superantigen. It is important to note, however, that the degree of apoptosis seen with T-cell populations from HIV-infected individuals varies greatly. This may be due to the variation in individual T-cell repertoires and the percentage of cells expressing the appropriate V_β molecule for stimulation by superantigens, as well as the level of class II MHC expression necessary for presentation of superantigens.

SUMMARY

Although the exact mechanisms by which superantigens may contribute to the pathogenesis of diseases are unknown, it seems increasingly likely that they have a role in the induction and pathogenesis of disease. The studies described here demonstrate that in several different diseases either bacterial or viral superantigens can be isolated from patients. There is also a preferential expansion of particular V_β T-cell subsets, which is a common feature of superantigen stimulation. From the work that has been done to date it can be hypothesized that superantigens may act in several ways. They may stimulate and activate T cells that are autoreactive and lead to the induction or exacerbation of autoimmune disease, as in RA. Alternatively, they may lead to the depletion of T-cell subsets based on V_β expression, thereby resulting in the severe reduction in lymphocytes in certain immunodeficiency diseases such as AIDS. But perhaps the most likely contribution of superantigens to disease pathogenesis is seen indirectly by their effect on the immune system—particularly the stimulation of large numbers of T lymphocytes expressing the same V_β domain. Thus it is likely that the direct effect of various T-cell–derived inflammatory mediators (i.e., interleukins and other cytokines) released by these activated T lymphocytes is the primary cause of disease pathology via response to superantigen stimulation.

In addition to the diseases discussed here, there are a number of other diseases in which a potential role for superantigens is being studied. These include autoimmune diseases seen after group A streptococcal infections in which the streptococcal M protein has been postulated to act as a superantigen[100, 101] such as scarlet fever, rheumatic heart disease, and poststreptococcal glomerulonephritis. Other diseases being studied include psoriasis,[102] lupus-like disease, and lymphoproliferative diseases (reviewed in Kotzin et al.[14]). In the coming years the exact role of superantigens and the specific mechanisms by which they contribute to disease should be more clearly defined. Our understanding of these molecules could also lead to new therapies for the treatment of these diseases.

REFERENCES

1. Herman A, Kappler J, Marrack P, et al: Superantigens: Mechanism of T-cell stimulation and role in immune responses. *Annu Rev Immunol* 9:745–772, 1991.
2. Festenstein H: Immunogenetic and biological aspects of in vitro lymphocyte allotransformation (MLR) in the mouse. *Transplant Rev* 15:62–88, 1973.
3. Dellabona P, Peccoud J, Kappler J, et al: Superantigens interact with MHC class II molecules outside of the antigen groove. *Cell* 62:1115–1121, 1990.
4. Fraser J: High affinity binding of staphylococcal enterotoxins A and B to HLA-DR. *Nature* 339:221–223, 1989.
5. Labrecque N, Thibodeau J, Sekaly R: Interactions between staphylococcal superantigens and MHC class II molecules. *Semin Immunol* 5:23–32, 1993.
6. Pullen A, Bill J, Kubo R, et al: Analysis of the interaction site for the self superantigen Mls-1[a] on T cell receptor Vβ. *J Exp Med* 173:1183–1192, 1991.
7. Scherer M, Ignatowicz L, Winslow G, et al: Superantigens: Bacterial and viral proteins that mannipulate the immune system. *Annu Rev Cell Biol* 9:101–128, 1993.
8. Lai E, Barth R, Hood L: Genomic organization of the mouse T-cell receptor β-chain family. *Proc Natl Acad Sci U S A* 84:3846–3850, 1987.
9. Kappler J, Staerz U, White J, et al: Self-tolerance eliminates T cells specific for Mls-modified products of the major histocompatibility complex. *Nature* 332:35–40, 1988.
10. MacDonald H, Schneider R, Lees R, et al: T-cell receptor V_β use predicts reactivity and tolerance to Mls[a]-encoded antigens. *Nature* 332:40–45, 1988.
11. Happ M, Woodland D, Palmer E: A third T-cell receptor β-chain vari

able region gene encodes reactivity to Mls-1a gene products. Proc Natl Acad Sci U S A 86:6293–6296, 1989.

12. Okada C, Holzmann B, Guidos C, et al: Characterization of a rat monoclonal antibody specific for a determinant encoded by the Vβ gene segment. Depletion of Vβ$^+$ T cells on mice with Mls-1a haplotype. *J Immunol* 144:3473–3483, 1990.
13. Waanders G, MacDonald H: Hierarchy of responsiveness *in vivo* and *in vitro* among T cells expressing distinct Mls-1a–reactive Vβ domains. *Eur J Immunol* 22:291–293, 1992.
14. Kotzin B, Leung D, Kappler J, et al: Superantigens and their role in human disease. *Adv Immunol* 54:99–166, 1993.
15. Frankel W, Rudy C, Coffin J, et al: Linkage of Mls genes to endogenous mammary tumor viruses of inbred mice. *Nature* 349:526–528, 1991.
16. Woodland D, Happ M, Gollob K, et al: An endogenous retrovirus mediating deletion of β cells? *Nature* 349:529–530, 1991.
17. Dyson P, Knight A, Fairchild S, et al: Genes encoding ligands for deletion of Vβ11 T cells cosegregate with mammary tumor virus genomes. *Nature* 349:531–532, 1991.
18. Marrack P, Kushnir E, Kappler J: A maternally inherited superantigen encoded by a mammary tumour virus. *Nature* 349:524–526, 1991.
19. Choi Y, Kappler J, Marrack P: A superantigen encoded in the open reading frame of the 3′ long terminal repeat of mouse mammary tumor virus. *Nature* 350:203–207, 1991.
20. Pullen A, Wade T, Marrack P, et al: Identification of the region of T cell receptor β chain that interacts with the self-superantigen Mls-1a. *Cell* 61:1365–1374, 1990.
21. Pullen A, Bill J, Kubo R, et al: Analysis of the interaction site for the self superantigen Mls-1a on T cell receptor Vβ. *J Exp Med* 173:1183–1192, 1991.
22. Cazenave P, Marche P, Jouvin-Marche E, et al: Vβ17-gene polymorphism in wild-derived mouse strains: Two amino acid substitutions in the Vβ17 region alter drastically T cell receptor specificity. *Cell* 63:717–728, 1990.
23. Davis M, Bjorkman P: T-cell antigen receptor genes and T-cell recognition. *Nature* 334:395–402, 1988.
24. von Boehmer H, Kieielow P: Self-nonself discrimination by T cells. *Science* 248:1369–1373, 1990.
25. Herzog M, Lafage M, Montano-Herose J, et al: Nucleocapsid-specific T and B cell responses in humans after rabies vacccination. *Virus Res* 24:77–89, 1992.
26. Higin A, Vacchio M, Morse H: A virus encoded superantigen in a retrovirus-induced immunodeficiency syndrome of mice. *Science* 252:424–427, 1991.
27. Laurence J, Hodtsev A, Posnett D: Superantigen implicated in depen-

dence of HIV-1 replication in T cells on TCR V beta expression. *Nature* 358:255–259, 1992.

28. Swaminathan S, Furey W, Pletcher J, et al: Crystal structure of staphylococcal enterotoxin B, a superantigen. *Nature* 359:801–806, 1992.
29. Peavy D, Adler W, Smith R: The mitogenic effects of endotoxin and staphylococcal enterotoxin B on mouse spleen cells and human peripheral lymphocytes. *J Immunol* 105:1453–1458, 1970.
30. Langford M, Stanton G, Johnson H: Biological effects of staphylococcal enterotoxin A on human peripheral lymphocytes. *Infect Immun* 22:62–68, 1978.
31. Janeway C, Yagi J, Conrad P, et al: T-cell responses to Mls and to bacterial proteins that mimic its behavior. *Immunol Rev* 107:61–88, 1989.
32. White J, Herman A, Pullen A, et al: The Vβ-specific superantigen staphylococcal enterotoxin B: Stimulation of mature T cells and clonal deletion in neonatal mice. *Cell* 56:27–35, 1989.
33. Dalidowicz J, Silverman S, Schantz E, et al: Chemical and biological properties of reduced and alkylated staphylococcal enterotoxin B. *Biochemistry* 5:2375–2381, 1966.
34. Spero W, Warren J, Metzger J: Effect of a single peptide bond scission by trypsin on the structure and activity of staphylococcal enterotoxin B. *J Biol Chem* 248:7289–7294, 1973.
35. Kappler J, Kotzin B, Herron L, et al: V beta-specific stimulation of human T cells by staphylococcal toxins. *Science* 244:811–813, 1989.
36. Callahan J, Herman A, Kappler J, et al: Stimulation of B10.BR T cells with superantigenic staphylococcal toxins. *J Immunol* 144:2473–2479, 1990.
37. Kappler J, Herman A, Clements J, et al: Mutations defining functional regions of the superantigen staphylococcal enterotoxin B. *J Exp Med* 175:387–396, 1992.
38. Irwin M, Hudson K, Fraser J, et al: Enterotoxin residues determining T-cell receptor V-beta binding specificity. *Nature* 359:841–843, 1992.
39. Hudson K, Robinson H, Fraser J: Two adjacent residues in staphylococcal enterotoxins A and E determine T cell receptor Vβ specificity. *J Exp Med* 177:175–184, 1993.
40. Mollick J, McMasters R, Grossman D, et al: Localization of a site on bacterial superantigens that determines T cell receptor B chain specificity. *J Exp Med* 177:283–293, 1993.
41. Fraser J, Urban R, Strominger J, et al: Zinc regulates the function of two superantigens. *Proc Natl Acad Sci U S A* 89:5507–5511, 1992.
42. Herman A, Labrecque N, Thibodeau J, et al: Identification of the staphylococcal enterotoxin A superantigen binding site in the β1 domain of the human histocompatibility antigen HLA-DR. *Proc Natl Acad Sci U S A* 88:9956–9958, 1991.

43. Karp D, Long E: Identification of HLA-DR1 β chain residues critical for binding staphylococcal enterotoxins A and E. *J Exp Med* 175:415–424, 1992.
44. Rauch AM: Kawasaki syndrome: Review of new epidemiologic and laboratory developments. *Pediatr Infect Dis J* 6:1016–1021, 1987.
45. Leung DYM: Immunologic aspects of Kawasaki disease. *J Rheumatol* 17:15–18, 1990.
46. Abe J, Kotzin BL, Jujo K, et al: Selective expansion of T cells expressing T-cell receptor variable regions $V_\beta 2$ and $V_\beta 8$ in Kawasaki disease. *Proc Natl Acad Sci U S A* 89:4066–4070, 1992.
47. Abe J, Kotzin BL, Meissner C, et al: Characterization of T cell repertoire changes in acute Kawasaki disease. *J Exp Med* 177:791–796, 1993.
48. Leung DYM, Meissmer HC, Fulton DR, et al: Toxic shock syndrome toxin–secreting *Staphylococcus aureus* in Kawasaki syndrome. *Lancet* 342:1385–1388, 1993.
49. Newburger JW, Takahashi M, Beiser AS, et al: A single intravenous infusion of gamma globulin as compared with four infusions in the treatment of acute Kawasaki syndrome. *N Engl J Med* 324:1633–1639, 1991.
50. Takei S, Arora YK, Walker SM: Intravenous immunoglobulin contains specific antibodies inhibitory to activation of T cells by staphylococcal toxin superantigens. *J Clin Invest* 91:602–607, 1993.
51. Todd J, Fishaut M, Dapral F, et al: Toxic-shock syndrome associated with phage-group-I staphylococci. *Lancet* 2:1116–1118, 1978.
52. Shands KN, Schmid GP, Dan BB, et al: Toxic-shock syndrome in menstruating women: Association with tampon use and *Staphylococcus aureus* and clinical features in 52 cases. *N Engl J Med* 303:1436–1432, 1980.
53. Reingold AL, Hargrett NT, Dan BB, et al: Nonmenstrual toxic shock syndrome: A review of 130 cases. *Ann Intern Med* 96:871–874, 1982.
54. Schlievert PM, Shands KN, Dan BB, et al: Identification and characterization of an exotoxin from *Staphylococcus aureus* associated with toxic-shock-syndrome. *J Infect Dis* 143:509–516, 1981.
55. Bergdoll MS, Crass BA, Reiser RF, et al: A new staphylococcal enterotoxin, enterotoxin F, associated with toxic-shock-syndrome *Staphylococcus aureus* isolates. *Lancet* 1:1017–1021, 1981.
56. Crass BA, Bergdoll MS: Toxin involvement in toxic shock syndrome. *J Infect Dis* 153:918–926, 1986.
57. Immerman RP, Greenman RL: Toxic shock syndrome associated with pyomyositis caused by a strain of *Staphylococcus aureus* that does not produce toxic-shock-syndrome toxin-1. *J Infect Dis* 156:505–507, 1987.
58. Schlievert PM: Staphylococcal enterotoxin B and toxic-shock syndrome toxin-1 are significantly associated with non-menstrual TSS. *Lancet* 1:1149–1150, 1986.
59. Fast DJ, Schlievert PM, Nelson RD: Toxic shock syndrome–associated staphylococcal and streptococcal pyrogenic toxins are potent in-

ducers of tumor necrosis factor production. *Infect Immun* 57:291–294, 1989.

60. Jupin C, Anderson S, Damais C, et al: Toxic shock syndrome toxin 1 as an inducer of human tumor necrosis factors and g interferon. *J Exp Med* 167:752–761, 1988.
61. Parsonnet J, Hickman RK, Eardley DD, et al: Induction of human interleukin-1 by toxic-shock-syndrome toxin-1. *J Infect Dis* 151:514–522, 1985.
62. Parsonnet J, Gillis ZA, Pier GB: Induction of interleukin-1 by strains of *Staphylococcus aureus* from patients with nonmenstrual toxic shock syndrome. *J Infect Dis* 154:55–63, 1986.
63. Poindexter NJ, Schlievert PM: Toxic-shock-toxin 1–induced proliferation of lymphocytes: Comparison of the mitogenic response of human, murine, and rabbit lymphocytes. *J Infect Dis* 151:65–72, 1985.
64. Uchiyama T, Kamagata Y, Yan X-J, et al: Study of the biological activities of toxic shock syndrome toxin-1. II. Induction of the proliferative response and the interleukin-2 production by T cells from human peripheral blood mononuclear cells stimulated with the toxin. *Clin Exp Immunol* 68:638–647, 1987.
65. Uchiyama T, Kamagata Y, Yan X-J, et al: Relative strength of the mitogenic and interleukin-2–production inducing activities of staphylococcal exotoxins presumed to be causative exotoxins of toxic shock syndrome: Toxic shock syndrome toxin-1 and enterotoxins A, B, C to murine and human T cells. *Clin Exp Immunol* 75:239–244, 1989.
66. Choi Y, Lafferty JA, Clements JR, et al: Selective expansion of T cells expressing $V_{\beta}2$ in toxic shock syndrome. *J Exp Med* 172:981–984, 1990.
67. Marrack P, Blackman M, Kushnir E, et al: The toxicity of staphylococcal enterotoxin B in mice is mediated by T cells. *J Exp Med* 171:455–464, 1990.
68. Miethke T, Duschek K, Wahl C, et al: Pathogenesis of the toxic shock syndrome: T cell mediated lethal shock caused by the superantigen TSST-1. *Eur J Immunol* 23:1494–1500, 1993.
69. Mourad W, Scholl P, Diaz A, et al: The staphylococcal toxic shock toxin 1 triggers B cell proliferation and differentiation via major histocompatibility complex–unrestricted cognate T/B cell interaction. *J Exp Med* 170:2011–2022, 1989.
70. Gregersen PK, Silver J, Winchester RJ: The shared epitope hypothesis. An approach to understanding the molecular genetics of susceptibility to rheumatoid arthritis. *Arthritis Rheum* 30:1205–1213, 1987.
71. Duke O, Panayi GS, Janossy G, et al: An immunohistological analysis of lymphocyte subpopulations and their microenvironment in the synovial membranes of patients with rheumatoid arthritis using monoclonal antibodies. *Clin Exp Immunol* 49:22–30, 1982.
72. Burmester GR, John B, Gramatzki M, et al: Activated T cells in vivo and in vitro: Divergence in expression of Tac and Ia antigens in the

nonblastoid small T cells of inflammation and normal T cells activated in vitro. *J Immunol* 133:1230–1234, 1984.

73. Stamenkovic I, Stegagno M, Wright EA, et al: Clonal dominance among T lymphocyte infiltrates in arthritis. *Proc Natl Acad Sci U S A* 85:1179–1183, 1988.
74. Cole BC, Daynes RA, Ward JR: Stimulation of mouse lymphocytes by a mitogen derived from *Mycoplasma arthritidis*. III. *Ir* gene control of lymphocyte transformation correlates with binding of the mitogen to specific Ia-bearing cells. *J Immunol* 129:1352–1359, 1982.
75. Cole BC, Daynes RA, Ward JR: Stimulation of mouse lymphocytes by a mitogen derived from *Mycoplasma arthritidis*. I. Transformation is associated with an H2 linked gene that maps to the I-E/IC subregion. *J Immunol* 127:1931–1936, 1981.
76. Lynch DH, Gurish MF, Cole BC, et al: T cell proliferative responses to a mitogen derived from *Mycoplasma arthritidis* are controlled by the accessory cell. *J Immunol* 131:1702–1706, 1983.
77. Cole BC, Kartchner DR, Wells DJ: Stimulation of mouse lymphocytes by a mitogen derived from Mycoplasma arthritidis (MAM). VIII. Selective activation of T cells expressing distinct V_βT cell receptors from various strains of mice by the superantigen MAM. *J Immunol* 144:425–431, 1990.
78. Friedman SM, Crow MK, Tumang JR, et al: Characterization of human T cells reactive with the *Mycoplasma arthritidis*–derived superantigen (MAM): Generation of a monoclonal antibody against $V_\beta17$, the T cell receptor gene product expressed by a large fraction of MAM-reactive human T cells. *J Exp Med* 174:891–900, 1991.
79. Cole BC, Thorpe RN, Hassell LA, et al: Toxicity but not arthritogenicity of *Mycoplasma arthritidis* for mice associates with the haplotype expressed at the major histocompatibility complex. *Infect Immun* 41:1010–1015, 1983.
80. Cannon GW, Cole BC, Ward JR, et al: Arthritogenic effects of Mycoplasma arthritidis T-cell mitogen in rats. *J Rheumatol* 14:735–741, 1988.
81. Baccala R, Smith LR, Vestberg M, et al: Mycoplasma arthritidis mitogen: V_β engaged in mice, rats, and humans, and requirement of HLA-DRa for presentation. *Arthritis Rheum* 35:434–442, 1992.
82. Haqqi TM, Anderson GD, Banerjee S, et al: Restricted heterogeneity in T-cell receptor V_β gene usage in the lymph nodes and arthritic joints of mice. *Proc Natl Acad Sci U S A* 89:1253–1255, 1992.
83. Cole BC, Balderas RA, Ahmed EA, et al: Genomic composition and allelic polymorphisms influence V_β usage by the Mycoplasma arthritidis superantigen. *J Immunol* 150:3291–3299, 1993.
84. Cole BC, Griffiths MM: Triggering and exacerbation of autoimmune arthritis by the *Mycoplasma arthritidis* superantigen MAM. *Arthritis Rheum* 36:994–1002, 1993.
85. Cromartie WJ, Craddock JG, Schwab JH, et al: Arthritis in rats after

systemic injection of streptococcal cells or cell walls. *J Exp Med* 146:1585–1602, 1977.
86. Clark RL, Cuttino JT, Anderle DK, et al: Radiologic analysis of arthritis in rats after systemic injection of streptococcal cell walls. *Arthritis Rheum* 22:25–35, 1979.
87. Dalldorf FG, Cromartie WJ, Anderle SK, et al: Relation of experimental arthritis to the distribution of streptococcal cell wall fragments. *Am J Pathol* 100:383–391, 1980.
88. Schwab JH, Brown RR, Anderle SK, et al: Superantigen can reactivate bacterial cell wall–induced arthritis. *J Immunol* 150:4151–4159, 1993.
89. Paliard X, West SG, Lafferty JA, et al: Evidence for the effects of a superantigen rheumatoid arthritis. *Science* 253:325–329, 1991.
90. Choi Y, Kotzin B, Herron L, et al: Interaction of *Staphylococcus aureus* toxin "superantigens" with human T cells. *Proc Natl Acad Sci U S A* 86:8941–8945, 1989.
91. Howell MD, Diveley JP, Lundeen KA, et al: Limited T-cell receptor β-chain heterogeneity among interleukin 2 receptor–positive synovial T cells suggests a role for superantigen in rheumatoid arthritis. *Proc Natl Acad Sci U S A* 88:10921–10925, 1991.
92. Mourad W, Mehindate K, Schall TJ, et al: Engagement of major histocompatibility complex class II molecules by superantigen induces inflammatory cytokine gene expression in human rheumatoid fibroblast-like synoviocytes. *J Exp Med* 175:613–616, 1992.
93. Imberti L, Sottini A, Bettinardi A, et al: Selective depletion in HIV infection of T cells that bear specific T cell receptor V_β sequences. *Science* 254:860–862, 1991.
94. Bisset LR, Opravil M, Ludwig E, et al: T cell response to staphylococcal superantigens by asymptomatic HIV-infected individuals exhibits selective changes in T cell receptor V_β-chain usage. *AIDS Res Hum Retroviruses* 9:241–246, 1993.
95. Brinchmann JE, Gaudernack G, Thorsby E, et al: Staphylococcal exotoxin superantigens induce human immunodeficiency virus type 1 expression in naturally infected $CD4^+$ T cells. *J Virol* 66:5924–5928, 1992.
96. Ameisen JC, Capron A: T-cell dysfunction and depletion in AIDS: The programmed cell death hypothesis. *Immunol Today* 12(4):102–105, 1991.
97. Meyaard L, Otto SA, Jonker RR, et al: Programmed death of T cells in HIV-1 infection. *Science* 175:331–338, 1992.
98. Gougeon M, Garcia S, Heeney J, et al: Programmed cell death in AIDS-related HIV and SIV infections. *AIDS Res Hum Retroviruses* 9:553–563, 1993.
99. Groux H, Torpier G, Monte D, et al: Activation-induced death by apoptosis in $CD4^+$T cells from human immunodeficiency virus–infected asymptomatic individuals. *J Exp Med* 175:331–340, 1992.

100. Tomai M, Kotb M, Majumdar G, et al: Superantigenicity of streptococcal M protein. *J Exp Med* 172:359–362, 1990.
101. Tomai MA, Aelion JA, Dockter ME, et al: T cell receptor V gene usage by human T cells stimulated with the superantigen streptococcal M protein. *J Exp Med* 174:285–288, 1991.
102. Leung DYM, Giorno R, Norris DA: A potential role for superantigens in the pathogenesis of psoriasis. *J Invest Dermatol* 100:225–228, 1993.

Index

B

C

F

G

I

N

O

P

T

U

V

The Year Books–

The best from 236,287 journal articles.

At Mosby, we subscribe to more than 950 medical and allied health journals from every corner of the globe. We read them all, tirelessly scanning for anything that relates to your field.

We send everything we find related to a given specialty to the distinguished editors of the **Year Book** in that area, and they pick out *the best*, the articles they feel *every practitioner in that specialty should be aware of.*

For the **1994 Year Books** we surveyed a total of 236,287 articles and found hundreds of articles related to your field. Our expert editors reviewed these and chose the developments you don't want to miss.

The best articles–condensed, organized, and with personal commentary.

Not only do you get the past year's most important articles in your field, you get them in a format that makes them easy to use.

Every article that the editors pick is condensed into a concise, outlined abstract, a summary of the article's most important points highlighted with bold paragraph headings. So you can quickly scan for exactly what you need.

In addition to identifying the year's best articles, the editors write concise commentaries following each article, telling whether or not the study in question is a reliable one, whether a new technique is effective, or whether a particular trend you've head about merits your immediate attention.

No other abstracting service offers this expert advice to help you decide how the year's advances will affect the way you practice.

With a special added benefit for Year Book subscribers.

In 1994, your **Year Book** subscription includes a new added benefit. Access to **MOSBY Document Express**, a rapid-response information retrieval service that puts copies of original source documents in your hands, in a little as a few hours.

With **MOSBY Document Express**, you have convenient, *around-the-clock-access to literally every article* upon which **Year Book** summaries are based. What's more, you can also order journal articles cited in references—or for that matter, virtually any medical or scientific article that can be located. Plus, at your direction, we will deliver the article(s) by FAX, overnight delivery service, or regular mail.

This new added benefit is just one of the enhanced services that makes your **Year Book** subscription an even better value—it's your key to the full breadth of health sciences information. For more details, see **MOSBY Document Express** instructions at the beginning of this book.